MCQs for
Master in Physiotherapy (MPT)
Entrance Examination

References from Standard Textbooks

Essential Orthopedics/Maheshwari/3rd Edition

Essential of Orthopedics for Physiotherapists/Ebnezar/1st Edition

Therapeutic Exercise/Kisner/5th Edition

Physical Rehabilitation/O'Sullivan/4th and 5th Edition

Joint Structure and Function/Norkins/4th Edition

Human Physiology/AK Jain/1st and 2nd Edition

Medicine/Davidson/20th Edition

Physiology/Sembulingam/3rd Edition

Human Anatomy/BD Chaurasia (Volume 1)/4th Edition

Essential Pediatrics/OP Ghai/6th Edition

Lippincott Williams and Wilkins Atlas of Anatomy/Thomas C William and Wilkins/1st Edition

Textbook of Physiotherapy/Dr BK Nanda/1st Edition

KD Tripathi/Essential Pharmacology/5th Edition

Essentials of Exercise Physiology/William D McArdle and Katch/2nd Edition

Grays Anatomy/42nd Edition

System of Orthopedics and Trauma/Apley and Soloman/7th Edition

Tidy's Physiotherapy/KM Varghese Company/12th Edition

Principal of Exercise Therapy/Dena Gardiner/4th Edition

The Orthopedic Physical Examination/Reider/1st Edition

MCQs for
Master in Physiotherapy (MPT) Entrance Examination

Third Edition

Suraj Kumar
BPT MPT PhD (Physiotherapy) MIAP SRF-ICMR
Professor
Centre for Physiotherapy and Rehabilitation Sciences
Jamia Millia Islamia
New Delhi, India

Foreword
Sunil Kumar

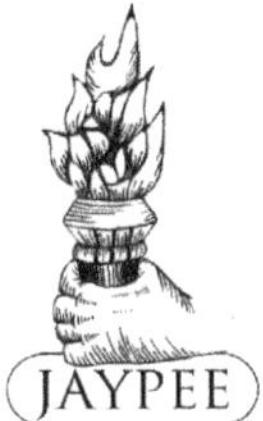

JAYPEE BROTHERS MEDICAL PUBLISHERS
The Health Sciences Publisher
New Delhi | London

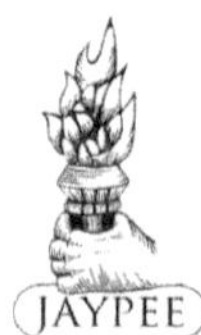

Jaypee Brothers Medical Publishers (P) Ltd.

Headquarters

Jaypee Brothers Medical Publishers (P) Ltd
EMCA House
23/23-B, Ansari Road, Daryaganj
New Delhi - 110 002, India
Landline: +91-11-23272143, +91-11-23272703
+91-11-23282021, +91-11-23245672
Email: jaypee@jaypeebrothers.com

Overseas Office

J.P. Medical Ltd
83 Victoria Street, London
SW1H 0HW (UK)
Phone: +44 20 3170 8910
Email: info@jpmedpub.com

Corporate Office

Jaypee Brothers Medical Publishers (P) Ltd
4838/24, Ansari Road, Daryaganj
New Delhi 110 002, India
Phone: +91-11-43574357
Fax: +91-11-43574314
Email: jaypee@jaypeebrothers.com

EU GPSR Authorised Representative

Logos Europe, 9 rue Nicolas Poussin
17000, La Rochelle, France
Phone: +33 (0) 6 67 93 73 78
E-mail: Contact@logoseurope.eu

Website: www.jaypeebrothers.com

Website: www.jaypeedigital.com

Inquiries for bulk sales may be solicited at: jaypee@jaypeebrothers.com

MCQs for Master in Physiotherapy (MPT) Entrance Examination

First Edition: 2012

Second Edition: 2020

Third Edition: **2023**

ISBN: 978-93-5696-376-4

Dedicated to

My parents, **Sri Raj Kumar Sinha**

and

Smt Manorma Sinha

both for forever encouraging me and for the prestigious guidance provided
in the limited resources.

CONTRIBUTORS

Anoop Aggarwal
Physiotherapist
Pandit Deen Dayal Institute for
the Physically Handicapped
New Delhi, India

Arvind Kumar
Lecturer in Physiotherapy
Department of Physical Medicine and Rehabilitation
CSM Medical University
Lucknow, Uttar Pradesh, India

CK Senthil
Director and Principal, NAISH
College No. 11
Koramangla, Bengaluru
Karnataka, India

G Venu Vendhan
Lecturer
Department of Physiotherapy
University Institute of Paramedical Sciences
CSJM University
Kanpur, Uttar Pradesh, India

Lalit Narayan
Superintendent Occupational Therapist
Pandit Deen Dayal Institute for the Physically Handicapped
New Delhi, India

Moazzam Hussain Khan
Assistant Professor
Centre for Physiotherapy and Rehabilitation Sciences
Jamia Millia Islamia
New Delhi, India

NK Sinha
Academic In-Charge
Bihar College of Physiotherapy
Viklang Bhawan, Patna, Bihar, India

Sandeep Babbar
Physiotherapist
Institute Rotatory Cancer Hospital
All India Institute of Health Sciences
New Delhi, India

Shohrab A Khan
Assistant Professor
Jamia Hamdard University, Delhi, India

Upendra Goswami
Physiotherapist
Postgraduate Institute of Medical Education and Research
Chandigarh, India

FOREWORD

This book is very well designed to evaluate the clinical understanding, reasoning capacity and analyzing skills of the professionals. The questions contained in this book have the potential to storm the brain of the reader and thoroughly examine his/her answering capabilities.

After reading one can easily discern how immensely the objective type questions arranged in the book will be helpful to the students of physiotherapy as well as professionals aiming to get admission in higher courses. This book contains meticulously designed questions distributed in different sections like exercise therapy, electrotherapy, biomechanics, orthopedics, and basic health sciences. Book has 20 sets of comprehensive model question papers with appropriate explanations at places wherever required, for encouraging and preparing the physiotherapy student. Book also contains supplementary bibliographic references to the most appropriate answers, so as to enhance their authenticity.

With my personal experience and the feedback received from various students and staff members I can state that Dr Suraj Kumar is a thoughtful teacher, an innovator and a person with a receptive brain, who is always willing to learn.

I wish the readers good luck in preparation for competitive examination and congratulate that he/she laid hand on the appropriate references.

Sunil Kumar
MS (Ortho)
Secretary (SOC)
Professor
Department of Orthopedics
Uttar Pradesh University of Medical Sciences
Saifai, Etawah, Uttar Pradesh, India

PREFACE TO THE THIRD EDITION

Encouraging feedback from the students was a great motivation to work on the third edition of *MCQs for Master in Physiotherapy (MPT) Entrance Examination*. As with any book, there is always a scope for improvement; changes and additions are made in third edition based on the feedback from enthusiastic literary critics.

This edition has been thoroughly updated, has 20 model question papers based on the latest examination pattern and references from standard books are given for better understanding.

This objective book is designed for physiotherapy students who wish to appear for the master level examinations as well as recruitment examination for various state government and central government jobs including recruitment examinations of railways, ESI hospitals, DSSSB, AYUSH, Homeopathy, Bhabha Atomic Research Centre (BARC), etc. The objective questions book consists of questions from exercise therapy, electrotherapy, orthopedics, medical, research analysis, PTM and PTS, biomechanics, and model questions.

Any constructive criticism is always welcome.

Suraj Kumar

PREFACE TO THE FIRST EDITION

The first edition of the *MCQs for Master in Physiotherapy (MPT) Entrance Examination* is written by Dr Suraj Kumar. The goal behind writing this book is to explain, in language easily understood by students, how the different entrance examinations, jobs, have been covered in single book. This task has been challenging and exciting because our rapidly increasing knowledge of physiotherapy continues to be growing.

As with any product, there is always scope for improvement; however, improvements are best made based on feedback from all professionals.

The decision to pursue the challenge of producing a high quality book on objective answers preparation after much deliberation. This objective book is designed for physiotherapy students who wish to appear for the master level examinations as well as recruitment examination for various state government and central government jobs including recruitment examinations of railways, ESI hospitals, DSSSB, AYUSH, Homeopathy, Bhaba Atomic Research Centre (BARC), etc. The objective questions book consists of questions from exercise therapy, electrotherapy, orthopedics, biomechanics, research methodology and model questions.

Suraj Kumar

ACKNOWLEDGMENTS

I am thankful to the Lord Almighty, who strengthen me with abundant blessing through enumerable means helping me in all accomplishments.

Many friends have helped me along the path of framing the objective questionnaire and shared their highly valuable knowledge for this book. My grateful thanks to everyone.

Special thanks to all those who have taught me—Dr Manda Chauhan, Dr Rajni Kalra, Dr Ramprabhu, Dr Ajay Bahl, Dr VP Sharma, Dr HK Tripathi, Dr Roshan Lal Meena, and Dr Tripta Ghai. I am grateful to my students for giving me the opportunity and privilege to frame the objective questionnaire with their valuable doubts regarding various issues that encouraged me to lay down the objective format questions for critically testing the in-depth physiotherapy related knowledge of the candidate. I express my special thanks to all those thousands of patients, treating and managing whom during last 10 years I have received innumerable opportunities to enhance the clinical and academic knowledge.

I would like to express my gratitude to my students specially Kratika Varshney, Sakshi Vishnoi, Deepjyoti Bajpeyi and Ajay Yadav, Ansh Gupta, Anuradha Gupta and Divyanshi, who helped me in the outcome of this book.

Finally I would express my sincere thanks to my mother, father, my son (Tejasvi) and my wife (Rina Ranjana), who have listened to and supported me throughout the period of preparing the questions and formulating the book.

I am very grateful to the whole team of M/s Jaypee Brothers Medical Publishers (P) Ltd, New Delhi, India, who helped and guided me, especially Shri Jitendar P Vij (Group Chairman), Mr Ankit Vij (Managing Director), Mr MS Mani (Group President), Dr Madhu Choudhary (Director–Educational Publishing), Ms Pooja Bhandari [Director–Production (Books and Journals)], Ms Sunita Katla (Executive Assistant to Group Chairman and Publishing Manager), Mr Ajay Kumar Sharma (Deputy General Manager), Ms Samina Khan (Executive Assistant to Director–Educational Publishing), Dr Sangeeta Yadav (Development Editor), Mr Rajesh Sharma (Production Coordinator), Ms Seema Dogra (Cover Visualizer), Mr Laxmidhar Padhiary (Proofreader), Mr Akshay Thakur (Typesetter), and their team members, for all their support to work in this project and make it a success. Without their cooperation, I could not have completed this project.

CONTENTS

Model Question Papers

1

CHAPTER

Exercise Therapy

Objective Questions with Answers

Orthosis and Prosthesis

Q 1. SOMI brace is:
[Sunder Textbook of Rehabilitation/2nd Ed./Pg. 122]
A. Sterno-occipital mandibular immobilization
B. Scapulo-occipital manubrium immobilization
C. Supraobturator muscle immobilization
D. Scapulo-occipital manipulation instrument

Q 2. The primary area of the residual limb used for weight bearing in a transtibial prosthesis is the:
[Essential of Orthopedics & Applied Physiotherapy Jayant Joshi/1st Ed.Pg. 239]
A. Patella tendon
B. Distal end of the residual limb
C. Lateral tibial condyle
D. Fibular head

Q 3. A therapist modifies a wheelchair to allow the rear wheels to be moved backward by approximately two inches. This type of modification would be most beneficial to a patient with:
[Physical Rehabilitation/O'Sullivan/4th Ed./Pg. 637]
A. Bilateral lower extremity amputations
B. Flaccid hemiplegia
C. Paraplegia
D. Tetraplegia

Q 4. Cock up splint is used in the management of:
[Essential Orthopaedics/Maheshwari/3rd Ed./Pg. 59]
A. Ulnar nerve palsy
B. Brachial plexus palsy
C. Radial nerve palsy
D. Combined Ulnar and Median nerve

Q 5. Von Rosen splint is used in:
[Essential Orthopaedics/Maheshwari/3rd Ed./Pg. 205]
A. CTEV
B. CDH
C. Fracture shaft of femur
D. Fracture tibia

Q 6. Milwaukee brace is used in:
[Essential Orthopaedics/Maheshwari/3rd Ed./Pg. 235]
A. Scoliosis
B. Fracture skull
C. Fracture tibia
D. CTEV

Q 7. For a patient having foot drop the orthosis recommended is:
A. KAFO
B. HKAFO
C. HFO
D. AFO

Q 8. Toe raising spring is indicated in:
A. Equinus deformity of foot
B. Foot drop
C. Flatfoot
D. Knee flexion deformity

Physiotherapy in Ortho

Q 9. In myositis ossificans traumatica at elbow:
[Therapeutic Exercise/Kisner/5th Ed./Pg. 574]
A. Forced passive mobilization should not be given
B. Forced passive mobilization should be given
C. Forced passive mobilization should be given after application of IFT
D. Forced passive mobilization should not be given under GA

Q 10. Putti platt surgical procedure to repair recurrent dislocation involves:
[Ebnezar/1st Ed./Pg. 88]
A. Shortening of scapularis muscle
B. Shortening of infraspinatus muscle
C. Shortening of supraspinatus muscle
D. Wedge osteotomy of humerus

Q 11. People having following tissue types are more prone to have rheumatic arthritis:
[Ebnezar/1st Ed./Pg. 392]
A. HLA – B34
B. HLA – DR4
C. HLA – B27
D. HLA – D27

Q 12. In talipes equinovarus foot is in:
[Ebnezar/1st Ed./Pg. 342]

Answer   1 A   2 A   3 B   4 C   5 B   6 A   7 D   8 B   9 A   10 A   11 B

A. Plantarflexion and eversion
B. Dorsiflexion and eversion
C. Plantarflexion and inversion
D. Dorsiflexion and inversion

Q 13. Which of the following HLA is positive in ankylosing spondylitis?

[Ebnezar/1st Ed./Pg. 402]

A. HLA DR3
B. HLA DR4
C. HLA B27
D. HLA DW

Q 14. Which of the following is true for carpal compression syndrome?

[Ebnezar/1st Ed./Pg. 237]

A. Ulnar compression at wrist
B. Ulnar compression at elbow
C. Median compression at wrist
D. Median compression at elbow

Q 15. Bilateral symmetrical pseudo fractures are seen most commonly in:

[Essential Orthopaedics/Maheshwari/3rd Ed./Pg. 264]

A. Multiple myeloma
B. Fibrous dysplasia
C. Osteomalacia
D. Paget's disease

Q 16. Complete diappearance of shadow of lesser trochanter in anteroposterior view of X-ray indicates:

[Essential Orthopaedics/Maheshwari/3rd Ed./Pg. 111]

A. Central dislocation of hip
B. Anterior dislocation of hip
C. Posterior dislocation of hip
D. Fracture neck of femur

Q 17. An old epileptic patient presented with a complaint of pain in both temporal regions and inability to close her mouth after episode of fits. The patient had similar problem 3 times in the past. Most probable diagnosis of the above case is:

[Therapeutic Exercise/Kisner/5th Ed./Pg. 433]

A. Fractured mandible
B. Dislocation of temporomandibular joint
C. Fracture of temporal bone
D. None of the above

Q 18. An old epileptic patient presented with a complaint of pain in both temporal regions and inability to close her mouth an after episode of fit. The patient had similar problem 3 times in the past, which of the following would be confirmatory for definite diagnosis:

[Lindsay/Neurology/4th Ed./Pg. 99]

A. History
B. Blood and urine examination
C. X-ray and CT scan
D. Ultrasound

Q 19. An old epileptic patient presented with a complaint of pain in both temporal regions and inability to close her mouth after episode of fit. The patient had similar problem 3 times in the past, treatment of choice for this is:

A. Closed reduction and plaster of paris cast
B. Closed reduction and bandage
C. Open reduction and internal fixation
D. Arthroplasty of TM joint

Q 20. All of the following are problems produced by multiple hereditary osteochondromatosis except:

[Churchill/12th Ed./Pg. 131]

A. Multiple bony swelling
B. Deformities
C. Dwarfism
D. Jaundice and anemia

Q 21. The fascia which is generally not involved in Duptren's contracture is:

[Ebnezar/1st Ed./Pg. 236]

A. Cleland's ligament
B. Greyson's ligament
C. Spiral band
D. All of the above

Q 22. Pitches with valgus extension overload syndrome are most symptomatic due to:

[Ebnezar/1st Ed./Pg. 27]

A. Loose bodies
B. Chondromalacia patellae
C. Osteophytes
D. Stress fractures

Q 23. Which of the following tendon is most commonly ruptured in rheumatoid disease?

[Therapeutic Exercise/Kisner/5th/Pg. 310]
[Ebnezar/1st Ed./Pg. 395]

A. Abductor pollicis longus
B. Extensor pollicis brevis
C. Extensor pollicis longus
D. Extensor indicis

Q 24. In the evaluation of an infant, Barlow's provocative test result is positive. This is an indication of:

[Essential Orthopaedics/Maheshwari/3rd Ed./Pg. 201]

A. Hip instability
B. Knee instability
C. Shoulder instability
D. Wrist instability

Q 25. The primary benefits of CPM after ligament reconstruction is:

[Therapeutic Exercise/Kisner/5th Ed./Pg. 61]

A. Pain management
B. Oedema reduction
C. Reduction of adhesion formation
D. Prevention of atrophy

Q 26. The etiology of periarthritis of shoulder is:

[Therapeutic Exercise/Kisner/5th Ed./Pg. 488]

A. Degenerative cartilage in glenoid cavity
B. Infection of shoulder joint
C. Fracture of surgical neck of humerus
D. Idiopathic

Q 27. Erb's palsy is due to injury of:

[Jayant Joshi/1st Ed./Pg. 253]

A. Head involving premotor area
B. Pelvis involving lumbosacral plexus
C. Thorax involving diaphragm
D. Upper roots of brachial plexus involving C5,6

Q 28. The following topical antibiotic agent is used in treatment of burn wounds:

[Physical Rehabilitation/O'sullivan/5th Ed./Pg. 1103]

A. Potassium permanganate
B. Betnovate
C. Silver sulfadiazine
D. Acetylsalcylate

Q 29. A man slipped while walking developed swelling immediately in the knee joint. Structure most probably injured is:

[Therapeutic Exercise/Kisner/5th Ed./Pg. 722]

A. Anterior cruciate ligament
B. Medial meniscus
C. Lateral Meniscus
D. Collateral ligaments

Answer	12 C	13 C	14 C	15 C	16 C	17 B	18 C	19 D	20 D	21 D	22 D	23 D
	24 A	25 C	26 D	27 D	28 C	29 A						

Q 30. The position of lower limb in osteoarthritis is:
[Essential Orthopaedics/Maheshwari/3rd Ed./Pg. 253]
A. Flexion adduction internal rotation
B. Extension adduction external rotation
C. Flexion abduction external rotation
D. Flexion adduction internal rotation

Q 31. Ganglion is most commonly seen over:
[Jayant Joshi/1st Ed./Pg. 29]
A. Dorsal aspect of wrist
B. Volar aspect of wrist
C. Over forehead
D. Dorsum of tongue

Q 32. Earliest movement to be impaired in TB hip is:
[Essential Orthopaedics/Maheshwari/3rd Ed./Pg. 182]
A. Flexion
B. Extension
C. Adduction
D. Abduction

Q 33. True about Dupuytren's contracture is:
[Ebnezar/1st Ed./Pg. 236]
A. More common in females
B. Palmar nodule is the earliest sign
C. Most common in orientals
D. Contracture of dermal tissue

Q 34. All are common with elbow dislocation except:
[Tidy's Physiotherapy/12th Ed./Pg. 35]
A. Myositis ossificans progressia
B. Median nerve palsy
C. Brachial artery injury
D. Volkmann's contracture

Q 35. Cob's angle is measured in:
[Ebnezar/1st Ed./Pg. 242]
A. Kyphosis
B. Scoliosis
C. Lordosis
D. Lateral flexion

Q 36. Myositis ossificans traumatica is commonest in which of the following joints?
[Therapeutic Exercise/Kisner/5th Ed./Pg. 574]
A. Hip
B. Knee
C. Elbow
D. Shoulder

Q 37. Myositis ossificans traumatica is most frequent in elbow dislocation in which of the following muscles?
[Therapeutic Exercise/Kisner/5th Ed./Pg. 574]
A. Triceps
B. Brachioradialis
C. Brachialis
D. Pronator teres

Q 38. A young adult sustained a closed fracture of both bones of right leg in a scooter accident. He was treated by closed reduction and above knee plaster cast for 3 months. His fracture united but on removal of plaster his knee was stiff.
A. Supracondylar fractures of humerus
B. Supracondylar fractures of femur
C. Rib fractures
D. Spine fractures

Q 39. All is true about multiple osteochondrometosis except:
A. Has hereditary predilection
B. Swelling stops growing after skeletal maturation
C. Produced dwarfism
D. Produced emanciation and anemia

Q 40. The attitude policeman taking tip indicates which of the following?
[BD Chaurasia/5th Ed./Pg. 53]
A. High brachial plexus injury
B. Low brachial plexus injury
C. Erb's palsy
D. Subscapularis paralysis

Q 41. Type of nerve lesion in Saturday night palsy most commonly is:
[Jayant Joshi/1st Ed./Pg. 258-259]
A. Axonotmesis
B. Neurotmosis
C. Neuropraxia
D. Traction injury

Q 42. X-ray characteristics of giant cell tumor:
[Essential Orthopaedics/Maheshwari/3rd Ed./Pg. 218-219]
A. Sun ray appearance
B. Onion peel appearance
C. Soap bubble
D. Ground glass appearance

Q 43. Prolonged immobilization can produce all of the following except:
[Therapeutic Exercise/Kisner/5th Ed./Pg. 66,890]
A. Osteoporosis
B. Joint stiffness
C. Kidney stones
D. Gallstones

Q 44. The best treatment in flail chest is:
A. Tracheostomy
B. Intercostal drainage
C. Positive pressure respiration
D. Chest binder

Q 45. Which of the following is correct in pulled elbow?
[Essential Orthopaedics/Maheshwari/3rd Ed./Pg. 88]
A. Dislocation of elbow joint
B. Sublaxation of elbow joint
C. Dislocation of radial head
D. Sublaxation of proximal radioulnar joint

Q 46. The basic cause of Volkmann's contracture is:
[Essential Orthopaedics/Maheshwari/3rd Ed./Pg. 85]
A. Muscle sequestrum formation in flexor policies longus and flexor profundus
B. Injury to ulnar and anterior interosseous nerves
C. Injury to vessels
D. Contracture of palmar fascia

Q 47. The finger deformities of Volkmann's ischemic contracture get corrected in which of the following position?
[Essential of Orthopaedics & Applied Physiotherapy/Jayanti Johsi/1st Ed./Pg. 100]
A. Wrist dorsiflexion
B. Wrist plantar flexion
C. Wrist neutral position
D. All of the above

Q 48. Post-traumatic avascular necrosis of scaphoid is most common in:
[Tidy's Physiotherapy/12th Ed./Pg. 20]
A. Proximal pole of scaphoid
B. Waist of scaphoid
C. Distal pole of scaphoid
D. None of the above

Answer										
	30 C	31 A	32 A	33 B	34 A	35 B	36 C	37 C	38 B	39 D	40 C	41 C
	42 C	43 D	44 D	45 C	46 C	47 A	48 B				

Q 49. Dupuytren's contracture is fibrosis of:
[Essential Orthopaedics/Maheshwari/3rd Ed./Pg. 882]
A. Palmar fascia
B. Forearm muscles
C. Sartorius fascia
D. None

Q 50. Most common nerve damage in shoulder dislocation:
[Essential Orthopaedics/Maheshwari/3rdEd./Pg. 76]
A. Radial nerve
B. Axillary nerve
C. Ulnar nerve
D. Median nerve

Q 51. In congenital dislocation of knee deformity seen is:
[Apley/Dutterworth/4th Ed./Pg. 309]
A. Varus
B. Valgus
C. Flexion
D. Extension

Q 52. Earliest visible change in osteoarthritis is:
[Essential Orthopaedics/Maheshwari/3rd Ed./Pg. 252]
A. Loss of water
B. Fibrillation
C. Decreased collagen content
D. Decreased hyaluronic acid level

Q 53. Earliest sign of Volkmann's ischemic contracture:
[Essential Orthopaedics/Maheshwari/3rd Ed./Pg. 85]
A. On passive extension there is pain
B. Obliteration of Radial pulse
C. Pale and cold hand
D. Warm and Red hand

Q 54. Most commonly the involved structure in Dupuytren's contracture is:
[Essential Orthopaedics/Maheshwari/3rd Ed./Pg. 257]
A. Natatory ligament
B. Pretendinous bands
C. Superficial transverse ligament
D. All of these

Q 55. The most common organism causing hematogenous osteomyelitis in children is:
[Essential Orthopaedics/Maheshwari/3rd Ed./Pg. 157]
A. *E. coli*
B. Tubercle bacillus
C. *Salmonella*
D. *Staphylococcus*

Q 56. Multiple hereditary osteochondrometosis presents all of the following problems except:
[Churchill/12th Ed./Pg. 131]
A. Bony swelling over body
B. Joint deformities
C. Leg length discrepancy
D. Anemia and toxemia

Q 57. Paraplegia in tuberculosis is most common in which region of the spine?
[Essential Orthopaedics/Maheshwari/3rd Ed./Pg. 1178]
A. Cervical spine
B. Dorsal spine
C. Lumbar spine
D. Sacral spine

Q 58. Gastrocnemius resection is done most commonly in:
[Essential Orthopaedics/Maheshwari/3rd Ed./Pg. 197]
A. CTEV
B. Residual polio
C. Cerebral palsy
D. Arthrogyposis multiplex

Q 59. Which of the following is correct female preponderance ratio in DDH?
[Essential Orthopaedics/Maheshwari/3rd Ed./Pg. 200]
A. Kyphosis
B. Scoliosis
C. Paraplegia
D. Hormonal

Q 60. All are the features of spinal tuberculosis except:
[Essential Orthopaedics/Maheshwari/3rd Ed./Pg. 178]
A. Kyphosis
B. Scoliosis
C. Paraplegia
D. Abscess

Q 61. Gastrocnemius resection is done most commonly in:
[Essential Orthopaedics/Maheshwari/3rd Ed./Pg. 191]
A. Residual polio
B. CTEV
C. Cerebral palsy
D. Arthrogryposis

Q 62. The expression knee movements 15–90 degree meant all of the following except:
A. Last 15 degree extension is absent
B. Last 30 degree flexion is absent
C. Free flexion from 15–90 degree
D. Full range of knee movement present

Q 63. A physical therapist examines a patient diagnosed with an acute posterior cruciate sprain. The mechanism of injury for the posterior cruciate is:
[Essential Orthopaedics/Maheshwari/3rd Ed./Pg. 128]
A. A forceful landing on the anterior tibia with the knee hyperflexed
B. An anteriorly directed force applied to the tibia when the foot is fixed
C. A valgus force applied to the knee when the foot is fixed
D. Hyperextension, medial rotation of the leg with lateral rotation body

Q 64. A patient diagnosed with right shoulder adhesive capsulitis is limited to 25 degrees of lateral rotation. Which mobilization technique would be indicated with this limitation?
[Therapeutic Exercise/Kisner/5th Ed./Pg. 124]
A. Lateral distraction and anterior glide
B. Medial distraction and posterior glide
C. Lateral distraction and posterior glide
D. Medial distraction and inferior glide.

Q 65. A therapist designs an exercise program for a patient rehabilitating from a lower extremity injury. The single most important factor in an exercise program designed to increase muscular strength is:
[Therapeutic Exercise/Kisner/5th Ed./Pg. 149]
A. The recovery time between exercise sets
B. The number of repetitions per set
C. The duration of the exercise session
D. The intensity of the exercise

Q 66. A patient involved in a motor vehicle accident sustains a fracture of the proximal fibula. The fracture damages the motor component of the common peroneal nerve.

Answer												
	49 A	50 B	51 D	52 B	53 A	54 D	55 D	56 D	57 B	58 A	59 D	60 B
	61 B	62 D	63 A	64 A	65 D							

Ankle dorsiflexion and eversion are tested as 2/5. The most appropriate intervention to assist patient with activities of daily living would be:

[Essential Orthopaedics/Maheshwari/3rd Ed./Pg. 59]

A. Electrical stimulation
B. An orthosis
C. An exercise
D. An exercise program
E. An aquatic program

Q 67. A therapist implements an aquatic program for a patient rehabilitating from a total hip replacement. During the treatment session the patient indicates how much easier it is to walk in the water compared to on land. What factor is responsible for the patient's ability to walk in water?

[Therapeutic Exercise/Kisner/5th Ed./Pg. 274]

A. Buoyancy
B. Pressure
C. Cohesion
D. Viscosity

Q 68. A therapist develops a list of behavioral objectives for a patient three weeks status post open reduction and internal fixation of the right femur. Which of the following would not be classified as a behavioral objective?

[Jayant Joshi/5th Ed./Pg. 156-157]

A. The patient will comprehend the difference between a two and a three-point gait pattern
B. The patient will provide two examples of appropriate exercise activities for his current condition
C. The patient will identify two appropriate assistive devices for ambulation
D. The patient will reform two sets of ten repetitions of shortening are quads and hell slides daily

Q 69. A patient is referred to physical therapy 24 hours after a total knee replacement. What exercise would be the most appropriate to begin treatment?

[Essential of Orthopaedics & Applied Physiotherapy/ Jayant Joshi/1st Ed./Pg. 213]

A. Quadriceps sets
B. Short arc quads
C. Standing leg curls
D. Straight leg raise

Q 70. A patient reports to her therapist that she completely tore one of the ligaments in her ankle. If the patient's comment is accurate, the injury to the ligament should be classified as a:

[Essential Orthopaedics/Maheshwari/ 3rd Ed./Pg. 4-5]

A. Grade I sprain
B. Grade III sprain
C. Grade I strain
D. Grade III strain

Q 71. A therapist reviews the medical chart of a patient admitted to the hospital two days age. The chart specifies the epidermal and dermal layers were completely destroyed and some of the subcutaneous tissue was damaged. This description best describes a ___ burn?

[Physical Rehabilitation/O'Sullivan/4th Ed./Pg. 850-851]

A. Superficial partial-thickness
B. Deep partial-thickness
C. Full-thickness
D. Subdermal

Q 72. Total joint replacements can allow individuals to achieve a significantly higher functional level. What is the primary indication for a total joint replacement?

A. Effusion
B. Limited range of motion
C. Muscle atrophy
D. Pain

Q 73. To test for possible anterior shoulder instability a physical therapist should move the humerus into:

[Orthopedic/Physical Assessment/Maggi/ 5th Ed./Pg. 279]

A. Abduction and medial rotation
B. Adduction and medial rotation
C. Abduction and lateral rotation
D. Adduction and lateral rotation

Q 74. A patient scheduled for total hip replacement surgery is referred to physical therapy for preoperative instruction. All of the following should be incorporated into the preoperative session except:

[Essential of Orthopaedics & Applied Physiotherapy Jayant Joshi/1st Ed./Pg. 205]

A. Deep breathing and coughing exercises
B. Gait training with an appropriate assistive device
C. Basic precautions for early bed mobility
D. Proper use of an adduction pillow

Q 75. A therapist examines a patient diagnosed with an Achilles tendon injury. Which clinical finding is not indicative of a ruptured Achilles tendon?

[Essential of Orthopaedics & Applied Physiotherapy/ Jayant Joshi/Pg. 562]

A. Negative Thompson test
B. Absent Achilles reflex
C. Lack of toe off during gait
D. A palpable defect in the musculotendinous unit

Q 76. A patient four weeks status post arthroscopic medial meniscectomy is limited in knee flexion range of motion. Which mobilization technique would be the most beneficial to increase knee flexion?

[Therapeutic Exercise/Kisner/5th Ed./Pg. 139]

A. Anterior glide of the tibia
B. Superior glide of the patella
C. Posterior glide of the tibia
D. Anterior glide of the fibula head

Q 77. Assuming normal development, which activity would typically not occur prior to nine months of age?

[Cash's Neurology/Pg. 43]

A. Rolling from prone to supine
B. Sitting independently
C. Use of a pincer grasp
D. Creeping

Q 78. A patient with a spinal cord injury positioned on a tilt table elevated to 60 degrees begins to complain of dizziness and nausea. The therapist's most immediate response should be to:

[Physical Rehabilitation/O'Sullivan/4th Ed./Pg. 884]

Answer   66 B   67 A   68 A   69 A   70 B   71 C   72 D   73 C   74 D   75 A   76 C   77 C

A. Lower the tilt table 10 degrees and take off the patient's abdominal binder

B. Leave the tilt table at 60 degrees and call for medical assistance

C. Monitor the patient's vital signs with the tilt table at 60 degrees and continue to elevate the table as tolerated

D. Lower the tilt table to horizontal and monitor the patient's vital signs

Q 79. A patient is referred to physical therapy with a C6 nerve root injury. Which of the following clinical findings would not be expected with this type of injury?

[Physical Rehabilitation/O'Sullivan/
4th Ed./Pg. 498]

A. Diminished sensation on the anterior arm and the index finger

B. Weakness in the biceps and supinator

C. Diminished brachioradialis reflex

D. Paresthesias of the long and ring fingers

Q 80. A therapist is concerned about the possibility of a patient developing a deep vein thrombosis following surgery. Which of the following special test would be useful to identify the presence of a deep vein thrombosis?

[Physical Rehabilitation/O'Sullivan/4th Ed./Pg. 588]

A. Bunnel-Littler test   B. Homans' sign

C. Kleiger test   D. Froment's sign

Q 81. A patient recovering into the hospital from a total knee replacement is examined by a physical therapist. Assuming an uncomplicated recovery, now much knee range of motion is realistic prior to discharge?

[Essential of Orthopaedics & Applied Physiotherapy
Jayant Joshi/1st Ed./Pg. 213]

A. 0-60 degrees   B. 0-90 degrees

C. 15-90 degrees   D. 15-105 degrees

Q 82. A therapist examines a 40 year old female diagnosed with rheumatoid arthritis. Which clinical finding is not characteristic of rheumatoid arthritis?

[Essential Orthopaedics/Maheshwari/3rd Ed./Pg. 245]

A. Ulnar deviation of the fingers

B. Swan neck deformity

C. Boutonniere deformity

D. Heberden's nodes

Q 83. While examining a patient diagnosed with Achilles tendonitis, a therapist, notes that the foot appears to be pronated in standing. Which motions combine to create pronation?

[Therapeutic Exercise/Kisner/5th Ed./Pg. 761]

A. Abduction, dorsiflexion, eversion

B. Adduction, dorsiflexion, inversion

C. Abduction, plantar flexion eversion

D. Adduction, plantar flexion inversion

Q 84. A patient status post motor vehicle accident is treated using skeletal traction. What bone when fractured is often associated with this type of traction?

[Essential Orthopaedics/Maheshwari/3rd Ed./Pg. 121]

A. Femur   B. Humerus

C. Tibia   D. Fibula

Q 85. A therapist examines a patient with bicipital tendonitis. Which clinical finding would you not expect the therapist to identify when examining the patient?

[Essential of Orthopaedics & Applied Physiotherapy
Jayant Joshi/1st Ed./Pg. 483]

A. Isometric resistance to the biceps brachii increases subjective pain levels

B. Referred pain in the c7-c8 dermatome

C. A painful arc is noted with active range of motion of the involved shoulder

D. Tenderness to palpation over the bicipital tendon

Q 86. A therapist examines a patient two days status post total hip replacement using a posterolateral approach. The patient is in bed with a sling-pulley system. Which exercise would be inappropriate for the patient assuming an uncomplicated postoperative course?

[Essential of Orthopaedics & Applied Physiotherapy
Janant Joshi/1st Ed./Pg. 208]

A. Active-assistive abduction and adduction with the thigh supported in the sling

B. Active knee flexion and extension in the suspension ling

C. Active exercise to the upper extremities

D. Bilateral ankle pumps

Q 87. A 25 year old male is diagnosed with a first degree acromioclavicular sprain. The injury occurred two days ago after being checked into the boards while playing hockey. Which of the following would you not expect to be true during the initial examination?

[Essential Orthopaedics/Maheshwari/
3rd Ed./Pg. 74]

A. Increased elevation of the clavicular end of the acromion

B. Inability to bring the arm completely across the chest

C. Inability to fully abduct the arm throughout the full range of motion

D. Point tenderness on palpation of the injury site

Q 88. Patella tracking dysfunction is a common problem in orthopedics. Dynamic factors for patella tracking dysfunction include:

[Therapeutic Exercise/Kisner/5th Ed./
Pg. 691,697/711]

A. Increase in the angulation between the quadriceps muscle and the patella tendon

B. A lateral femoral condyle that is not sufficiently prominent anteriorly

C. Vastus medialis oblique muscle insufficiency

D. Shallow trochlear groove

Q 89. A therapist instructs a patient in residual limb wrapping. Which bandage would be the most appropriate to utilize for a patient with a transfemoral amputation?

[Tidy's Physiotherapy/12th Ed./Pg. 211]

A. Two inch   B. Four inch

C. Six inch   D. Eight inch

Answer   78 D   79 D   80 C   81 B   82 D   83 A   84 A   85 B   86 A   87 A   88 C   89 C

Q 90. A patient with an amputation must be competent with residual limb care. The most objective long term goal for bandaging would be:

[Tidy's Physiotherapy/12th Ed./Pg. 211]

A. The patient will possess general knowledge regarding bandaging of the residual limb
B. The patient will attempt to bandage the residual limb twice a day
C. The patient will observe three styles of residual limb bandaging
D. The patient will perform proper bandaging of the residual limb 100% of the time

Q 91. A therapist provides preoperative training for a patient scheduled for thoracic surgery. Which activity would be most appropriate to deep vein thrombosis postsurgery?

[Tidy's Physiotherapy/12th Ed./Pg. 216]

A. Deep breathing   B. Incentive spirometry
C. Coughing   D. Ankle pumps

Q 92. A patient rehabilitating from cardiac surgery is monitored using an arterial line. The primary purpose of an arterial line is to:

[Refer to text]

A. Measure right arterial pressure
B. Measure heart rate and oxygen saturation of the blood
C. Measure pulmonary artery pressure
D. Measure blood pressure

Q 93. A therapist alerts a nurse to skin breakdown on a patient's right heel. Which position would leave the patient most susceptible to additional tissue damage?

*[Physical Rehabilitation/O'sullivan/
4th Ed./Pg. 883]*

A. Right side-lying   B. Left side-lying
C. Prone   D. Supine

Q 94. A therapist reminds a patient of postoperative contraindications following hip replacement surgery. Which statement would not be considered good advice?

*[Essential of Orthopaedics & Applied Physiotherapy
Jayant Joshi/1st Ed./Pg. 208]*

A. When turning, pivot to the affected side
B. Do not cross your legs
C. Avoid low chairs
D. Keep a pillow between your legs while sleeping

Q 95. Based on the "rule of nines", an adult who has burns on the anterior right arm, the anterior of the thorax, and the genital region would be classified as having burns over ____ percent of body?

[Tidy's Physiotherapy/12th Ed./Pg. 304]

A. 19   B. 2.5
C. 23.5   D. 28

Q 96. A patient is referred to physical therapy for range of motion and strengthening exercises after sustaining an anterior dislocation of the shoulder. The patient was immobilized in a sling and swathe for four weeks and it has been five weeks since the injury date. Which activity would

be the most appropriate for the patient to begin strengthening of the involved shoulder?

*[Essential of Orthopaedics & Applied Physiotherapy
Jayant Joshi/1st Ed./Pg. 2]*

A. Medial and lateral rotation in side-lying with two pound weights within the available range of motion
B. Medial and lateral rotation using elastic tubing with the arm at the patient's side and elbow at 90 degrees
C. Isokinetic medial and lateral rotation at speeds less than 120 degrees per second
D. Isometric strengthening exercise with the arm positioned at the patient's side

Q 97. A patient status postradical mastectomy secondary to breast cancer is referred to physical therapy. Typical intervention includes all of the following except:

[Tidy's Physiotherapy/12th Ed./Pg. 380]

A. Monitoring postoperative circumferential measurements
B. Passive and active-assistive range of motion
C. Elevation and positioning of the upper extremity
D. Providing pain medication

Q 98. A 36-year-old female is limited to 30 degrees of lateral rotation at the right shoulder. Which shoulder mobilization technique would be the most beneficial to increase lateral rotation?

[Therapeutic Exercise/Kisner/5th Ed./Pg. 124]

A. Anterior glide of the humeral head
B. Posterior glide of the humeral head
C. Inferior glide of the humeral head
D. Superior glide of the humeral head

Q 99. Which progressive resistive exercise would function to strengthen the infraspinatus and teres minor?

[Daniel/7th Ed./Pg. 108]

A. Extension of the shoulder with dumbbell weights
B. Flexion of the shoulder with dumbbell weights
C. Lateral rotation of the shoulder with elastic tubing
D. Medial rotation of the shoulder with elastic truing

Q 100. Dependent bed mobility is a realistic goal for a patient with C6 tetraplegia. In order to achieve this goal, a physical therapist should initiate strengthening to all of the following muscles except the:

[Physical Rehabilitation/O'Sullivan/4th Ed./Pg. 895]

A. Teres major   B. Flexor carpi ulnaris
C. Biceps brachii   D. Anterior deltoid

Q 101. A physical therapist examines a 16-year-old male diagnosed with left knee anterior cruciate ligament insufficiency. During the examination a Lachman test is performed. Ideally, the therapist should perform the test with the knee in:

[Essential Orthopaedics/Maheshwari/3rd Ed./Pg. 313]

A. Complete extension   B. 15-20 degrees
C. 25-35 degrees   D. 35-40 degrees

Q 102. A patient with a full-thickness burn over the entire anterior aspect of the neck is examined in physical therapy. The physical therapist must plan a treatment program based on the anticipation of a possible ______ contracture:

[Tidy's Physiotherapy/12th Ed./Pg. 300]

Answer   90 D   91 D   92 D   93 D   94 A   95 C   96 D   97 D   98 A   99 C   100 B   101 C

A. Flexion
B. Extension
C. Rotation with extension
D. Rotation with side bending

Q 103. Proper position of the affected area is essential for patients with burns. Proper positioning should be maintained:
[Tidy's Physiotherapy/12th Ed./Pg. 307]
A. Not less than twelve hours per day
B. Until skin grafts have been performed
C. Only when the patient is sleeping
D. Consistently throughout the day

Q 104. A patient with a transfemoral amputation begins gait training with prosthesis. What effect will a hip flexion contracture have on the patient's gait?
[Tidy's Physiotherapy/KM Varghese/12th Ed./Pg. 269]
A. The patient will demonstrate increased stability in the prosthetic knee
B. The patient's step length on the prosthetic side will be increased.
C. The hip flexion contracture will not affect the patient's gait pattern
D. The patient will not begin to ambulate until normal range of motion is restored

Q 105. A physical therapist examines a patient with a suspected acutely torn medial meniscus. Which symptom is not commonly associated with a medial meniscus tear?
[Essential Orthopaedics/Maheshwari/3rd Ed./Pg. 129]
A. Tenderness along the medial point line
B. Moderation to severe pain
C. Joint locking
D. Hamstrings atrophy

Q 106. A physical therapist treats a 32 year old female diagnosed with thoracic outlet syndrome. While exercising the patient begins to complain of feeling light headed and dizzy. The therapist immediately pushes the patient to a nearby chair and begins to monitor her vital signs. The therapist measure the patient's respiration rate as 10 breaths per minute, pulse rate of 45 beats per minute, and blood pressure of 115/85 mm Hg. Which of the following statements is most accurate?
[Reider/1st Ed./Pg. 61]
A. Pulse rate and respiration rate are below normal levels
B. Pulse rate and blood pressure are above normal levels
C. Blood pressure and respiration rate are above normal levels
D. The patient's vital signs are within normal limits

Q 107. In designing a wheelchair for a patient with bilateral transfemoral amputations, the axle should be moved in what direction?
[Refer to text]
A. Two inches laterally
B. Two inches backward
C. Two inches forward
D. Standard position is appropriate

Q 108. Which aquatic exercise would be the most effective in reducing tone in a patient with a spinal cord injury?
[Cash's Neurology/4th Ed./Pg. 348]
A. Slow passive movements of the neck and upper extremities with the patient floating in supine
B. Passive abduction and adduction of the upper extremities with the patient in short sitting
C. Approximation of the trunk with the patient floating in supine
D. Gentle rocking of the trunk with the patient in short sitting

Q 109. A therapist prepares to treat a patient in isolation by donning a mask. Which of the following solution categories would require only the use of a mask?
[Refer to text]
A. Strict isolation
B. Contact isolation
C. Respiratory isolation
D. Enter precautions

Q 110. A 14 year old girl presents with a twenty-five degree left thoracic scoliotic curvature. All of the following are appropriate immediate forms of treatment except:
[Essential Orthopaedics/Maheshwari/3rd Ed./Pg. 234-235]
A. Use of corset/orthotics
B. Postural exercise
C. Deep breathing
D. Surgical intervention

Q 111. A therapist examines a patient referred to physical therapy diagnosed with bicipital tendonitis. Which of the following special tests would be the most useful to confirm the patient's diagnosis?
[Orthopaedic Physical Assessment/5th Ed./Pg. 309]
A. Halstead maneuver
B. Apprehension test
C. Drop arm test
D. Yergasn's test

Q 112. When wrapping the residual limb of a patient with a transfemoral amputation a therapist should adhere to all of the following except:
[Tidy's Physiotherapy/12th Ed./Pg. 264]
A. The bandage should provide increased pressure proximally
B. The bandage should be smooth and wrinkle free
C. The bandage should be applied using diagonal turns
D. The bandage should be applied to encourage proximal joint extension

Q 113. Which surgical technique is commonly performed on a shoulder to repair a defect in the glenoid labrum?
[Essential Orthopaedics/Maheshwari/3rd Ed./Pg. 76]
A. Acromioplasty
B. Bankart
C. Inferior capsular shift
D. Magnuson

Q 114. A physical therapist assists a patient with C7 tetraplegia into a prone on elbows position on a mat. The therapist instructs the patient to push his elbows down, tuck his chin, and lift his trunk off of the mat while rounding out the shoulders. This exercise is helpful in strengthening the:
[Physical Rehabilitation/O'Sullivan/4th Ed./Pg. 414]
A. Serratus anterior and scapular muscles
B. Serratus anterior
C. Latissimus dorsi and scapular muscles
D. Sacrospinalis and semispinalis

**Q 115. A physical therapist instructs a 67-year-old female, four weeks status post total hip replacement in a home exercise

---

Answer 102 A 103 D 104 B 105 D 106 A 107 B 108 A 109 C 110 D 111 D 112 A 113 B
114 A

program. Which exercise description would be inappropriate for the patient?

[Essential of Orthopaedics & Applied Physiotherapy/ Jayant Joshi/Elesiver/1st Ed./Pg. 208]

A. Lie on your involved side and lift the involved leg towards the ceiling.
B. Place a rolled up towel under your knee. Rest the weight of the thigh on the towel roll. Lift the heel off the table so that you straighten the knee.
C. Lie on your back with the opposite knee bent. Tighten the thigh muscle, keeping the leg straight and lift the leg toward the ceiling
D. Lie on your back with knees bent. Raise you buttocks off the table

Q 116. A 16-year-old basketball player is anxious to return to athletic competition following rehabilitation from an Achilles tendon rupture. The athlete is objectively ready to return to competition, however continues to demonstrate a severe preoccupation with reinjury. The most appropriate response is the:

[Essential of Orthopaedics & Applied Physiotherapy/ Jayant Joshi/1st Ed./Pg. 562-563]

A. Allow the patient to return to basketball without restriction
B. Information patient that he should not participate in basketball this season
C. Design a functional progression for basketball which allows the patient to progress to higher level activities in a gradual fashion
D. Discuss other less demanding athletic activities with the patient

Q 117. A patient is referred to physical therapy after sustaining a Colles' fracture. A Colles' fracture refers to an injury of the:

[Essential Orthopaedics/Maheshwari/3rd Ed./Pg. 192]

A. Ulna
B. Radius
C. Olecranon
D. Scaphoid

Q 118. A physical therapist treats a patient with incomplete L4 paraplegia. The therapist uses proprioceptive neuromuscular facilitation techniques to strengthen the abdominals and improve trunk stability in sitting. The most appropriate technique to improve strength and control include:

[Therapeutic Exercise/Kisner/5th Ed./Pg. 202]

A. Hold-relax alternating movement in sitting
B. D1 flexion in quadruped
C. D1 flexion in supine
D. Alternating isometrics and timing for emphasis in sitting

Q 119. A patient two weeks status post transtibial amputation is instructed by his physician to remain at rest for two days after contracting bronchitis. The most appropriate position for the patient in bed is:

[Essential of Orthopaedics & Applied Physiotherapy/ Jayant Joshi/1st Ed./Pg. 231]

A. Supine with a pillow under the patient's knees
B. Supine with a pillow under the patient's thigh and knee
C. Supine with the legs extended
D. Side-lying in the fetal position

Q 120. A 21-year-old male suffers a primary dislocation of the right shoulder playing football. The athlete is referred to physical therapy after three weeks of immobilization. A physical therapist might elect to begin treatment with all of the following except:

[Essential of Orthopaedics & Applied Physiotherapy/ Jayant Joshi/1st Ed./Pg. 79, 81]

A. Isometric shoulder exercises
B. Passive range of motion exercises
C. Active-assistive range of motion exercises
D. High speed isokinetic exercises

Q 121. A patient with a C3 spinal cord injury is positioned in supine. Which area is most susceptible to pressure in this position?

[Physical Rehabilitation/O'Sullivan/4th Ed./Pg. 883]

A. Greater trochanter
B. Anterior iliac crest
C. Medial malleolus
D. Sacrum

Q 122. A therapist identifies excessive femoral neck anteversion during an examination of a patient diagnosed with trochanteric bursitis. This structural finding commonly results in:

[Joint Structure and Function/Norkin/ 3rd Ed./Pg. 323]

A. An increase in hip lateral rotation
B. An increase in hip medial rotation
C. An increase in hip extension
D. An increase in hip flexion

Q 123. The most common mechanism for an anterior talofibular ligament sprain is:

[Essential of Orthopaedics & Applied Physiotherapy Jayant Joshi/Pg. 556]

A. Inversion and dorsiflexion
B. Inversion an plantar flexion
C. Inversion
D. Pronation, eversion, and dorsiflexion

Q 124. A patient is referred to physical therapy diagnosed with right hip trochanteric bursitis. Which clinical finding is usually not associated with trochanteric bursitis?

[Essential of Orthopaedics & Applied Physiotherapy/ Jayant Joshi/1st Ed./Pg. 33]

A. Resisted abduction reproduces symptoms
B. Full hip active range of motion
C. Positive Ober's test
D. Joint play motions are limited in a capsular pattern

Q 125. A patient status post large rotator cuff repair surgery is referred to physical therapy. Which of the following motions would you initially expect to be the most restricted?

[Essential of Orthopaedics & Applied Physiotherapy/ Jayant Joshi/1st Ed./Pg. 478 -479]

A. Extension
B. Abduction
C. Medial rotation
D. Lateral rotation

Q 126. A physical therapist performs passive range of motion to a patient with C7 tetraplegia. The patient's bilateral straight leg raise is measured passively to 90 degrees. What should

---

Answer   115 A   116 C   117 B   118 D   119 C   120 D   121 D   122 B   123 B   124 D   125 D

the physical therapist conclude about the patient's ability to perform activities of daily living?

[Physical Rehabilitation/O'Sullian/4th Ed./Pg. 898]

A. The patient requires a straight leg raise of 110–120 degrees in order to perform long sit and activities of daily living
B. The patient is at a functional range to perform long sit and activities of daily living
C. The patient's range of motion is beyond the expected limit for long sit and activities of daily living
D. The patient requires a straight leg raise of 150 degrees in order to perform long sit and activities of daily living

Q 127. A patient with one week status post left total hip replacement is diagnosed with an acute deep vein thrombosis in the left calf. The physical therapist's role in the care of a deep vein thrombosis is:

[Physical Rehabilitation/O'sullivan/4th Ed./Pg. 798]

A. Continued gait training with an assistive device and partial weight bearing
B. Progressive resistive exercise for bilateral lower extremities
C. Patient is on bedrest with no active therapy to the left leg
D. Postural drainage and diaphragmatic breathing

Q 128. To calculate % TBSA (according to the rules of nines) left lower extremity is given weightage of:

[Physical Rehabilitation/O'Sullivan/4th Ed./Pg. 853]

A. 9%   B. 9.9%
C. 27%   D. 18%

Q 129. A 15-year-old boy has pain over the tibial tubercle and clinically very prominent. The pain has been for 4 months with no history of injury and systemic illness. He most probably has:

[Essential Orthopaedics/Maheshwari/3rd Ed./Pg. 269]

A. Osgood-Schlatter disease
B. Ruptured quadriceps tendon
C. Fracture of tibial tubercle
D. Anterior cruciate ligament instability

Q 130. The carpal tunnel located on the volar aspect of the wrist contains:

[Therapeutic Exercise/Kisner/5th Ed./Pg. 370]

A. 9 tendons and median nerve
B. 11 tendons and ulnar nerve
C. 11 tendons and radial nerve
D. 7 tendons and median nerve

Q 131. A patient with a full-thickness burn receives a skin graft. Immediately after the procedure the graft site requires:

[Physical Rehabilitation/O'Sullivan/4th Ed./Pg. 801]

A. Temporary immobilization
B. Long term immobilization of one month
C. Active-assistive range of motion
D. Aggressive passive range of motion

Q 132. A patient with a history of rheumatoid arthritis is referred to physical therapy diagnosed with acute glenohumeral joint pain. Which treatment technique would be inappropriate for the patient?

[Therapeutic Exercise/Kisner/5th Ed./Pg. 115]

A. Passive range of motion in pain free range
B. Grade iii and iv mobilization
C. Periodic immobilization in a sling
D. Gentle joint oscillation techniques

Q 133. A patient diagnosed with an incomplete spinal cord lesion that presents with muscle paralysis on the ipsilateral side of the lesion and a loss of pain, temperature, and sensitivity on the contralateral side of the lesion describes:

[Physical Rehabilitation/O'Sullivan/4th Ed./Pg. 874-875]

A. Stinert's disease
B. Central cord syndrome
C. Interior spinal artery syndrome
D. Brown-Sequard's syndrome

Q 134. The physical therapist's initial priority for an acute burn patient is:

[Physical Rehabilitation/O'Sullivan/4th Ed./Pg. 861]

A. Functional examination of bed mobility and transfers
B. Correct positioning of burned and unaffected body parts
C. Cognitive screening to determine the patient's level of understanding
D. Diversional therapy to assess the patient's level of pain

Q 135. The tendon of the _____________ muscle is commonly compressed against the bottom of the acromion process in a patient diagnosed with impingement syndrome?

[Essential of Orthopaedics & Applied Physiotherapy/ Jayant Joshi/1st Ed./Pg. 477]

A. Supraspinatus   B. Infraspinatus
C. Teres minor   D. Subscapularis

Q 136. Bed positioning is important for patient's status post amputation. The prone position or prone lying is recommended for thirty minutes several times a day. This position is of particular importance for _____ amputations?

[Essential of Orthopaedics & Applied Physiotherapy/ Jayant Joshi/1st Ed./Pg. 231]

A. Transfemoral   B. Transtibial
C. Syme's   D. Hip disarticulation

Q 137. A physical therapist observes a patient with a transfemoral amputation during gait training. The therapist identifies marked lateral rotation of the prosthesis at heel strike. Which of the following would not be a contributing factor to the patient's gait deviation?

[Essential of Orthopaedics & Applied Physiotherapy/ Jayant Joshi/Elesiver/1st Ed./Pg. 244]

A. Weak hip medial rotators
B. Inadequate suspension
C. Excessive toe-out built into the prosthesis
D. Prosthesis is too short

Q 138. A physical therapist is concerned with a patient's lateral knee discomfort. The therapist attempts to determine if contracture tensor fasciae latae or iliotibial band could be contributing to the patient's symptoms. Which special test might help to identify a restriction in this area?

[Essential of Orthopaedics & Applied Physiotherapy/ Jayant Joshi/5th Ed./Pg. 693-694]

Answer   126 A   127 C   128 D   129 A   130 A   131 A   132 B   133 D   134 C   135 A   136 A   137 D

A. Ober
B. Thomas
C. Apley's compression
D. Thomson

Q 139. A physical therapist instructs a patient diagnosed with rotator cuff tendonitis in transverse plane resistive exercises. Which motions would be appropriate based on the given information?

[Essential of Orthopaedics & Applied Physiotherapy/ Jayant Joshi/1st Ed./Pg. 480]

A. Abduction and adduction
B. Flexion and extension
C. Medial and lateral rotation
D. Pronation and supination

Q 140. A therapist hypothesizes that patient's persistent shoulder pain is caused by an injury to a specific upper extremity muscle. What selective tissue tension assessment would provide the therapist with the most useful information to test the hypothesis?

[Therapeutic Exercise/Kisner/5th Ed./Pg. 168-170]

A. Active range of motion
B. Active-assistive range of motion
C. Passive range of motion
D. Resisted isometrics

Q 141. A therapist attempts to gain information on the ligamentous integrity of the knee. Which of the following special tests would not provide the therapist with the desired information?

[Essential Orthopaedics/Maheshwari/3rd Ed./Pg. 313]

A. Anterior drawer test
B. Apprehension test
C. Lachman's test
D. Pivot shift test

Q 142. A therapist modifies a wheelchair to allow the rear wheels to be moved backward by approximately two inches. This type of modification would be most beneficial to a patient with:

[Physical Rehabilitation/O'Sullivan/4th Ed./Pg. 637]

A. Bilateral lower extremity amputations
B. Flaccid hemiplegia
C. Paraplegia
D. Tetraplegia

Q 143. A therapist performs a talar tilt test on a 22-year-old female rehabilitating from an inversion ankle sprain. Which ligament does the talar tilt test examine?

[Maggi/5th Ed./Pg. 890-893]

A. Anterior tibiofibular
B. Calcaneofibular
C. Deltoid
D. Posterior tibiofibular

Q 144. What is the first functional task that should be taught to a patient with a T2 spinal cord injury?

[Physical Rehabilitation/O'Sullivan/4th Ed./Pg. 906]

A. Rolling
B. Self range of motion
C. Ambulation with long leg braces
D. Bed to wheelchair transfer

Q 145. A patient rehabilitating from knee surgery is examined in physical therapy. The patient's involved knee range of motion begins at 15 degrees of flexion and ends at 90 degrees of flexion. The total available range of motion for this patient is _______ degrees?

[Norkin's Goniometry/3rd Ed./Pg. 33]

A. 60
B. 75
C. 90
D. 105

Q 146. A patient is able to actively hyperextend the right knee 5 degrees. Assuming the patient's total knee range of motion is 65 degrees, which of the following recordings would be the most representative of the patient's actual range of motion?

[Norkin's Goniometry/3rd Ed./Pg. 31]

A. 5-0-60
B. 5-0-65
C. 5-60
D. 5-65

Q 147. A therapist instructs a patient diagnosed with rotator cuff tendonitis in a home exercise program. The most important consideration when designing a home exercise program is to:

[Therapeutic Exercise/Kisner/5th Ed./Pg. 23]

A. Focus the program on the individual needs of the patient
B. Limit the length of the program to 10 minutes
C. Provide written instructions that detail the frequency and duration of each exercise
D. Provide written instructions that detail the frequency and duration of each exercise
E. Limit the amount of equipment required to complete the program

Q 148. A patient rehabilitating from a spinal cord injury works on self-range of motion activities in sitting. Suddenly, the patient begins to demonstrate signs and symptoms of autonomic dysreflexia. The most appropriate therapist action is to:

[Physical Rehabilitation/O'Sullivan/ 4th Ed./Pg. 883-884]

A. Keep the patient in sitting, monitor blood pressure, and check the bowel and bladder for impairment
B. Lie the patient flat, monitor blood pressure, and check the bowel and bladder for impairment
C. Lie the patient flat, monitor blood pressure, and give the patient fluids
D. Keep the patient sitting, monitor blood pressure, wait for medical assistance

Q 149. A therapist palpates proximally along the second metacarpal. Which carpal bone does not articulate with the second metacarpal?

[BD Chaurasia]

A. Capitate
B. Hamate
C. Trapezoid
D. Trapezium

Q 150. A therapist palpates the proximal row of carpals in a patient diagnosed with carpal tunnel syndrome. Which of the following bones does not articulate with the proximal row of carpals?

[Therapeutic Exercise/Kisner/5th Ed./Pg. 590]

Answer   138 A   139 C   140 D   141 B   142 A   143 B   144 A   145 B   146 A   147 A   148 A   149 B

A. Hamate
B. Radius
C. Trapezium
D. Ulna

Q 151. A therapist develops a physical therapy problem list after competing an initial examination on a patient diagnosed with right shoulder impingement. Which of the following entries would not typically belong in the physical therapy problem list?

[Refer to text]
A. Decreased active right shoulder lateral rotation
B. Decreased strength of the right upper trapezius and middle deltoid
C. Increased pain with right shoulder active movement
D. Increased stress secondary to financial problems

Q 152. Which clinical observation is not usually characteristic with a rotator cuff tear?

[Essential of Orthopaedics & Applied Physiotherapy/ Jayant Joshi/1st Ed./Pg. 478]
A. The patient is less than 40 years old
B. The patient is often unable to move the arm actively without pain
C. Scapulohumeral rhythm is altered
D. Night pain is a common patient complaint

Q 153. Earliest sign of Volkmann's ischemic contracture is:

[Essential Orthopaedics/Maheshwari/3rd Ed./Pg. 85]
A. Pain
B. Numbness
C. Paresthesia
D. Pallor

Q 154. Claw hand is seen in:
A. Ulnar nerve injury
B. Carpal tunnel syndrome
C. Syringomyelia
D. Cervical rib

Q 155. Nerve abscess is seen in the .... nerve.

[Essential Orthopaedics/Maheshwari/3rd Ed./Pg. 51]
A. Median
B. Ulnar
C. Lateral fibular
D. Sciatic

Q 156. Tardy ulnar nerve palsy is due to:

[Essential Orthopaedics/Maheshwari/3rd Ed./Pg. 87]
A. Cubitus valgus
B. Fixation of nerve in the groove by osteoarthritis
C. Excision of elbow joint
D. Fracture of internal condyle

Q 157. Myositis ossificans is commonly seen at in the......... joint:

[Therapeutic Exercise/Kisner/5th Ed./Pg. 574]
A. Knee
B. Elbow
C. Shoulder
D. Hip

Q 158. Duptyren's contracture is:

[Essential Orthopaedics/Maheshwari/3rd Ed./Pg. 256]
A. Thickening of palmar fascia
B. Base of little finger involved first
C. Seen in cirrhotics
D. Seen in epileptics on hydantoin
E. All of the above

Q 159. Calcification of menisci is seen in:

[Essential Orthopaedics/Maheshwari/3rd Ed./Pg. 251]
A. Hyperparathyroidism
B. Pseudogout
C. Renal osteodystrophy
D. Acromegaly

Q 160. Clubfoot in a newborn is treated by:

[Essential Orthopaedics/Maheshwari/3rd Ed./Pg. 196]
A. Surgery
B. Manipulation by the mother
C. Dennis Brown splint
D. Strapping

Q 161. Tardy ulnar nerve palsy is not seen in:

[Essential Orthopaedics/Maheshwari/3rd Ed./Pg. 87]
A. Cubitus valgus
B. Dislocation of elbow
C. Fracture scaphoid
D. B and C

Q 162. Commonest cause of wrist drop is:

[Essential Orthopaedics/Maheshwari/3rd Ed./Pg. 86]
A. Intramuscular injection
B. Fracture humerus
C. Dislocation of elbow
D. Dislocation of shoulder

Q 163. Distance from elbow in forearm amputation is..... inches.

[Tidy/KM Varghese/12th Ed./Pg. 273]
A. 5
B. 7
C. 8
D. 9

Q 164. Distance from the acromion in arm amputation is..... inches.

[Tidy/KM Varghese/12th Ed./Pg. 273]
A. 5
B. 7
C. 8
D. 9

Q 165. Distance from the tip of greater trochanter in thigh amputation is.....inches.

[Tidy's Physiotherapy/12th Ed./Pg. 260]
A. 5
B. 7
C. 9
D. 11

Q 166. Distance from the knee joint in below knee amputation is......inches.

[Tidy/KM Varghese/12th Ed./Pg. 260]
A. 4
B. 5.5
C. 6
D. 7

Q 167. Musculoskeletal abnormalities in neurofibromatosis is:

[Essential Orthopaedics/Maheshwari/3rd Ed./Pg. 269]
A. Hypertrophy of limb
B. Scoliosis
C. Pseudoarthrosis
D. All

Q 168. Commonest cause of paraplegia:

[Essential Orthopaedics/Maheshwari/3rd Ed./Pg. 153]
A. Tuberculosis
B. Trauma
C. Secondaries
D. Transverse myelitis

Q 169. Myositis ossificans is most common around the joint:

[Therapeutic Exercise/Kisner/5th Ed./Pg. 574]
A. Knee
B. Elbow
C. Wrist
D. Hip

Q 170. Treatment of CTEV should begin:

[Essential Orthopaedics/Maheshwari/3rd Ed./Pg. 193]

Answer

150 D	151 D	152 A	153 A	154 A	155 B	156 A	157 B	158 E	159 B	160 B	161 D
162 C	163 B	164 C	165 D	166 B	167 D	168 B	169 B				

A. Soon after birth   B. After discharge from hospital
C. After one month   D. At 2 years

Q 171. Soft tissue calcification around the knee is seen in:
[Essential Orthopaedics/Maheshwari/3rd Ed./Pg. 251]
A. Scurvy   B. Scleroderma
C. Hyperparathyroidism   D. Pseudogout

Q 172. In De Quervain's syndrome the following tendons are inflamed:
[Essential Orthopaedics/Maheshwari/3rd/Pg. 257]
A. Extensor pollicis longus and extensor pollicis brevis
B. Extensor carpi radialis longus and opponens
C. Extensor pollicis brevis and abductor pollicis longus
D. Abductor pollicis and extensor carpi radialis brevis

Q 173. Commonest site of myositis ossificans traumatica is:
[Therapeutic Exercise/Kisner/5th Ed./Pg. 79]
A. Brachialis   B. Extensor carpi radialis longus
C. Triceps brachii   D. Brachioradialis

Q 174. In pseudogout features include:
[Essential Orthopaedics/Maheshwari/3rd Ed./Pg. 251]
A. Involvement of smaller joints and uric acid crystals
B. Involvement of large joints and calcium pyrophosphate crystals
C. Involvement of large joints and hypercalcemia
D. Involvement of large joins and uric acid crystals

Q 175. The mallet finger results from injury to:
[Essential Orthopaedics/Maheshwari/3rd Ed./Pg. 100]
A. Abductor digiti minimi
B. Extensor carpi radialis longus
C. Extensor carpi ulnaris
D. Extensor tendons of the terminal phalanx of finger

Q 176. Perthe's disease is characterized by:
[Essential Orthopaedics/Maheshwari/3rd Ed./Pg. 269]
A. Painful hip in childhood and avascular necrosis of femoral head
B. Fracture displacement of neck of femur in an adolescent
C. Congenital dislocation of hip
D. Femoral anteversion in childhood

Q 177. Greenstick fracture generally occurs in:
[Essential Orthopaedics/Maheshwari/3rd Ed./Pg. 47]
A. Children   B. Osteoporosis
C. Very old persons   D. Infected bones

Q 178. Most important pathology in club foot is:
[Essential Orthopaedics/Maheshwari/3rd Ed./Pg. 194]
A. Congenital talonavicular dislocation
B. Tightening of ttendo-Achilles
C. Calcaneal fracture
D. Lateral derangement

Q 179. The most important sign in Volkmann's ischemic contracture is
[Essential Orthopaedics/Maheshwari/3rd Ed./Pg. 185]
A. Pain   B. Pallor
C. Numbness   D. Obliteration of radial pulse

Q 180. Painful arc syndrome is due to:
[Essential Orthopaedics/Maheshwari/3rd Ed./Pg. 76]
A. Chronic supraspinatus tendinitis
B. Subacromial bursitis
C. Fracture greater tubercle
D. All of the above

Q 181. Which of the following is characteristic feature of Charcot's joint?
[Essential Orthopaedics/Maheshwari/3rd Ed./Pg. 166}
A. Acutely painful swollen joint
B. Painless swollen stiff joint
C. Painless swollen hypermobile joint
D. Red hot ankylosed joint

Q 182. Which of the following crystals are present in gouty arthritis?
[Essential Orthopaedics/Maheshwari/3rd Ed./Pg. 251]
A. Monosodium urate dehydrate
B. Monosodium urate monohydrate
C. Calcium hydroxyappetite
D. Purine nucleotide

Q 183. The commonest deformity at hip in post polio residual paralysis is:
[Essential Orthopaedics/Maheshwari/3rd Ed./Pg. 268]
A. Flexion deformity
B. Extension deformity
C. Flexion adduction deformity
D. Flexion abduction deformity

Q 184. McMurray's test is most frequently positive in which of the following injuries?
[Essential Orthopaedics/Maheshwari/3rd Ed./Pg. 313]
A. Torn anterior cruciate ligament
B. Torn posterior cruciate ligament
C. Torn medial semilunar cartilage
D. Torn lateral semilunar cartilage

Q 185. A young adult sustained a closed fracture of both bones of right leg in a scooter accident. He was treated by closed reduction and above knee plaster cast for 3 months. His fracture united but on removal of plaster his knee was stiff. The treatment of choice to regain the knee movements is:
[Therapeutic Exercise/Kisner/5th Ed./Pg. 61-62]
A. Active and assisted movements
B. CPM
C. Arthroscopic surgery
D. Open surgery

Q 186. Meniscal calcification is a feature of:
[Essential Orthopaedics/Maheshwari/3rd Ed./Pg. 25]
A. Gout   B. Hyperparathyroidism
C. Pseudogout   D. Ankylosing spondylitis

Q 187. Recurrent clubfoot is due to failure of development of:
[Essential Orthopaedics/Maheshwari/3rd Ed./Pg. 198]
A. Tendocalcaneus   B. Peroneal muscles
C. Plantar fascia   D. Tibialis anterior

Answer	170 A	171 D	172 C	173 A	174 B	175 D	176 A	177 A	178 A	179 D	180 D	181 C
	182 A	183 D	184 C	185 B	186 C	187 A						

Q 188. The early feature of Pott's paraplegia is:
[Essential Orthopaedics/Maheshwari/3rd Ed./Pg. 178-179]
A. Flexor spasm
B. Increased tendon jerk
C. Muscular atrophy
D. Sensory loss

Q 189. Maximum weight used for skin traction is:
[Essential Orthopaedics/Maheshwari/3rd Ed./Pg. 21]
A. 5 kg
B. 7 kg
C. 10 kg
D. 15 kg

Q 190. K-wire is used in:
[Essential Orthopaedics/Maheshwari/3rd Ed./Pg. 15]
A. Cerclage
B. Fixing forearm hones
C. Prior to plating
D. All the above

Q 191. Triangular relation of elbow is in:
[Essential Orthopaedics/Maheshwari/3rd Ed./Pg. 80]
A. Fracture ulna
B. Anterior dislocation of elbow
C. Posterior dislocation of elbow
D. Supracondylar fracture

Q 192. Treatment of acute myositis ossificans is:
[Essential Orthopaedics/Maheshwari/3rd Ed./Pg. 42]
A. Active mobilization
B. Passive mobilization
C. Infrared therapy
D. Immobilization

Q 193. Tardy ulnar nerve palsy is seen with:
[Essential Orthopaedics/Maheshwari/3rd Ed./Pg. 57]
A. Lateral humeral condyle fracture
B. Supracondylar fracture
C. Medial humeral condyle fracture
D. Fracture capitulum

Q 194. Anterior dislocation of shoulder causes all except:
[Essential Orthopaedics/Maheshwari/3rd Ed./Pg. 74]
A. Circumflex artery injury
B. Avascular necrosis head of femur
C. Brachial plexus injury
D. Hip bone fractures

Q 195. Trendelenburg's sign is not seen in:
[Essential Orthopaedics/Maheshwari/3rd Ed./Pg. 305]
A. Tuberculous arthritis
B. Rheumatoid arthritis
C. Posterior dislocation hip
D. Torn smith arthritis

Q 196. Infection in Ring Finger in acute Tenosynovitis is most likely to spread to
[Essential Orthopaedics/Maheshwari/3rd Ed./Pg. 256]
A. Dorsum of hand
B. Thenar space
C. Parona's space
D. Palmar space

Q 197. Medial meniscal tear is more common than that of lateral meniscus tear because of its decreased:
[Essential Orthopaedics/Maheshwari/3rd Ed./Pg. 29]
A. Nerve supply
B. Vascularity
C. Mobility
D. Fibroelasticity

Q 198. Total Claw hand is caused by injury to:
[Essential Orthopaedics/Maheshwari/3rd Ed./Pg. 53-54]
A. Radial nerve
B. Ulnar and radial nerve
C. Ulnar and medial nerve
D. Radial and medial nerve

Q 199. Most common cause of scoliosis in children is:
[Essential Orthopaedics/Maheshwari/3rd Ed./Pg. 233]
A. Unequal limb length
B. Postpoliomyelitis
C. Hemivertebrae
D. Marfan's syndrome

Q 200. Peripheral nerves can withstand ischemia up to:
[Essential Orthopaedics/Maheshwari/3rd Ed./Pg. 56]
A. 30 minutes
B. 1 hour
C. 2 hours
D. 4 hours

Q 201. Most common cause of neuropathic joints:
[Refer to text]
A. Diabetes
B. Leprosy
C. Syphilis
D. Rheumatoid arthritis

Q 202. In a newborn child, abduction and internal rotation produces a click sound. It is known as:
[Essential Orthopaedics/Maheshwari/3rd Ed./Pg. 201]
A. Otorolani's sign
B. Telescoping sign
C. McMurray's sign
D. Lachman's sign

Q 203. Club foot seen in a 15-year-old could be treated successfully by:
[Essential Orthopaedics/Maheshwari/3rd Ed./Pg. 195]
A. Appropriate foot wear
B. Soft tissue operation
C. Triple arthrodesis
D. Quadruple fusion

Q 204. Trigger finger is most likely to be associated with:
[Essential Orthopaedics/Maheshwari/3rd Ed./Pg. 252]
A. Diabetes
B. Trauma
C. Gout
D. Rheumatoid arthritis

Q 205. Pointing index is due to:
[Essential Orthopaedics/Maheshwari/3rd Ed./Pg. 52]
A. Ulnar nerve injury
B. Radial nerve injury
C. Median nerve injury
D. Injury to flexor digitorum profundus tendon

Q 206. Radial nerve injury of this type recovers with conservative management:
[Essential Orthopaedics/Maheshwari/3rd Ed./Pg. 51]
A. Neurotmesis
B. Crush injury
C. Neuropraxia
D. Chemical injury

Q 207. Convex foot arch is seen in:
[Essential Orthopaedics/Maheshwari/3rd Ed./Pg. 205]
A. Elderly
B. Children
C. Obese
D. Congenital vertical talus

Q 208. In correction of clubfoot by manipulation, which deformity should be corrected first?
[Essential Orthopaedics/Maheshwari/3rd Ed./Pg. 193]
A. Forefoot adduction
B. Varus
C. Eqinus
D. Internal tibial torsion

Q 209. Stiffness in knee is maximum when traction is at:
[Essential Orthopaedics/Maheshwari/3rd Ed./Pg. 71]
A. Skin
B. Lower end femur
C. Upper end tibia
D. Calcaneum

Answer

188 A	189 A	190 D	191 D	192 D	193 A	194 D	195 C	196 D	197 C	198 C	199 B
200 B	201 A	202 A	203 C	204 A	205 C	206 C	207 D	208 A	209 A		

Q 210. Bryant's triangle is useful in diagnosis of following except:
[Essential Orthopaedics/Maheshwari/3rd Ed./Pg. 310]
A. Supratrochanteric shortening
B. Intratrochanteric shortening
C. Anterior dislocation hip
D. Posterior dislocation hip

Q 211. Pathognomonic sign of traumatic fracture:
[Essential Orthopaedics/Maheshwari/3rd Ed./Pg. 1]
A. Swelling
B. Tenderness
C. Redness
D. Crepitus

Q 212. Most common mode of metastasis in osteogenic sarcoma:
[Essential Orthopaedics/Maheshwari/3rd Ed./Pg. 218]
A. Subperiosteal spread
B. Hematogenous
C. Lymphatic
D. Transcortical

Q 213. Commonest deformity in congenital dislocation of hip:
[Essential Orthopaedics/Maheshwari/3rd Ed./Pg. 111]
A. Small head of femur
B. Angle of torsion
C. Decreased neck shaft angle
D. Shallow acetabulum

Q 214. All are seen in osteogenesis imperfecta except:
[Essential Orthopaedics/Maheshwari/3rd Ed./Pg. 268]
A. Joint dislocation
B. Ligament laxity
C. Osteoporosis
D. Blue sclera

Q 215. Dashboard injury cases:
[Essential Orthopaedics/Maheshwari/3rd Ed./Pg. 111]
A. Anterior dislocation of the hip
B. Posterior dislocation of the hip
C. Central dislocation of hip
D. Fracture neck femur

Q 216. Carrying angle is decreased in:
[Essential Orthopaedics/Maheshwari/3rd Ed./Pg. 85]
A. Cubitus varus
B. Cubitus valgus
C. Genu valgum
d. Genu varum

Q 217. Treatment in the early stage of myositis ossificans is:
[Essential Orthopaedics/Maheshwari/3rd Ed./Pg. 42]
A. Immobilization
B. Massage
C. Excision of the bone
D. Active joint movements

Q 218. Most common complication of Colle's fracture is:
[Essential Orthopaedics/Maheshwari/3rd Ed./Pg. 95]
A. Non union
B. Stiffness of finger
C. Vascular injury
D. Sudeck's dystrophy

Q 219. Most common complication of clavicle fracture is:
[Essential Orthopaedics/Maheshwari/3rd Ed./Pg. 73]
A. Malunion
B. Nonunion
C. Injury to brachial plexus
D. Stiffness of shoulder

Q 220. Most common bone fractured during birth:
[Essential Orthopaedics/Maheshwari/3rd Ed./Pg. 73]
A. Scapula
B. Humerus
C. Clavicle
D. Radius

Q 221. A child with upper leg swelling with pulmonary nodule most probable diagnosis is:
[Essential Orthopaedics/Maheshwari/3rd Ed./Pg. 218]
A. Osteoclastoma
B. Chondrosarcoma
C. Osteosarcoma
D. Chondroblastoma

Q 222. Calcium content of bone is increased in:
[Essential Orthopaedics/Maheshwari/3rd Ed./Pg. 260]
A. Prolonged immobilization
B. Glucocorticoid administration
C. Hyperparathyroidism
D. Estrogen supplementation in postmenopausal women

Q 223. Bone dysplasia is due to:
[Refer to text]
A. Faulty nutrition
B. Faulty development
C. Vitamin deficiency
D. Hormonal imbalance

Q 224. Adventitious bursa is:
[Refer to text]
A. Found normally over any joint
B. Due to degeneration of connective tissue overlying a joint
C. Found over bony prominences
D. Can turn into malignancies

Q 225. Volkmann's ischemic contracture the muscle commonly involved is:
[Essential Orthopaedics/Maheshwari/3rd Ed./Pg. 85]
A. Palmaris longus
B. Flexor indicis
C. Flexor digitorum profundus
D. Flexor pollicis

Q 226. What is the position of immobilization in fracture of both bones of the forearm in an adult male?
[Essential Orthopaedics/Maheshwari/3rd Ed./Pg. 91]
A. Prone
B. Midprone
C. Full supine
D. 10 degree supine

Q 227. Common injury to baby is:
[Essential Orthopaedics/Maheshwari/3rd Ed./Pg. 3]
A. Fracture humerus
B. Fracture clavicle
C. Fracture radius and ulna
D. Fracture femur

Q 228. Most common joint to undergo dislocation is:
[Essential Orthopaedics/Maheshwari/3rd Ed./Pg. 74]
A. Shoulder
B. Radioulnar
C. Hip
D. Patellofemoral

Q 229. A football player, while playing, twists his knee over the ankle. He still continues to play. After 2 days he noticed painful swelling of the knee joint. The diagnosis is:
[Essential Orthopaedics/Maheshwari/3rd Ed./Pg. 129]
A. Medial meniscus tear
B. Anterior cruciate ligament tear
C. Medial collateral ligament injury
D. Posterior cruciate ligament injury

Q 230. A 3-year-old child falls from 2 meter height. On X-ray no abnormality of lower leg as seen. After 2 years, the child presents with calcaneal valgus. Probable cause is:
[Essential Orthopaedics/Maheshwari/3rd Ed./Pg. 141]

Answer	210 B	211 D	212 B	213 B	214 A	215 B	216 A	217 A	218 B	219 D	220 C	221 C
	222 D	223 B	224 B	225 C	226 B	227 B	228 A	229 B				

A. Undiagnosed
B. Tibial epiphyseal plate injury
C. Avascular necrosis of talus
D. Rocker bottom foot

Q 231. A patient with recurrent dislocation of shoulder presents to the hospital. The doctor tries to abduct his arm and to extend the elbow and external rotation, but the patient doesn't allow to do so. This test is called:
[Essential Orthopaedics/Maheshwari/3rd Ed./Pg. 75]
A. Duga's test
B. Hamilton's test
C. Callway's test
D. Apprehension test

Q 232. If the greater tuberosity of the humerus is lost, which of the following movements will be affected?
[Essential Orthopaedics/Maheshwari/3rd Ed./Pg. 76]
A. Adduction and flexion
B. Abduction and lateral rotation
C. Medial rotation and adduction
D. Flexion and medial rotation

Q 233. A lady present with a history of fracture radius, which was put on plaster of Paris cast for 4 weeks. After that she developed swelling of hands with shiny skin. What is the most likely diagnosis?
[Essential Orthopaedics/Maheshwari/3rd Ed./Pg. 41]
A. Rupture of extensor pollicis longus tendon
B. Myositis ossificans
C. Reflex sympathetic dystrophy
D. Malunion

Q 234. All are related to recurrent shoulder dislocation except:
[Essential Orthopaedics/Maheshwari/3rd Ed./Pg. 74]
A. Hill Sach's defect
B. Bankart lesion
C. Lax capsule
D. Rotator cuff injury

Q 235. Best diagnostic procedure for ACL injury
[Refer to text]
A. Lachman's test
B. Pivot shift test
C. Anterior drawer test
D. McMurray's test

Q 236. Sprengel's shoulder is due to deformity:
[Essential Orthopaedics/Maheshwari/3rd Ed./Pg. 204]
A. Scapula
B. Humerus
C. Clavicle
D. Vertebra

Q 237. Stress fracture is most common in:
[Essential Orthopaedics/Maheshwari/1st Ed./Pg. 74]
A. Shoulder joint
B. Patella
C. Clavicle
D. Neck of femur

Q 238. Which one of the following structures is at least risk of damage in knee dislocation?
[Essential Orthopaedics/Maheshwari/3rd Ed./Pg. 130]
A. Cruciate ligaments
B. Common peroneal nerve
C. Patella
D. Popliteal artery

Q 239. Which one of the following is not a radiological feature of osteoarthritis?
[Essential Orthopaedics/Maheshwari/3rd Ed./Pg. 252]
A. Widening of the joint space
B. Osteophyte formation
C. Subchondral sclerosis
D. Cyst formation

Q 240. Which pain is improving with exercise?
[Essential Orthopaedics/Maheshwari/3rd Ed./Pg. 251]
A. Osteoarthritis
B. Ankylosing spondylitis
C. Neurogenic joint
D. Rheumatoid arthritis

Q 241. An adult sustained a fracture of the both bones of mid forearm at the same level. After manipulation the position of immobilisation of the forearm in the plaster would be:
[Essential Orthopaedics/Maheshwari/3rd Ed./Pg. 91]
A. Full supination
B. 10° supination
C. Full pronation
D. Mid prone

Q 242. Rheumatoid arthritis can cause many symptoms in its later stages. Which of the following symptoms would most likely be common in a patient who has had rheumatoid arthritis for a long period of time?
[Essential Orthopaedics/Maheshwari/3rd Ed./Pg. 249]
A. Radial deviation of the fingers
B. Enlargement of Heberden's nodes
C. Ulnar deviation of the fingers
D. Increased muscle strength

Q 243. You are treating a patient who is complaining of right shoulder pain. The patient has been diagnosed with a frozen adhesive capsulated shoulder. Which of the following would describe the capsular pattern of the glenohumeral joint?
[Therapeutic Exercise/Kisner/Pg. 489]
A. External rotation, abduction, internal rotation
B. External rotation, internal rotation, abduction
C. Internal rotation, abduction, external rotation
D. Abduction, external rotation, internal rotation

Q 244. The hip musculature involves several muscle groups for different actions. Hip abduction takes place with nerve innervation from the superior gluteal nerve. Which muscles compose the hip abductor group?
[Therapeutic Exercise/Kisner/5th Ed./Pg. 672]
A. Psoas major, iliacus, sartorius
B. Gluteus medius, gluteus minimus, tensor fasciae latae
C. Gluteus medius, gluteus minimus, sartorius
D. Gluteus medius, gracilis, pectineus

Q 245. Which is not function of patella?
[Therapeutic Exercise/Kisner/5th Ed./Pg. 689]
A. Protection of knee joint
B. Increase the leverage
C. Convergence of muscle force
D. Increases the stride length

Q 246. Ortolani's test is done for:
[Essential Orthopaedics/Maheshwari/3rd Ed./Pg. 261]
A. Congenital dislocation of hip
B. Congenital dislocation of knee
C. Acquired dislocation of hip
D. Both B and C

Massage

Q 247. In effleurage the hands move:
[Concise Exercise therapy/Roshan Lal Meena/1st Ed./Pg. 139]

Answer

| 230 C | 231 D | 232 B | 233 C | 234 C | 235 A | 236 A | 237 C | 238 B | 239 A | 240 B | 241 D |
| 242 C | 243 A | 244 B | 245 D | 246 A | | | | | | | |

A. In the direction of gravity
B. In the direction of lymph and venous flow from medial
C. To lateral direction
D. From posterior to anterior direction

Q 248. A therapist designs a treatment plan for a patient with myositis ossificans. Which treatment would be contraindicated during the acute stage?
[Essential Orthopaedics/Maheshwari/3rd Ed./Pg. 92]
A. Rest
B. Active assistive range of motion
C. Isometrics
D. Massage

Q 249. Transverse friction massage is a valuable treatment technique in a variety of common musculoskeletal disorders. Which of the following statements does not accurately describe the application technique of transverse friction massage?
[Concise Exercise Therapy/Roshan Lal Meena/
1st Ed./Pg. 152]
A. The therapist moves the skin back and forth in a direction perpendicular to the normal orientation of the fibers
B. A lubricant is used to prevent excessive skin friction
C. Fingers that are not involved directly in the massage are used to provide stabilization
D. The rate of movement is 2–3 cycles per second and rhythmical

Q 250. Kneading, wringing, and rolling are all specific variations of which basic massage technique?
[Concise Exercise Therapy/Peepee/Roshan Lal Meena/
1st Ed./Pg. 143]
A. Effeurage
B. Vibration
C. Petrissage
D. Tapotement

Q 251. Which type of joint receptor would a therapist expect to be most sensitive to high frequency vibration deep pressure, and velocity changes in joint position?
[Physical Rehabilitation/O'sullivan/4th Ed./
Pg. 138-140]
A. Free nerve endings
B. Golgimazzoni corpuscles
C. Pacinian corpuscles
D. Ruffini endings

Physiotherapy In Medical Condition

Q 252. The lateral segment of the right lower lobe is drained by the postural drainage technique with the patient:
[Therapeutic Exercise/Kisner/5th Ed./Pg. 873]
A. Lying on the left side with the foot end of the bed raised by 18 inches
B. Lying on the right side with the foot end of the bed raised by 18 inches
C. Prone lying with foot end of the bed raised by 24 inches
D. Semi prone lying without raising the foot end of the bed

Q 253. While treating a patient in ward for chest care through coughing it should be ensured that:
[Therapeutic Exsercise/Kisner/5th Ed./Pg. 864]
A. Sputum is not expectorated
B. The patient is in supine lying position

C. The diaphragmatic breathing is not used
D. The bronchospasm is not induced

Q 254. In tracheal stimulation to elicit the cough reflex the therapist places his finger/thumb on:
[Therapeutic Exercise/Kisner/5th Ed./Pg. 870]
A. Manubrium sternum
B. Sternoclavicular joint
C. List below the xiphisternum
D. Just above the suprasternal notch

Q 255. The mitral valve of the heart controls the:
[AK Jain/Physiology/3rd Ed./Pg. 292]
A. The amount of the blood from left. Atrium to the left. Ventricle
B. The amount of the blood from left. Atrium to the right. Ventricle
C. The amount of the blood from left. Ventricle to the right. Ventricle
D. The amount of the blood to pulmonary artery

Q 256. A obstructive lung disease characterized by permanent dilation of the medium sized bronchi usually the fourth to ninth generations and repeat infections in these areas is known as:
[Therapeutic Exercise/Kisner/5th Ed./Pg. 208]
A. Bronchial asthma
B. Empyema
C. Emphysema
D. Bronchiectasis

Q 257. In rehydration therapy ORS used is:
[Essential Pediatrics/O.P. Ghai/6th Ed./Pg. 272]
A. Oxygen replacement therapy
B. Oxygenated respiratory solution
C. Oral rehydration solution
D. Optimal recovery set

Q 258. Which of the following stages of physiotherapy program is suitable for cardiac rehabilitation?
[Therapeutic Exercise/Kisner/5th Ed./Pg. 243]
A. Stage 1
B. Stage 2
C. Stage 3
D. Stage 4

Q 259. A physical therapist designs an exercise program for a patient rehabilitating from cardiac surgery. During the treatment session the therapist monitors the patient's oxygen saturation rate. Which of the following would be most representative of a normal oxygen saturation rate?
[Refer to text]
A. 45%
B. 60%
C. 80%
D. 95%

Q 260. A therapist reviews the results of a pulmonary function test of a patient with chronic obstructive pulmonary disease. Which of the following results is typical of a patient with COPD?
[Therapeutic Exercise/Kisner/5th Ed./
Pg. 875]
A. Decreased functional residual capacity
B. Increased vital capacity

Answer
247 B   248 D   249 B   250 C   251 C   252 B   253 D   254 D   255 A   256 D   257 C   258 D
259 D

C. Increased residual volume

D. Increased forced expiratory volume in one second

Q 261. A therapist working in an acute care hospital examines a patient that sustained a CVA two-day ago. The therapist positions the patient in side-lying on the hemiplegic side. Which of the following is not a benefit of positioning on the hemiplegic side?

[Physical Rehabilitation/O'Sullian/4th Ed./Pg. 550]

A. Reduces spasticity through elongation of the hemiplegic side

B. Allows the unaffected extremity to reach and perform functional tasks

C. Increases the influence of tonic neck and labyrinthine reflexes

D. Enhances proprioceptive awareness of the hemiplegic side through weight bearing

Q 262. A 12-year-old female that became anoxic in a near drowning performs dynamic activities in quadruped. The next posture to attain in the developmental sequence is:

[Physical Rehabilitation/O'sullivan/4th Ed./Pg. 419]

A. Half kneeling   B. Tall kneeling

C. Plantigrade   D. Standing

Q 263. An order is received to perform chest physical therapy on a patient status postabdominal surgery. A chart review identifies right atelectasis. The most appropriate exercise to teach the patient is:

[Therapeutic Exercise/Kisner/5th Ed./Pg. 863-869]

A. Reflex cough techniques

B. Codman's pendulum exercise

C. Segmental breathing

D. Quick paced shallow breathing

Q 264. A therapist attempts to obtain information on a patient's endurance level by administering a low level exercise test on a treadmill. Which of the following measurement methods would provide the therapist with an objective measurement of endurance?

[Therapeutic Exercise/Kisner/5th Ed./Pg. 891]

A. Facial color

B. Facial expression

C. Rating on a perceived exertion

D. Respiration rate

Q 265. A physical therapist examines a neurological patient with a flaccid left side. In order to facilitate muscular activity, the treatment plan should include:

[Physical Rehabilitation/O'Sullivan/4th Ed./Pg. 378-379]

A. Weight bearing, tapping, elevation

B. Vibration, tapping, prolonged stretch

C. Weight bearing, tapping, approximation

D. Approximation, elevation, prolonged stretch

Q 266. A therapist instructs a patient with pulmonary disease in energy conservation techniques. Which of the following techniques would be the most effective when assisting a patient to complete a selected activity without dyspnea?

[Therapeutic Exercise/Kisner/5th Ed./Pg. 893]

A. Diaphragmatic breathing   B. Pacing

C. Pursed lip breathing   D. Ventilatory muscle training.

Q 267. A therapist attempts to assist a patient to clear secretions after performing postural drainage techniques. What position would allow the patient to produce the most forceful cough?

[Therapeutic Exercise/Kisner/5th Ed./Pg. 868]

A. Prone   B. Side-lying

C. Supine   D. Upright sitting

Q 268. A therapist examines the viscosity and color of a sputum sample after competing postural drainage activities. The sputum is a yellowish-greenish color and is very thick. The therapist can best describe the sputum as:

[Tidy/KM Varghes/12th Ed./Pg. 172]

A. Fetid   B. Frothy

C. Mucoid   D. Purulent

Q 269. A physical therapist designs a treatment plan for an eight-year-old boy with cystic fibrosis. A major component of the treatment plan will include education the patient's family in appropriate bronchial drainage techniques. Which of the following lung segments would be inappropriate for bronchial drainage?

[Tidy's Physiotherapy/12th Ed./Pg. 200]

A. Left middle lobe

B. Apical segments of the upper lobes

C. Another basal segments of the lower lobes

D. Anterior segments of the upper lobes

Q 270. A therapist conducts reflex testing on a patient with a traumatic brain injury. Which stimulus should the therapist utilize to test for clonus at the ankle?

[Physical Rehabilitation/O'sullivan/4th Ed./Pg. 183]

A. Active-assistive dorsiflexion of the ankle

B. Active dorsiflexion of the ankle

C. Passive, rapid dorsiflexion of the ankle

D. Passive, slow dorsiflexion of the ankle

Q 271. A patient diagnosed with pure athetoid cerebral palsy would most likely demonstrate:

[Cash's Neurology/4th Ed./Pg. 520]

A. Disturbed sense of balance and faulty depth perception

B. Hypertonicity, contractures, and clonus

C. Show, involuntary, uncontrolled movements

D. Severe intention tremor

Q 272. A patient status post CVA rocks back and forth in a supine position with legs flexed and arms clasped around his knees. Expected therapeutic outcomes include all of the following except:

[Physical Rehabilitation/O'Sullivan/ 4th Ed./Pg. 552-553]

A. Decreased extensor spasticity in the lower extremities

B. Inhibition of flexor spasticity in the upper extremities

C. Protraction of the scapula

D. Facilitation of extensor tone in the trunk

Q 273. A development examination is completed on an eight month old infant. Findings from the examination include: the patient brings hands to mouth, requires assistance for ring sitting, presents with slight head lag, and does not reach across midline for objects. This child appears:

[Cash's Neurology/4th Ed./Pg. 51-55]

Answer   260 C   261 C   262 B   263 C   264 C   265 C   266 B   267 D   268 D   269 A   270 C   271 C
272 D

A. Appropriate with normal development
B. Developmentally delayed
C. Developmentally accelerated
D. To present with cerebral palsy

Q 274. Facilitation of muscle tone is performed through all of the following except:
[Therapeutic Exercise/Kisner/5th Ed./Pg. 197]
A. Approximation
B. Maintained pressure
C. Vibration
D. Quick icing

Q 275. A patient with moderate chronic obstructive pulmonary disease performs an exercise test that will stress the patient to the point of limitation. During the test the therapist monitors the patient's physiologic response to exercise. Which of the following findings would not require cessation of the testing session?
A. A 20 mm Hg decrease in diastolic blood pressure with an increase in workload
B. Systolic hypertension greater than 160 mm Hg
C. A PO2 of less than 55 mm Hg
D. Maximal shortness of breath

Q 276. A patient involved in a cardiac rehabilitation program exercises on a treadmill. While exercising the patient reports his level of perceived exertion as a 7 on Borg's ten-point scale. Which words best describe the patient's rate of perceived exertion?
A. Weak
B. Moderate
C. Strong
D. Very strong

Q 277. A therapist examines a patient's breath sounds though auscultation. The therapist classifies the breath sounds in a selected lung segment as absent. Which condition is not typically associated with absent breath sound?
[Tidy's Physiotherapy/12th Ed./Pg. 207-208]
A. Pleural effusion
B. Pneumothorax
C. Obesity
D. Consolidation

Q 278. A therapist completes an initial examination on a patient diagnosed with complete C7 tetrapegia. The patient problem list includes the following: inability to complete an independent bed to wheelchair transfer, decreased passive lower extremity range of motion tissue breakdown over the ischial tuberosities, and decreased upper extremity strength. Which of the following treatment activities should be given the highest priority?
[Physical Rehabilitation/O'sullivan/4th Ed./Pg. 883]
A. Pressure relief activities
B. Transfer training using a sliding board
C. Self-range of motion activities
D. Upper extremity strengthening exercise

Q 279. A cardiac rehabilitation phase I program should begin 1–4 days after the patient's infarct and should consist of all of the following prior to discharge except:
[Tidy/KM Varglere/12th Ed/Pg. 243]
A. Progressive resistive exercise program for the upper and lower extremities
B. Monitor heart rate and blood pressure during exercise

C. Patient and family education
D. Submaximal low level treadmill test

Q 280. A physical therapist from a home care agency examines a 50-year-old patient diagnosed with chronic bronchitis. The patient is overweight and presents with cyanosis at the fingertips and shallow breathing. The most immediate goal would be to:
[Tidy's Physiotherapy/12th Ed./Pg. 187]
A. Implement a low level exercise program
B. Implement breathing exercises and postural drainage technique
C. Prescribe a wheelchair for mobility
D. Complete a manual muscle test of the upper and lower extremities

Q 281. A patient with an IV in the antecubital region is treated in physical therapy. The therapist would like to instruct the patient in upper extremity active range of motion exercises, but is concerned about placing excessive pressure on the infusion site. Which of the following exercises would not be indicated?
A. Shoulder abduction and adduction
B. Shoulder flexion and extension
C. Elbow flexion and extension
D. Wrist flexion and extension

Q 282. An 18-year-old female diagnosed with left-sided congestive heart failure is referred to physical therapy. Which objective finding is most commonly associated with left-sided heart failure?
[Tidy/KM Varghese/12th Ed./Pg. 230]
A. Distended neck veins
B. Liver and spleen congestion
C. Peripheral edema
D. Pulmonary edema

Q 283. A patient in a phase I cardiac rehabilitation program begins walking with assistance. Which following monitoring techniques would not be necessary in a phase I program?
[Tidy's Physiotherapy/12th Ed./Pg. 465]
A. Blood pressure
B. Electrocardiography
C. Electromyography
D. Heart rate

Q 284. A therapist completes a developmental assessment on a five-month-old infant. If the therapist elects to examine the infant's palmar grasp reflex, which of the following stimuli is the most appropriate?
[Cash's Neurology/4th Ed./Pg. 43]
A. Contact to the ball of the foot in upright standing
B. Maintained pressure to the palm of the hand
C. Noxious stimulus to the palm of the hand
D. Sudden change in the position of the hand

Q 285. Secretion removal techniques are an integral component of a pulmonary rehabilitation program. What is the simplest method to clear secretions from the upper airway?
[Therapeutic Exercise/Kisner/5th Ed./Pg. 868]
A. Cough
B. Percussion
C. Shaking
D. Vibration

Answer 273 B   274 B   275 B   276 D   277 D   278 A   279 A   280 B   281 C   282 D   283 C   284 B
285 A

Q 286. A therapist instructs a patient to expire maximally after taking a maximal inspiration. The therapist can use these instructions to measure the patient's:
[Therapeutic Exercise/Kisner/5th Ed./Pg. 856]
A. Expiratory reserve volume inspiratory reserve volume
B. Inspiratory reserve volume
C. Total lung capacity
D. Vital capacity

Q 287. A therapist instructs a patient in diaphragmatic breathing exercises. Which of the following instructions would not be helpful in teaching diaphragmatic breathing?
[Therapeutic Exercise/Kisner/5th Ed./Pg. 863]
A. Place your dominant handover your midrectus area
B. Place your nondominant handover your midsternal area
C. Inspire slowly through your nose
D. As you expire watch your lower hand rise

Q 288. A therapist volunteers to assist participants at the finish line in a 10K rod race. The race takes place on a hot and humid day and some of the race organizers are concerned about the potential for heat related disorders such as heat exhaustion and heat stroke. The most significant variables to different between heat exhaustion and heat stroke are:
A. Blood pressure and pulse rate
B. Coordination and level of fatigue
C. Mental status and skin temperature
D. Pupil dilation and blood pressure

Q 289. A therapist monitors patient vital signs while exercising in a phase I cardiac rehabilitation program. The patient is status postmyocardial infarction and has progressed without difficulty while involved in the program. Which of the following vital sign recordings would exceed the typical limits of a phase I program?
A. Heart rate elevated 18 beats/minute above resting level
B. Respiration rate = 25 breaths/minutes
C. Systolic blood pressure decreases by 20 mm Hg from resting level
D. Diastolic blood pressure less than 100 mm Hg

Q 290. A therapist examines a patient status post-traumatic brain injury. Then examining neurologic tone the most appropriate method is:
[Physical Rehabilitation/O'Sullivan/4th Ed./Pg. 183-184]
A. Active range of motion of the involved extremities
B. Passive range of motion of the involved extremities
C. Passive range of motion of the involved and uninvolved extremities
D. Resisted motion of the involved extremities

Q 291. A therapist completes a developmental assessment on a three month old child. Which reflex is simulated by the head suddenly dropping into extension?
[Cash's Neurology/4th Ed./Pg. 142]
A. Moro   B. Grasp
C. Tonic labyrinthine   D. Extensor thrust

Q 292. When treating a patient with hemiplegia in tall kneeling, which treatment technique would be the least effective?
[Tidy/KM Varghese/12th Ed./Pg. 329]

A. Proprioceptive neuromuscular facilitation "chopping" in D1, D2
B. Reaching across midline with the unaffected arm
C. Reaching across midline with the hands in prayer position
D. Straight plane motion with the unaffected arm

Q 293. A physical therapist a one month old infant. During the treatment session the therapist strokes the cheek of the infant causing the infant to turn its mouth towards the stimulus. This action best defines the __________ reflex?
[Cash's Neurology/4th Ed./Pg. 43]
A. Moro   B. Rooting
C. Startle   D. Righting

Q 294. A therapist performs upper extremity passive range of motion exercises to a patient with an IV connected to the dorsum of his right hand. During the treatment session the therapist notices a small amount of blood which has backed up in the IV line. The therapist's most immediate response should be to:
A. Turn off the IV
B. Removed the IV
C. Reposition the peripheral IV line
D. Contact the primary physician

Q 295. A therapist examines a patient referred to physical therapy diagnosed with peripheral vascular disease. Which of the following would be the most valid indicator that the patient is not a candidate for an active exercise program?
[Therapeutic Exercise/Kisner/5th Ed./Pg. 830]
A. Cool skin
B. Resting claudication
C. Decreased peripheral pulses
D. Decreased vital capacity

Q 296. A patient status postspinal fusion is referred for chest physical therapy. The therapist instructs patient in diaphragmatic breathing exercises. Instructions are given to the patient to place his dominant handover the mid rectus abdominis area and his nondominant handover the midstream area. As the patient inhales slowly through the nose the therapist encourage the patient to:
[Therapeutic Exercise/Kisner/5th Ed./Pg. 862]
A. Direct air so that the nondominant hand rises during inspiration
B. Direct air so that the dominant hand rise during inspiration
C. Direct air so that both hands rise equally during inspiration
D. Direct air so that both hands do not move during inspiration

Q 297. Which illness is characterized by bronchial hyper-irritability that is triggered by a number of stimuli resulting in narrowing of the air passages?
[Tidy's Physiotherapy/12th Ed./Pg. 192]
A. Asthma   B. Pneumonia
C. Bronchitis   D. Pleurisy

Q 298. The treatment plan for a patient with hemiplegia includes reinforcing normal movement through key points of control and avoiding all reflex movement patterns and associated reactions. This approach most closely resembles:
[Cash's Neurology/4th Ed./Pg. 157]

Answer   286 D   287 D   288 C   289 C   290 C   291 A   292 D   293 D   294 C   295 D   296 B   297 A

A. Bobath
B. Kabat
C. Trendelenburg
D. Brunnstrom

Q 299. Which statement concerning the APGAR newborn assessment is not true?
A. The test is administered at 1 and 5 minutes after birth
B. The maximum score is 5
C. A score of less than 4 is indicative of respiratory distress
D. The score for each assessed item range from 0-2

Q 300. The ratio of chest compressions to breaths during two man cardiopulmonary resuscitation is:
A. 5:1
B. 10:1
C. 15:1
D. 15:2

Q 301. The most appropriate standard position for bronchial drainage to the posterior basal segment of the lower lobes is:
[Therapeutic Exercise/Kisner/5th Ed./Pg. 873]
A. Patient lying prone with lower extremities declined six inches
B. Patient in side-lying with a six inch elevation at the foot of the bed
C. Patient in side-lying with a twenty inch elevation at the foot of the bed
D. Patient lying in prone with a twenty inch elevation at the foot of the bed

Q 302. A patient with cardiac disease rates the intensity of exercise as 12 using Borg's Original Rate of Perceived Exertion Scale. A rating of 12 on the perceived exertion scale would correspond to approximately ___ percent of the patient's age-adjusted maximum heart rate?
A. 50
B. 60
C. 75
D. 85

Q 303. A therapist position a patient in preparation for postural drainage activities. Which of the following lung segments would not require the foot of the bed to be elevated?
[Therapeutic Exercise/Kisner/5th Ed./ Pg. 872-833]
A. Anterior segments of the upper lobes
B. Right middle lobe
C. Anterior basal segments of the lower lobes
D. Lateral basal segments of the lower lobes

Q 304. A physical therapist examines a patient with multiple sclerosis. The therapist documents that the patient presents with dysdiadochokinesia. Which objective finding is most representative of dysdiadochokinesia?
[Physical Rehabilitation/O'Sullivan/4th Ed./ Pg. 740]
A. Inability to perform rapid alternating movements
B. Inability to discriminate selected tactile input
C. Difficulty with speech articulation
D. Presence of involuntary, rhythmic, and oscillatory movements at rest

Q 305. Which of the following developmental milestones is usually not observed when examining a four month old infant?
[Cash's Neurology/4th Ed./Pg. 147]
A. Eyes follow objects 180 degrees
B. Infant laughs
C. Transfers blocks from one hand to the other
D. Holds head erect when held in a sitting position

Q 306. The intermittent use of tone reducing lower extremity bivalve casting for children with cerebral palsy hypothesizes that casting may:
[Cash's Neurology/4th Ed./Pg. 547]
A. Increase compensatory stabilizing efforts
B. Cause flexion of the toes which inhibits the plantar grasp response
C. Facilitate trunk stability by reducing contractures of the foot
D. Inhibit the use of extensor thrust by preventing plantar flexion

Q 307. A phase IV cardiac rehabilitation program can best be described as:
A. A program of maintenance designed to allow the patient to continue a lifelong routine of exercise and education
B. A program that is monitored by electrocardiogram to determine the patient's maximal heart rate and exercise tolerance
C. A program that allows for independent progression of exercise at home
D. A two to four month program based solely on exercise which allows the patient to attain the appropriate maximal heart rate for his/her age group

Q 308. A therapist treats a patient status post CVA. Which action would be most likely to facilitate elbow extension in a patient with hemiplegia?
A. Turn the head o the affected side
B. Turn the head to the unaffected side
C. Extend the lower extremities
D. Flex the lower extremities

Q 309. A patient with hemiplegia lying in supine demonstrates a synergistic pattern of movement when attempting to move his affected leg. The patient's hip is abducted and externally related knee flexed, ankle plantar flexed and inverted, toes plantar flexed and classified as:
[Physical Rehabilitation/O'sullivan/4th Ed./Pg. 532]
A. Purely extension
B. Purely flexion
C. A combination of flexion and extension on a pattern with
D. Isolated active movement

Q 310. A 35-year-old patient, six months status post CVA and right hemiparesis, attends physical therapy on an outpatient basis. As the patient lies supine on the mat, the therapist applies resistance to right elbow flexion. The therapist notes mass flexion of the right lower extremity as the resistance applied. The therapist should document this as:
[Physical Rehabilitation/O'Sullivan/14th Ed./Pg. 571]
A. Raimiste's phenomenon
B. Souque's phenomenon
C. Coordination synkinesis
D. Homolateral synkinesis

Q 311. A child with athetoid cerebral palsy is referred to physical therapy. Which of the following characteristics would

---

a physical therapist typically identify when examining the child?

[Cash's Neurology/4th Ed./Pg. 520]

A. Continuous low tone and intermittent tonic spasms
B. Small range movements with full control within the range
C. Disorganized movement with fluctuating muscle tone
D. Little to no influence from tonic neck reflexes

Q 312. A patient is examined following a pneumectomy secondary to lung cancer. All of the following may be seen postoperatively except:

[Tidy's Physiotherapy/12th Ed./Pg. 207]

A. An ineffective cough
B. Increased chest expansion with inhalation
C. Decreased endurance with activities of daily living
D. Pain with inhalation

Q 313. A patient begins to demonstrate signs and symptoms of a seizure including uncontrollable muscular movements, convulsions, and confused behavior. Appropriate intervention would include:

[Tidy's Physiotherapy/12th Ed./Pg. 470]

A. Attempt to check airway breathing and circulation
B. Place a soft object between the patient's teeth
C. Hold or restrain the patient
D. Protect the victim from injury, but do not restrain

Q 314. A physical therapist examines a six-month-old infant with spina bifida. The infant suddenly begins to act strangely at the conclusion of treatment. A primary survey reveals the infant is not breathing, but does have a pulse. The most immediate response would be to:

A. Begin chest compressions
B. Begin mouth to mouth breathing
C. Begin mouth to nose breathing
D. Begin mouth to mouth and nose breathing

Q 315. A physical therapist conducts an initial examination on a patient diagnosed with Parkinson's disease. Which of the following clinical findings would you expect the therapist to identify?

[Cash's Neurology/4th Ed./Pg. 421]

A. Aphasia
B. Ballistic movements
C. Severe muscle atrophy
D. Cogwheel rigidity

Q 316. Therapists often elevate the foot of a treatment table to maximize the electiveness of specific postural drainage techniques. Standard postural drainage positioning of the __________ would not require elevation of the treatment table?

[Therapeutic Exercise/Kisner/5th Ed./Pg. 872]

A. Anterior segments of the upper lobes
B. Lateral basal segments of the lower lobes
C. Posterior basal segments of the lower lobes
D. Right middle lobe

Q 317. A therapist develops a treatment program for a patient diagnosed with cystic fibrosis. Which of the following treatment activities would be the most essential to improve ventilation?

[Tidy's Physiotherapy/12th Ed./Pg. 201]

A. Gait training
B. Family education
C. Postural drainage
D. Home adaptations

Q 318. A therapist monitors a patient's blood pressure during exercise. Which of the following responses would be considered normal?

A. Diastole pressure increases 5 mm Hg during exercise
B. Systolic pressure does not decline as the intensity of exercise declines
C. Systolic pressure does not increase during active exercise
D. Systolic pressure declines during exercise before the intensity of the exercise declines

Q 319. In order to maximize the effectiveness of postural drainage techniques for the right middle lobe a therapist should elevate the foot of the bed ______ inches?

[Therapeutic Exercise/Kisner/5th Ed./Pg. 872]

A. 4
B. 8
C. 16
D. 24

Q 320. A therapist performs percussion over a selected area on the chest wall of a patient diagnosed with chronic obstructive pulmonary disease. The therapist documents the sound as dull. Which structure would typically yield this type of sound?

[Therapeutic Exercise/Kisner/5th Ed./Pg. 859]

A. Lung
B. Liver
C. Heart
D. Viscera

Q 321. A therapist utilizes the results of a symptom-limited exercise treadmill test to determine the intensity of exercise for a patient who previously sustained a cardiac event. Which of the following guidelines would be the most appropriate when determining an appropriate exercise intensity for the patient?

A. 20 percent of the maximal heart rate obtained on the treadmill test
B. 20 percent of the maximal heart rate obtained on the treadmill test
C. 60 percent of the maximal heart rate obtained on the treadmill test
D. 80 percent of the maximal heart rate obtained on the treadmill test

Q 322. A therapist assesses a patient's voice sounds as part of a respiratory examination. Which condition is typically associated with increases voice sounds?

[Therapeutic Exercise/Kisner/5th Ed./Pg. 860-861]

A. Pneumothorax
B. Consolidation
C. Atelectasis
D. Pleural effusion

Q 323. A 63-year-old female status post stroke is screened for admission into a rehabilitation hospital. A part of the screen the therapist utilizes a standardized instrument to document the extent of the patient's impairments and disabilities. Which of the following standardized instruments would be most beneficial to provide an assessment of motor function?

[Physical Rehabilitation/O'Sullivan/4th Ed./Pg. 543]

A. Barthel Index
B. Functional Independence Measure
C. Fugl-Meyer Assessment
D. Rivermead Mobility Index

Answer 311 C 312 B 313 D 314 D 315 D 316 A 317 C 318 A 319 C 320 A 321 C 322 B
323 C

Q 324. A physical therapist reviews an initial examination of a patient diagnosed with an upper motor neuron disease. The examination documents the existence of a positive Babinski reflex. A positive Babinski reflex is characterized by:

[Cash's Neurology/4th Ed./Pg. 115]

A. Extension of the great toe   B. Flexion of the great toe
C. Abduction of the great toe   D. Adduction of the great toe

Q 325. A physical therapist examines a patient with lower extremity hypertonicity. All of the following could be used by the therapist to temporarily reduce tone except:

[Cash's Neurology/4th Ed./Pg. 190-191]

A. Gentle rocking   B. Cryotherapy
C. Approximation   D. Sustained stretch

Q 326. Restrictive lung diseases limit to varying degrees the maximum volume of air that can be inhaled and exhaled. Examples of restrictive diseases include all of the following except:

[Therapeutic Exercise/Kisner/5th Ed./Pg. 876]

A. Emphysema   B. Pleural effusion
C. Pneumonia   D. Bony abnormality of the chest

Q 327. A physical therapist positions a patient with hemiplegia in a plantigrade position to promote weight bearing through the affected upper extremity. The most appropriate hand position on the plinth is:

[Physical Rehabilitation/O'Sullivan/4th Ed./Pg. 420]

A. Total palmar contact with the fingers fully extended
B. Total palmar contact with fingers flexed
C. Weight bearing on a closed fist
D. Palmar contact with support of the palmar arches and weight through the heel of the hand

Q 328. A physical therapist's emphasis when treating a child with __________ is aggressive bronchial drainage, chest vibration and percussion?

[Tidy's Physiotherapy/12th Ed./Pg. 200]

A. Cystic fibrosis
B. Chronic asthma
C. Respiratory muscle weakness
D. Pneumothorax

Q 329. A patient demonstrates unilateral neglect to the left. The physical therapist's short term goals for the patient include reducing the patient's neglect. Which treatment technique would not be effective in improving the patient's condition?

[Cash's Neurology/4th Ed./Pg. 260]

A. Have the patient participate in bilateral tasks to increase total body awareness
B. Place the patient's food on the right side of the tray so the patient can eat by himself
C. Have the patient observe himself massaging his left upper extremity
D. Have the patient use a mirror while dressing

Q 330. A physical therapist performs a vertebral artery test on a patient prior to using traction and mobilization techniques in upper cervical spine. During the test the patient begins to demonstrate nystagmus and blurred vision. The therapist should:

[Orthopaedic Physical Assessment/Magee/5th Ed./Pg. 171]

A. Repeat the vertebral artery test to confirm the original results
B. Proceed cautiously with traction and mobilization techniques in the upper cervical spine
C. Avoid traction or mobilization techniques in the upper cervical spine
D. Discharge the patient from physical therapy

Q 331. A physical therapist attempts to have a patient status post CVA reach for a cone by moving her trunk away from midline. The most appropriate type of manual contact to assist the patient with the movement is:

[Cash's Neurology/4th Ed./Pg. 236]

A. Firm deep touch   B. Light, intermittent touch
C. Maintained touch   D. No manual contact

Q 332. A physical therapist would not expect a seven month old infant to have completed which of the following developmental milestones?

[Cash's Neurology/4th Ed./Pg. 49-51]

A. Hold head erect when sitting
B. Crawl forward
C. Sit unsupported
D. Roll from supine to prone

Q 333. During an examination of a patient with a traumatic brain injury a therapist notes the patient mumbling phrases which are nonpurposeful in nature. As the physical therapist initiates passive range of motion to the patient's lower extremities, the patient attempts to strike the therapist in the head. According to the Ranchos Los Amigos levels of cognitive functioning, the patient would be best described at level:

[Physical Rehabilitation/O'Sullivan/4th Ed./Pg. 787]

A. II   B. III
C. IV   D. V

Q 334. Exercise causes a significant increase in the body's cardiac output. During mild to moderate exercise what redistribution of the available cardiac output would you expect?

[Refer to text]

A. An increase in cerebral and coronary blood flow
B. A decrease in cerebral and active skeletal muscle blood flow
C. An increase in coronary and active skeletal muscle blood flow
D. A decrease in cerebral and coronary blood flow

Q 335. A patient with right hemiplegia is observed during gait training. The patient performs side stepping towards the hemiplegic side. The physical therapist may expect the patient to compensate for weakened abductors by:

*[Physical Rehabilitation/O'Sullivan/
4th Ed./Pg. 544]*

A. Hip hiking of the unaffected side
B. Lateral trunk flexion towards the hemiplegic side
C. Lateral trunk flexion towards the unaffected side
D. Hip extension of the hemiplegic side

Answer   324 A   325 C   326 A   327 D   328 A   329 B   330 C   331 B   332 B   333 C   334 C   335 C

Q 336. The rate of pin rolling tremors in Parkinson's disease is:
[Tidy's Physiotherapy/12th Ed./Pg. 332]
A. 1–2 times per second
B. 20–30 times per second
C. 16 times per second
D. 6–8 times per second

Q 337. Thromboangiitis obliterans is also known as:
[Therapeutic Exercise/Kisner/5th Ed./Pg. 826]
A. Trendelenburg's disease
B. Thomas and Andy's disease
C. Buerger's disease
D. Philip's disease

Q 338. A patient in a pulmonary rehabilitation program is positioned in supine with a pillow under the knees. The therapist claps between the clavicle and nipple on each side. This technique is utilized for postural drainage of the:
[Therapeutic Exercise/Kisner/5th Ed./Pg. 872]
A. Anterior segments of the upper lobes
B. Anterior basal segments of the lower lobes
C. Superior segments of the lower lobes
D. Posterior basal segment of the lower lobes

Q 339. A therapist identifies that a child is unable to roll from prone to supine. Which reflex could most interfere with the child's ability to roll?
[Neurology/Cash's/4th Ed./Pg. 44]
A. Asymmetrical tonic neck reflex
B. Moro reflex
C. Galant reflex
D. Symmetrical tonic neck reflex

Q 340. A therapist develops a plan of care for a patient with hemiplegia. What is the primary purpose of using a sling in the management of a subluxed shoulder?
[Physical Rehabilitation/O'Sullian/4th Ed./Pg. 538]
A. Correct the cause of the subluxation
B. Decrease muscle spasticity
C. Facilitate movement patterns
D. To hold the upper extremity in proper alignment

Q 341. A therapist reviews a laboratory report for a 41-year-old male diagnosed with chronic obstructive pulmonary disease. Which of the following would be considered a normal hemoglobin value?
[Physiology/AK Jain/3rd Ed./Pg. 56]
A. 10 g/DL
B. 15 g/DL
C. 20 g/DL
D. 25 g/DL

Q 342. A therapist applies a hot pack to the lumbar region of a patient rehabilitating from a lumbar laminectomy. Which mode of heat transmission is utilized with hot packs?
[Tidy's Physiotherapy/12th Ed./Pg. 458]
A. Conduction
B. Convection
C. Evaporation
D. Radiation

Q 343. A physical therapist reviews the initial examination of a patient diagnosed with a cerebellar CVA. The therapist might expect the patient's primary impairment to be:
[Physical Rehabilitation/O'Sullivan/4th Ed./Pg. 544]
A. Visual field cuts
B. Gait disturbances
C. Impaired speech
D. Impaired comprehension skills

Q 344. A therapist completes an examination on a young girl with spastic cerebral palsy. The therapist determines that the girl has involvement in all four extremities as well as the head, neck, and trunk. What type of cerebral palsy classification best describes the girl's condition?
[Neurology/Cash's/4th Ed./Pg. 519]
A. Spastic diplegia
B. Spastic hemiplegia
C. Spastic tetraplegia
D. Spastic triplegia

Q 345. A therapist positions a patient in prone with two pillows under the hips in preparation for bronchial drainage. If the therapist's goal is to perform bronchial drainage to the superior segments of the lower lobes, which area should the therapist's force be directed.
[Therapeutic Exercise/Kisner/5th Ed./Pg. 823]
A. Between the clavicle and nipple on each side
B. Over the area between the clavicle and top of the scapula on each side of the spine
C. Over the lower ribs on each side
D. Over the middle of the back at the tip of the scapula on each side of the spine

Q 346. Secretion removal techniques are often a necessary component of a pulmonary rehabilitation program. Which pulmonary disease is usually associated with a change in the composition of secretions?
[Tidy's Physiotherapy/12th Ed./Pg. 200]
A. Asthma
B. Bronchiectasis
C. Chronic bronchitis
D. Cystic fibrosis

Q 347. A therapist performs a respiratory assessment on a patient with restrictive lung disease. If the therapist records the respiration rate as 22 breaths per minute, which term is most appropriate to classify the patient's respiration rate?
[Therapeutic Exercise/Kisner/5th Ed./Pg. 858]
A. Eupnea
B. Tachypnea
C. Bradypnea
D. Hyperpnea

Q 348. A therapist treats a 15-year-old female of Spanish descent. The patient speaks only a few words of English and has significant difficulty understanding the therapist's instructions. The most appropriate therapist action is to:
[Refer to next]
A. Speak strongly and directly to the patient
B. Encourage frequent feedback from the patient
C. Utilize an interpreter
D. Emphasize nonverbal communication

Q 349. A physical therapist prepares a patient for ambulation. The patient has been in the hospital for six-weeks with pneumonia and has only recently had enough strength to begin ambulation training. Which of the following treatment activities would be the last to occur?
*[Physical Rehabilitation/O'Sullivan/4th Ed./
Pg. 421-422]*

Answer   336 D   337 C   338 A   339 A   340 D   341 B   342 A   343 B   344 C   345 D   346 D   347 B
348 C

A. Development of standing balance
B. Development of sitting balance
C. Training in a specific gait pattern
D. Training with weight shifting in a standing position

Q 350. Assuming normal development which of the following activities should a child first accomplish?
[Neurology/Cash's/4th Ed./Pg. 222]
A. Rolling from prone to supine
B. Rolling from supine to prone
C. Turning from side to supine
D. Turning from supine to side

Q 351. A therapist attempts to auscultate over the aortic valve. Which of the following areas is the most appropriate to isolate the desired valve?
[Refer to text]
A. Second left intercostal space at the left sternal border
B. Second right intercostals space at the right sternal border
C. Fourth left intercostals space along the lower left sternal border
D. Fifth left intercostals space at the midclavicular line

Q 352. A therapist completes a pulmonary function test on a male patient admitted to the hospital three days age. Assuming normal valves, the patient's residual volume should be approximately_______ percent of the total lung capacity?
[AK Jain/Physiology/3rd Ed./Pg. 435-436]
A. 10   B. 25
C. 35   D. 50

Q 353. A therapist positions a patient for bronchial drainage to the anterior segments of the upper lobes. The most appropriate patient position is:
[Therapeutic Exercise/Kisner/5th Ed./Pg. 872]
A. Supine with a pillow under the knees
B. Supine with the head of the bed elevated 16 inches
C. Supine with the foot of the bed elevated 16 inches
D. Supine with the foot of the bed elevated 16 inches
E. Prone with the head of the bed elevated 12 inches

Q 354. A therapist attempts to estimate the energy expenditure in calories for a cardiac patient performing a selected activity for 15 minutes. Assuming the therapist has a metabolic equivalent value for the activity, what other variables are necessary in order to obtain an estimate of the patient's energy expenditure?
[Refer to text]
A. Patient's height and weight
B. Patient's weight and oxygen consumption
C. Patients stroke volume and heart rate
D. Patient's residual volume and heart rate

Q 355. A therapist outlines a walking program for a patient rehabilitating from a prolonged illness. Which of the following recommendations would not be beneficial to the patient?
[Refer to text]
A. Wear comfortable, loose fitting clothing appropriate for the present temperature and weather
B. Walk at a rate designed to bring the heart to target levels

C. Walk continuously; frequent stops interfere with aerobic training
D. When walking up steep hills lean back ward slightly and lengthen your stride

Q 356. A therapist designs a general fitness program for a senior citizen group. Which of the following guidelines is not accurate?
[Tidy/KM Varghese/12th Ed./Pg. 415]
A. Allow participants the opportunity to reduce the intensity of exercise
B. Exercise intensity should be at a level which will provide a training effect
C. Exercise should be performed daily for at least 30 minutes
D. Exercise activities should include a warm-up and cool-down period

Q 357. A patient diagnosed with Parkinson's disease has difficulty initiating movement. What proprioceptive neuromuscular facilitation technique would be most appropriate to treat this problem?
[Therapeutic Exercise/Kisner/5th Ed./Pg. 202]
A. Contract relax   B. Rhythmic initiation
C. Rhythmic stabilization   D. Slow reversal

Q 358. A physical therapist instructs a patient to move from sitting through quadruped to tall kneeling. By moving through the developmental sequence a patient gains ____ control during movement and __ during static positioning?
[Therapeutic Exercise/Kisner/5th Ed./Pg. 169]
A. Isometric, isotonic   B. Isotonic, isometric
C. Isometric, isokinetic   D. Isokinetic, isotonic

Q 359. The long-term goal of a patients status post CVA is to walk to work. Which of the following conditions would serve as the largest obstacle to the patient achieving the goal?
[Physical Rehabilitation/O'Sullivan/4th Ed./Pg. 571]
A. Homonymous hemianopia
B. Expressive aphasia
C. Agraphia
D. Dysarthria

Q 360. A physical therapist examines a patient with right hemiplegia four days status post CVA. All of the following would be appropriate short term goals excepts:
[Physical Rehabilitation/O'Sullivan/4th Ed./Pg. 544-545]
A. Improve sitting balance
B. Initiate activities of daily living with assistance
C. Demonstrate awareness of the hemiplegic side through positioning
D. Perform lower extremity exercises without assistance

Q 361. A patient status post CVA with abnormal tone on the right side lies supine in bed. The patient's physical therapist is-courage her from lying supine for long periods of time because:
[Physical Rehabilitation/O'Sullivan/4th Ed./Pg. 549]
A. The position can cause shoulder-hand syndrome
B. The position increases an inferior subluxation
C. The position encourages tonic neck and labyrinthine reflexes
D. The position increase stone in the pectoralis

Answer   349 D   350 C   351 B   352 B   353 A   354 B   355 D   356 C   357 B   358 B   359 A   360 D
361 C

Q 362. On chest X-ray the silhouette sign presents as:
[Refer to text]

A. The two separate structures adjacent to each other are not identified because of lack of difference in bone densities
B. Paralysis of diaphragm over shadows the lung
C. Enlargement of cardiac field in the transverse direction
D. A sharp contrast between two adjacent

Q 363. PEEP in chest care physiotherapy refers to:
[Refer to text]

A. Peak expiratory exercise performance
B. Positive end expiratory pressure
C. Positive endurance exercise for pulmonary performance
D. Peak myography and electrocardiography of pulmonary performance

Q 364. The ratio of chest compression to manual ventilation for a single rescuer in CPR is:
[Refer to text]

A. 15:2
B. 10:2
C. 12:2
D. 5:1

Q 365. Blind nasal intubation is indicated in:
[Refer to text]

A. Traumatic quadriplegia
B. Cervical spondylosis
C. Fracture mandible
D. T.M. joint ankylosis

Passive and Active Exercise

Q 366. Active repetitive exercises, usually of the ankles or wrist performed to maintain or improve circulation in the extremities are also known as:
[Therapeutic Exercise/Kisner/5th Ed./Pg. 894]

A. Buerger's exercises
B. Phelp's exercises
C. Pumping exercises
D. Functional exercises

Q 367. Reliable method of increasing central excitation to stimulate motor units in largest proportion of muscle is by:
[Therapeutic Exercise/Kisner/5th Ed./Pg. 197]

A. Application of assistance to voluntary movement
B. Application of resistance to voluntary movement
C. Voluntary movement eliminating gravity
D. None of these

Q 368. A therapist attempts to obtain information on the ability of noncontractile tissue to allow motion at a specific joint. Which selective tissue tension assessment would provide the therapist with the most valuable information?
[Therapeutic Exercise/Kisner/5th Ed./Pg. 44]

A. Active range of motion
B. Active-assistive range of motion
C. Passive range of motion
D. Resisted isometrics

Q 369. A therapist completes a selected resistive test as part of an initial examination. The patient reports feeling pain during the test, however strength is normal. Which of the following conclusions is most likely?
[Magee/5th Ed./Pg. 39]

A. Capsular or ligamentous laxity
B. A minor lesion of the muscle or tendon
C. A complete rupture of the muscle or tendon
D. Intermittent claudication may be present

Q 370. A therapist determines the maximum load patient can squat ten time is 240 lbs. The patient's ten repetition maximum should be recorded as:
[Therapeutic Exercise/Kisner/5th Ed./Pg. 161]

A. 10 lbs
B. 24 lbs
C. 120 lbs
D. 240 lbs

Q 371. A physical therapist examines a patient with unilateral lower extremity weakness. As the patient performs hip flexion in supine, the therapist helps the patient complete the full range of motion. This would best be described as:
[Gardiner/4th Ed./Pg. 41]

A. Active exercise
B. Passive exercise
C. Resistive exercise
D. Active-assistive exercise

Q 372. In Delorme and Watkins technique of progressive resisted exercise the RM is
[Therapeutic Exercise/Kisner/5th Ed./Pg. 207]

A. Progressively increased
B. Progressively decreased
C. Kept constant
D. Decided by the patient

Q 373. A therapist employed in a nursing home routinely treats patients in excess of 70 years of age. The therapist has noted several consistent postural changes in her patients. Which of the following does not accurately describe the postural changes associated with aging?
[Joint Structure and Function/Norkin/Pg. 429-430]

A. Forward head
B. Rounded shoulders
C. Increased hip extension
D. Increased knee flexion

Physiotherapy Assessment

Q 374. In supraspinatus tendinitis the painful arc syndrome ranges from:
[Ebnezar/1st Ed./Pg. 232]

A. 45°–60°
B. 60°–120°
C. 135°–150°
D. 0°–90°

Q 375. Positive rose water test is suggestive of:
[Refer to text]

A. Psoriatic arthritis
B. Gouty arthritis
C. Tubercular arthritis
D. Rheumtoid arthritis

Q 376. Radiologically bamboo spine sign is seen in which of the following?
[Ebnezar/1st Ed./Pg. 403]

A. Fluorosis
B. Ankylosing spondylitis
C. Hyperparathyroidism
D. Osteoporosis

Q 377. Thomas knee flexion test is used to detect:
[Norkin's Goniometry/3rd Ed./Pg. 206]

A. Lumber lordosis
B. Obliquity of pelvis
C. Hip flexion deformity
D. Knee flexion deformity

Q 378. Thomas knee flexion test is performed by:
[Norkin's Goniometry/3rd Ed./Pg. 206]

A. Abducting diseased hip
B. Adducting diseased hip
C. Flexing diseased hip
D. Flexing normal hip

Answer	362 A	363 B	364 A	365 D	366 C	367 B	368 C	369 B	370 D	371 D	372 D	373 D
	374 B	375 D	376 B	377 C	378 D							

Q 379. Ape thumb deformity is produced by injury to which of the following nerves?
[Therapeutic Exercise/Kisner/5th Ed./Pg. 356]
A. Ulnar
B. Median
C. Radial
D. Circumflex

Q 380. Mallet finger is produced in which of the following injuries?
[Therapeutic Exercise/Kisner/1st Ed./Pg. 625]
[Orthopaedics of Applied Physiotherapy/Jayant Joshi/ 1st Ed./Pg. 120]
A. Avulsion of extensor tendon at the base of middle phalanx
B. Avulsion of flexor profundus tendon at the base of terminal phalanx
C. Avulsion of extensor tendon at the base of terminal phalanx
D. None of the above

Q 381. Gower's sign is seen in:
[Cash's Neurology/4th Ed./Pg. 581]
A. Herpes zoster
B. Sciatic nerve palsy
C. Duchenne muscular dystrophy
D. Marfan's syndrome

Q 382. Thomas test is done for identifying which deformity?
[Norkin/Goniometry/3rd Ed./Pg. 206]
A. Fixed flexion deformity
B. Fixed extension deformity
C. Spinal deformities
D. Rotational deformity

Q 383. Modified Allen's test is used for:
A. Radial artery
B. Brachial artery
C. Popliteal artery
D. Dorsalis pedis artery

Q 384. Positive Froment's test suggests involvement of which nerve?
[Essential Orthopaedics/Maheshwari/3rd Ed./Pg. 56]
A. Ulnar
B. Median
C. Radial
D. Musculocutaneous

Q 385. Krukenberg's amputation is done for problems of which of the following?
[Essential Orthopaedics/Maheshwari/ 3rd Ed./Pg. 279]
A. Thigh
B. Arm
C. Leg
D. Forearm

Q 386. Swan neck deformity of fingers absence of Bunnel's intrinsic test is likely due to:
[Essential Orthopaedics/Maheshwari/Pg. 245-246]
A. Contracture of intrinsic muscles
B. Paralysis of extensors of finger
C. Paralysis of long flexors of finger
D. Volar subluxation of PIP joint

Q 387. Purpose of the heel knee test is to
[Refer to text]
A. Determine active range of motion
B. Assess functional ability
C. Rule out degenerative disc disease
D. Assesses coordination of movement of lower extremities

Q 388. A therapist attempts to assess the integrity of the L4 spinal level. Which deep tendon reflex would provide the therapist with the most useful information?
[Physical Rehabilitation/O'Sullian/4th Ed./Pg. 185]
A. Lateral hamstrings
B. Medial hamstrings
C. Patellar reflex
D. Achilles reflex

Q 389. A physical therapist performs a manual muscle test on a patient with unilateral lower extremity weakness. The therapist should test the patient's hip adductors with the patient positioned in:
[Daniel/7th Ed./Pg. 206]
A. Prone
B. Side-lying
C. Standing
D. Supine

Q 390. A patient is limited to 55 degrees in an active straight leg raise. A therapist should apply the contract-relax technique to the _______ to improve the patient's active range of motion?
[Therapeutic Exercise/Kisner/5th Ed./Pg. 85]
A. Abductors and hip flexors
B. Hamstrings and hip extensors
C. Quadriceps and hip flexors
D. Adductors and hip extensors

Q 391. A therapist position a patient in supine prior to performing a manual muscle test of the supintor. To isolate the supinator and minimize the action of the biceps the therapist should position the patient's elbow in:
[Daniel/7th Ed./Pg. 125]
A. 30 degrees of elbow flexion
B. 60 degrees of elbow flexion
C. 90 degrees of elbow flexion
D. Terminal elbow flexion

Q 392. A therapist completes a vertebral artery test on a patient diagnosed with a cervical strain. Which component of the vertebral artery test is most likely to assess the patency of the intervertebral foramen?
[Magee/5th Ed./Pg. 17]
A. Rotation
B. Lateral flexion
C. Flexion
D. Extension

Q 393. A therapist instructs a patient to close her eyes and hold out her hand. The therapist places a series of different weights in the patient's hand one at a time. The patient is then asked to identify the comparative weight of the objects. This method of sensory testing is used to examine:
[Physical Rehabilitation/O'Sullivan/ 4th Ed./Pg. 147]
A. Barognosis
B. Graphesthesia
C. Recognition of texture
D. Stereognosis

Q 394. A therapist attempts to have a patient quantify his pain using a subjective pain scale. The therapist explains to the patient that he should assign a numerical value between zero and ten to describe the pain. Which of the following would best describe a score of ten?
[Saunders/Magee/4th Ed./Pg. 5]
A. No pain
B. Mild pain
C. Moderate pin
D. Most severe pain

Answer

| 379 B | 380 D | 381 C | 382 A | 383 A | 384 A | 385 D | 386 D | 387 D | 388 C | 389 B | 390 B |
| 391 D | 392 D | 393 A | 394 D | | | | | | | | |

Q 395. A therapist attempts to gather information on the ligamentous integrity of a patient's knee. Which special test would be inappropriate based on the desired objective?

[Essential Orthopaedics/Maheswari Mehta/3rd Ed./Pg. 313]

A. Posterior sag sign
B. Anterior drawer test
C. McMurray test
D. Lachman test

Q 396. A therapist identifies signs and symptoms of neurovascular compression after examining a patient with an upper extremity injury. Which of the following special tests would not be helpful in identifying the presence of neurovascular compression?

[Magee/5th Ed./Pg. 440-441]

A. Find's sign
B. Froment's sign
C. Phalen's test
D. Bunnel-Lutler test

Q 397. A physical therapist attempts to measure a patient's shoulder lateral rotation. Proper positioning the upper extremity in supine would be described by which of the following?

[Refer to text]

A. Shoulder abducted to 90 degrees, elbow flexed to 90 degrees
B. Shoulder abducted to 90 degrees, elbow fully extended
C. Shoulder abducted to 90 degrees, elbow flexed to 45 degrees
D. Shoulder in neutral, elbow flexed to 90 degrees

Q 398. A physical therapist examines a patient with a limited straight leg raise of 40 degrees due to inadequate hamstrings length. Which proprioceptive neuromuscular techniques would be most appropriate in increase the patient's hamstrings length?

[Therapeutic Exercise/Kisner/5th Ed./Pg. 85]

A. Contract-relax
B. Rhythmic initiation
C. Rhythmic stabilization
D. Rhythmic rotation

Q 399. A therapist performs a muscle screening examination on a 43-year-old female diagnosed with carpal tunnel syndrome. The therapist attempts to pull the patient's fingers from a position of adduction to abduction. This action is used to test the:

[Daniel/7th Ed./Pg. 152]

A. Finger extensors
B. Opponens pollicis
C. Dorsal interossei
D. Palmar interossei

Q 400. A patient demonstrates mild dizziness during vertebral artery testing. The therapist should pay particular attention when treating the patient to avoid positioning the neck in:

[Reider/1st Ed./Pg. 61]

A. Extension and extremes of rotation
B. Flexion and extremes of rotation
C. Flexion and side bending
D. Extension and side bending

Q 401. A therapist can obtain valuable information during an examination by using special orthopedic tests. Which of the following tests in not performed with the patient in supine?

[Essential Orthopaedics/Maheswari/3rd Ed./Pg. 313]

A. Anterior drawer test
B. Apley's compression test
C. McMurray test
D. Patella Patellar apprehension test

Q 402. Closed packed position of hip joint is:

[Norkin/3rd Ed./Pg. 245]

A. Full flexion, external rotation and abduction
B. Full flexion, internal rotation and abduction
C. Full extension, internal rotation and abduction
D. Full flexion, external rotation and abduction

Q 403. Ober test is used to test contracture of the:

[Magee/Elesiver/5th Ed./Pg. 693-694]

A. Rectus femoris
B. Gluteus medius
C. Piriformis
D. Iliotibial band

Q 404. Berg balance test for balance assessment is most suitable in which age group patients?

[Refer to text]

A. 60–70
B. 20–25
C. 5–10
D. More

Q 405. Which test is concerned with tennis elbow?

[Essential of Orthopaedics & Applied Physiotherapy/Maheshwari/3rd Ed./Pg. 313]

A. McMurray test
B. Allen's test
C. Apley's test
D. Corevis test

Q 406. A therapist examines a patient referred to physical therapy with thoracic outlet syndrome. Which of the following special tests would not assist the therapist to confirm the physician's diagnosis?

[Magee/5th Ed./Pg. 308]

A. Adson's maneuver
B. Allen test
C. Halstead Maneuver
D. Speed's maneuver

Q 407. Pointing Index sign is seen in nerve:

[Essential Orthopaedics/Maheshwari/3rd Ed./Pg. 52]

A. Ulnar
B. Radial
C. Median
D. Axillary

Q 408. McMurray's test is performed to clinically identify:

[Essential Orthopaedics/Maheshwari/3rd Ed./Pg. 313]

A. Torn muscle around knee
B. Synovial effusion of the knee
C. Torn meniscus
D. Torn ligamentum patellae

Q 409. Duga's test is helpful in:

[Essential Orthopaedics/Maheshwari/3rd Ed./Pg. 75]

A. Dislocation of hip
B. Scaphoid fracture
C. Fracture neck of femur
D. Anterior dislocation of shoulder

Q 410. Phalan's test is positive in:

[Essential of Orthopaedics & Applied Physiotherapy/Jayant Joshi/Elesiver/1st Ed./Pg. 265]

A. Ulnar bursitis
B. Tennis elbow
C. Carpal tunnel syndrome
D. De Quervain's disease

Q 411. Patient with pain in cervical region, is immediately referred from physical therapy department to a higher orthopedic specialty center. Possibly which of following test was found positive by therapist during assessment?

[Refer to text]

Answer

| 395 C | 396 D | 397 A | 398 A | 399 D | 400 C | 401 B | 402 C | 403 D | 404 A | 405 D | 406 D |
| 407 C | 408 C | 409 D | 410 C | | | | | | | | |

A. Bakody sign
B. Tineis test
C. Sharp purcursor test
D. Foramina compression test

Q 412. Gower's sign is apparent during which of following position?

[Refer to text]

A. Lying
B. Sit to standing
C. Walking
D. Running

Assistive Devices

Q 413. A therapist prepares to instruct a patient in a three-point gait pattern using axillary crutches. The most appropriate initial step to facilitate patient learning is to.
[Physical Rehabilitation/O'sullivan/4th Ed./Pg. 430]
A. Distinguish a three-point gait pattern from other gait patterns
B. Demonstrate a three-point gait pattern
C. Provide the patient with direct feedback on his/her performance.
D. Provide a written handout which illustrates the use of a three-point gait pattern

Q 414. A therapist instructs a patient in ambulation activities in the parallel bars. Which of the following activities would be the most appropriate to initiate treatment?
[Physical Rehabilitation/O'sullivan/4th Ed./Pg. 422]
A. Assuming the standing position
B. Instructing/demonstrating
C. Lateral weight shifting
D. Stepping forward and backward

Q 415. A physical therapist prepares a patient for ambulation. The patient has been in the hospital for six weeks with pneumonia and has only recently had enough strength to begin ambulation training. Which of the following treatment activities would be the last to occur?
[Physical Rehabilitation/O'Sullivan/4th Ed./Pg. 421-422]
A. Development of standing balance
B. Development of sitting balance
C. Training is a specific gait pattern
D. Training in weight shifting in a standing position

Q 416. A therapist provides exercise guidelines for a group of expectant mothers. Contraindications for exercise during pregnancy include all of the following except.
[Therapeutic Exercise/Kisner/5th Ed./Pg. 811]
A. Maternal diabetes
B. Placenta prievia
C. Incompetent cervix
D. Diastasis recti

Proprioceptive Neuromuscular Facilitation

Q 417. A patient completes a D1 extension pattern for the upper extremity. The prime movers of the scapula during this pattern are the:
[Therapeutic Exercise/Kisner/5th Ed./Pg. 196]
A. Trapezius and middle deltoid
B. Pectoralis minor and pectoralis major
C. Serratus anterior, pectoralis major, and anterior deltoid
D. Rhomboids, pectoralis minor, and levator scapulae

Q 418. A physical therapist treats a patient with quadriceps weakness using repeated contractions. This proprioceptive neuromascular facilitation technique should be applied:
[Therapeutic Exercise/Kisner/5th Ed./Pg. 195]
A. At the initiation of movement
B. At the point where the desired muscular response begin to diminish
C. At the end of the available range of motion
D. Only after a manual stretch to the hamstrings

Q 419. A therapist instructs a patient in a D2 flexion pattern. Which of the following most accurately describes the scapula components of a D2 flexion pattern?
[Therapeutic Exercise/Kisner/5th Ed./Pg. 196]
A. Scapular elevation, adduction, upward rotation
B. Scapular elevation, abduction, upward rotation
C. Scapular depression, adduction downward rotation
D. Scapular depression abduction, downward rotation

Q 420. A physical therapist uses proprioceptive neuromuscular facilitation to increase join range of motion using the hold-relax technique. This technique utilizes an ______ contraction, which is at the end point of the available range of motion?
[Therapeutic Exercise/Kisner/5th Ed./Pg. 205]
A. Isotonic
B. Isometric
C. Isokinetic
D. Eccentric

Q 421. A physical therapist use proprioceptive neuromuscular facilitation techniques to increase muscular strength. The therapist instructs the patient to actively perform a pattern of hip extension, abduction, and medial rotation. This pattern emphasizes strengthening of the:
[Therapeutic Exercise/Kisner/5th Ed./Pg. 200]
A. Psoas major and minor, iliacus
B. Tensor fasciae latae, biceps femoris
C. Gluteus maximus, medius, and minimus
D. Gluteus maximus, piriformis, adductor magnus

Q 422. Rhythmic stabilization is an ______ technique that can be implemented to increase join stability?
[Therapeutic Exercise/Kisner/5th Ed./Pg. 1116]
A. Isometric
B. Isotonic
C. Isokinetic
D. Eccentric

Q 423. A therapist attempts to strengthen the serratus anterior by utilizing proprioceptive neuromuscular facilitation techniques. Which pattern would be the most beneficial to strengthen the serratus anterior?
[Therapeutic Exercise/Kisner/5th Ed./Pg. 198]
A. D2 flexion
B. D2 extension
C. D1 flexion
D. D1 extension

Q 424. A therapist to improve a patient's lower extremity strength. Which proprioceptive neuromuscular facilitation technique would be the most appropriate to achieve the therapist's goals?
[Therapeutic Exercise/Kisner/5th Ed./Pg. 202]
A. Contract relax
B. Repeated contraction
C. Rhythmic stabilization
D. Hold-relax

Answer
411 C   412 B   413 B   414 B   415 D   416 B   417 D   418 B   419 A   420 B   421 C   422 A
423 C   424 B

Neuromuscular Coordination

Q 425. In Frenkel's exercises the progression is made by:
[Suraj Kumar/Exercise Therapy/1st Ed./Pg. 212]
A. Gradually increasing the speed of the movements
B. Rapidly increasing the speed of the movements
C. Increase speed on first day and decrease the speed on second day. Then progress on alternate days
D. Decrease the speed of the movements progressively

Q 426. A physical therapy record indicates a patient exhibits dysdiadochokinesia. Based on the patient's documented deficit, which test would you expect to be the most difficult for the patient?
[Physical Rehabilitation/O'Sullivan/4th Ed./Pg. 160]
A. Alternate supination/pronation of the forearm
B. State balance assessment
C. March in place
D. Walk along a straight line

Q 427. A therapist designs an exercise program for a patient rehabilitating from a prolonged illness. Which of the following exercises is indicated for coordination training?
[Physical Rehabilitation/O'Sullivan/4th Ed./Pg. 730-731]
A. Buerger-Allen exercises
B. Codman's exercise
C. DeLorme's exercise
D. Frenkel's exercises

Q 428. A physical therapist treating a patient in supine elects to reinforce active movement of the lower extremity in a flexion, adduction, and lateral rotation pattern. This proprioceptive neuromuscular facilitation technique pattern is termed:
[Therapeutic Exercise/Kisner/5th Ed./Pg. 196]
A. D1 flexion
B. D1 extension
C. D2 flexion
D. D2 extension

Manual Therapy

Q 429. What is Maitland's 2nd degree of mobilization:
[Therapeutic Exercise/Kisner/5th Ed./Pg. 116]
A. Large amplitude of movement performed up to limit of range
B. Small amplitude of movement performed up to limit of range
C. Large amplitude of movement performed within the free range but not moving into any resistance or stiffness
D. Small amplitude of movement performed at the beginning of range

Q 430. Contraindication for manipulation is:
[Therapeutic Exercise/Kisner/5th Ed./Pg. 114]
A. Locked joint
B. Acute nerve root compression
C. Pain free stiff joint
D. None of the above

Q 431. Which of the following is contraindication for manual stretching?
[Therapeutic Exercise/Kisner/5th Ed./Pg. 68]
A. Decreased ROM because of adhesion's
B. Muscle weakness

C. Muscle shortening
D. Bony block to joint motion

Q 432. Manual therapies can be applied to:
[Exercise Therapy/Dina Gardiner/4th Ed./Pg. 135]
A. Joints
B. Muscles
C. Neural structures
D. All of the above

Q 433. A patient two months status post total knee replacement is referred to physical therapy for range of motion and strengthening exercise. Which treatment techniques would be inappropriate for the patient?
[Jayant Joshi/1st Ed./Pg. 212]
A. Active stretching using the contract relax technique
B. Joint mobilization to increase joint play
C. Exercise on a stationary bicycle against mild resistance
D. Performing straight leg raising short are extension, and knee flexion exercises using leg weights

Q 434. A patient is referred to physical therapy with a twenty degree restriction in wrist extension which mobilization technique would facilitate wrist extension?
[Therapeutic Exercise/Kisner/5th Ed./Pg. 132]
A. Dorsal glide of the carpals
B. Stabilize lunate, volar glide radius
C. Stabilize capitate, volar glide lunate
D. Stabilize radius, volar glide scaphoid

Q 435. A treatment program is designed to include late morning sessions involving aggressive stretching moderate exercise, energy conservation, and stress management techniques. This program would be most appropriate for which diagnosis?
[Cash's Neurology/4th Ed./Pg. 403-404]
A. Guillain-Barre syndrome
B. Myasthenia gravis
C. Osgood-Schlatter disease
D. Multiple sclerosis

Q 436. A therapist prepares to treat a patient with limited ankle range of motion using joint mobilization techniques. If the therapist elects to mobilize the talocrural joint in the resting position, the therapist should position the ankle in:
[Therapeutic Exercise/Kisner/5th Ed./Pg. 142]
A. 5 degrees dorsiflexion, 5 degrees inversion
B. 5 degrees plantar flexion 5 degrees inversion
C. 10 degrees plantar flexion, midway between inversion and eversion
D. 15 degrees plantar flexion, 5 degrees eversion

Q 437. A therapist performs manual muscle test on a patient with unilateral upper extremity weakness. The patient is able to complete 75% of the available range of motion with gravity eliminated. The therapist should record the muscle grade as:
[Muscle Testing/Daniel/7th Ed./Pg. 7]
A. Poor plus
B. Poor
C. Poor minus
D. Trace plus

Q 438. A physical therapist performs a manual muscle test on a patient hip flexor. The therapist attempts to complete the test in supine, but the patient has difficulty holding the

---

Answer   425 D   426 A   427 D   428 A   429 B   430 B   431 D   432 D   433 B   434 D   435 B   436 C
437 C

limb in the test position. What alternate test position would be appropriate to test the patient's hip flexors?

[Daniel/7th Ed./Pg. 183]

A. Prone
B. Side-lying
C. Sitting
D. Standing

Q 439. A therapist completes a manual muscle test on the right lower trapezius muscle. In order to properly assess the muscle, the therapist should position the patient in:

[Muscle Testing/Daniel/7th Ed./Pg. 78]

A. Supine
B. Prone
C. Right side-lying
D. Left side-lying

Q 440. A physical therapist examines a patient with shoulder subluxation secondary to a flaccid upper extremity. The therapist's short term goal is to prevent further subluxation. The following techniques would be beneficial in treating the flaccid upper extremity except:

[Therapeutic Exercise/Kisner/5th Ed./Pg. 195-192]

A. Distraction and stretching techniques
B. Approximation techniques
C. Neuromuscular electrical stimulation
D. Arm support when sitting and standing

Q 441. A therapist assesses the strength of a patient's right hip adductors by positioning the patient in right side-lying. During resting the patient is unable to move the extremity through the available range of motion. The most appropriate position to retest the hip adductors is:

[Daniel/7th Ed./Pg. 207]

A. Sitting
B. Prone
C. Supine
D. Left side-lying

Q 442. A manual muscle test is conducted on the medial portion of the deltoid. The muscle is able to move through the full range of motion with gravity eliminated, but cannot function against gravity. The results of the manual muscle test should be recorded as:

[Daniel/7th Ed./Pg. 97]

A. Trace
B. Poor
C. Fair
D. Good

Q 443. A therapist completes a manual muscle test where resistance is applied toward plantar flexion eversion. This description best describes a manual muscle test of the:

[Daniel/7th Ed./Pg. 241]

A. Tibialis anterior
B. Tibialis posterior
C. Peroneus longus
D. Peroneus brevis

Q 444. A physical therapist performs a manual muscle test on the primary hip abductor. The therapist should perform the test while palpating the:

[Daniel/7th Ed./Pg. 199]

A. Rectus femoris
B. Gluteus medius
C. Sartorius
D. Gluteus minimus

Q 445. A manual muscle test of the triceps reveals evidence of slight contractility without any active range of motion. The muscle should be graded as:

[Daniel/7th Ed./Pg. 121]

A. Zero
B. Trace
C. Poor
D. Fair

Q 446. A therapist records a manual muscle test grade of poor for right hip adduction. The most appropriate patient position to conduct the test would be:

[Daniel/7th Ed./Pg. 200]

A. Supine
B. Prone
C. Right side-lying
D. Left side-lying

Q 447. A physical therapist performs a test to measure the strength of a patient's lower abdominal muscles. The most appropriate technique to examine the strength of the abdominals is:

[Therapeutic Exercise/Kisner/5th Ed./Pg. 149]

A. Partial sit-up
B. Full sit-up with rotation
C. Single leg lowering teste.
D. Double leg lowering test

Q 448. A therapist assigns a grade of good after completing a manual muscle test of the extensor digitorum. The most appropriate patient position to conduct the test would be:

[Muscle Testing/Daniel/7th Ed./Pg. 150]

A. Supine
B. Prone
C. Side-lying
D. Standing

Q 449. A therapist completes a manual muscle test on a muscle that inverts the foot and assists in plantar flexion of the ankle joint. This description best describes the:

[Muscle Testing/Daniel/7th Ed./Pg. 238]

A. Tibialis anterior
B. Tibialis posterior
C. Peroneus longus
D. Peroneus tertius

Q 450. Muscles that flex or extend in the sagittal plane against gravity are tested in the _____________ plane for gravity eliminated testing?

[Norkin/3rd Ed./Pg. 6]

A. Coronal
B. Frontal
C. Sagittal
D. Transverse

Q 451. A patient is found to have limited knee extension. Which of the following mobilization techniques would be indicated?

[Therapeutic Exercise/Kisner/5th Ed./Pg. 139]

A. Lateral glide of the patella
B. Caudal glide of the patella
C. Posterior glide of the tibia
D. Anterior glide of the tibia

Q 452. A physical therapist performs a manual muscle test on a patient's shoulder medial rotators. Which muscle would not be involved in this test?

[David/5th Ed./Pg. 693-694]

A. Pectoralis major
B. Subscapularis
C. Teres major
D. Teres minor

Q 453. Proper technique is essential to obtain accurate results when performing a manual muscle test. Which of the following manual muscle testing instructions is not accurate?

[Daniel/7th Ed./Pg. 6]

A. Have the patient perform the movement actively
B. Stabilize proximal to the joint
C. Check the passive range of motion of the joint being moved
D. Apply pressure at the proximal end of the moving part

Q 454. A physical therapist performs a manual muscle test on a patient with bilateral upper extremity weakness. The

Answer	438 B	439 B	440 A	441 C	442 B	443 D	444 B	445 B	446 A	447 D	448 A	449 B
	450 D	451 D	452 D	453 C								

therapist should test the patient's scapular adductors with the patient positioned in:

[Daniel/7th Ed./Pg. 74]

A. Prone
B. Side-lying
C. Standing
D. Supine

Q 455. To check peak muscle strength of the rectus femoris the patient should be placed in:

[Daniel/7th Ed./Pg. 124]

A. Crook lying
B. Half lying
C. Sit lying
D. High sitting

Q 456. The grade of muscle power in ankle dorsiflexors is zero in which of the following?

[Daniel/7th Ed./Pg. 235]

A. Absent dorsiflexion movement eliminating gravity
B. Absent dorsiflexion movement against gravity
C. Absent dorsiflexion movement against resistance
D. Absent visible or palpable muscle contraction

Q 457. The best method to examine the grade 2 power of elbow flexors is:

[Daniel/7th Ed./Pg. 116]

A. Patient lying supine
B. Patient lying prone
C. Patient sitting with shoulder neutral
D. Patient sitting with shoulder 90 degree abducted

General Exercise

Q 458. Cooling down exercises are performed for a period of:

[Therapeutic Exercise/Kisner/5th Ed./Pg. 241]

A. 5 to 8 minutes
B. 1 to 2 minutes
C. 15 to 20 minutes
D. 30 to 45 seconds

Q 459. High intensity and high velocity resistance exercise characterized by a resisted eccentric muscle contraction followed by rapid concentric contraction followed by a rapid concentric contraction and designed to increase the muscle power and contraction is also known as:

[Therapeutic Exercise/Kisner/5th Ed./Pg. 208]

A. Plyometric training
B. Stress endurance exercise
C. Hold relax exercises
D. VC training

Q 460. A therapist reviews the results of a complete blood count taken on a 65-year-old male recently admitted to the hospital. Which of the following blood test values may be considered a precaution for therapeutic exercise?

A. White blood cell count: 6.2×10^3 μL
B. Hematocrit: 46 mL/dL
C. Hemoglobin: 8 g/dL
D. Platelet count: 250×10^3 μL

Q 461. A physical therapist uses rhythmic initiation to assist a patient in learning to roll from supine to prone. The physical therapist's initial command should be:

[Therapeutic Exercise/Kisner/5th Ed./Pg. 202]

A. Slowly roll over by yourself
B. Help me roll you over
C. Stop me from rolling you over
D. Relax and let me move you

Q 462. A physical therapist instructs a patient to perform a quadriceps setting exercise. This exercise is considered to be an _________ exercise?

[Therapeutic Exercise/Kisner/5th Ed./Pg. 169]

A. Eccentric
B. Isokinetic
C. Isometric
D. Isotonic

Q 463. A female distance runner complains of recurrent friction blisters whenever she increases the intensity of her training regimen. Appropriate physical therapy care of friction blisters includes all of the following except:

[Tidy/KM Varghese/12th Ed./Pg. 284]

A. Pad the blister with a pressure pad
B. Use of skin tougheners with astringents
C. Soak regularly in ice water after activity
D. Make a large incision along the periphery of the blister with a sterile instrument

Q 464. Effective measures to prevent decubitus ulcers include all of the following except:

[Tidy/KM Varghese/12th Ed./Pg. 278]

A. Frequent inspection of the skin for redness and signs of skin breakdown
B. Turning and position changes every 4 hours
C. Early ambulation when possible
D. Passive range of motion exercises

Q 465. What massage technique is commonly used at the beginning and conclusion of treatment and may be used during transitional periods prior to changing massage techniques?

[Concise Exercise therapy/Roshan Lal Meena/1st Ed./Pg. 139]

A. Effleurage
B. Petrissage
C. Tapotement
D. Vibration

Q 466. A therapist instructs a patient diagnosed with rotator cuff tendonitis in a home exercise program. The most important consideration when designing a home exercise program is to:

[Therapeutic Exercise/Kisner/5th Ed./Pg. 23]

A. Focus the program on the individual needs of the patient
B. Limit the length of the program to 10 minutes
C. Provide written instructions that detail the frequency and duration of each exercise
D. Limit the amount of equipment required to complete the program

Others

Q 467. Hydrocortisone process all of the following properties except:

[KD Tripthi/Essential Pharmacology/5th Ed./Pg. 254]

A. Antiallergic
B. Antirheumatic
C. Antidiabetic
D. Antifibrotic

Q 468. The acronym HARM used for the management of acute sports injuries stands for:

[Refer to text]

A. Help athlete regain mobility
B. Help to ambulate with rapid motion

Answer   454 A   455 C   456 D   457 D   458 A   459 A   460 C   461 D   462 C   463 D   464 B   465 A
         466 C   467 C

C. Do not use heat, alcohol, running and massage

D. Hot packs, aerobics, resisted exercises and mobilization

Q 469. Renal stones are most frequently seen in:
[Essential Orthopaedics/Maheshwari/3rd Ed./Pg. 266]

A. Neurofibromatosis   B. Deficiency rickets

C. Fibrous dysplasia   D. Hyperparathyroidism

Q 470. The optimal position for a patient who begins to demonstrate signs of orthostatic hypotension is:
[O'Sullivan/4th Ed./Pg. 884]

A. Supine   B. Sitting upright

C. Standing   D. Walking

Q 471. A patient is referred to physical therapy following a work related lifting injury. The patient complains of acute back pain and has obvious muscle spasms throughout the paraspinal region. Which treatment option would be the most appropriate for the patient:

A. Hot packs and ultrasound

B. Extension exercises

C. Flexion exercise

D. Unable to determine based on the information given

Investigation

Q 472. Which of the following is most dependable in the diagnosis of prolapsed intervertebral disc?
[Ebnezar/1st Ed./Pg. 315]

A. X-ray   B. Myelogram

C. Bone scan   D. MRI

Q 473. Which of the following procedures is most commonly used to determine activity tolerance after myocardial infarction?
[Medicine/Davidson/20th Ed./Pg. 593]

A. Graded exercise test   B. MUGA

C. Echocardiography   D. All of the above

Q 474. Earliest changes in Perthes disease is seen by:
[Essential Orthopaedics/Maheshwari/3rd Ed./Pg. 269-270]

A. X-ray   B. CT

C. MRI   D. US

E. Nuclear scan

Q 475. Percentage of positively of HLA-B27 in ankylosing spondylosis:
[Tidy's Physiotherapy/12th Ed./Pg. 128]

A. 10%   B. 96%

C. 78%   D. 100%

Q 476. A 16-year-old high school track participant returns to physical therapy after a physician appointment. The patient indicates that magnetic resonance imaging revealed a tear in the medial meniscus of the left knee. As you look back on the initial examination, which of the following special tests would you expect to have been position?
[Essential Orthopaedics/Maheshwari/3rd Ed./Pg. 313]

A. Lachman   B. Pivot shift

C. McMurray   D. Apprehension

Q 477. Laboratory testing reveals that a patient postchemotherapy has a platelet count of 60,000 mm³. Which activity would be the most appropriate for the patient based on the platelet value?
[Therapeutic Exercise/Kisner/5th Ed./Pg. 220]

A. Strict bed rest

B. Active range of motion

C. Light activities of daily living

D. Stationary cycling

Q 478. Group exercise is commonly used to treat individuals of similar diagnoses. Which of the following is not true when discussing group exercise?
[Dina Gardiner/Exercise Therapy/17th Ed./Pg. 264]

A. Groups of equal ability inevitably need more time than groups of mixed ability

B. Groups should be used for the benefit of patients and not due to staff shortage

C. All patients should be thoroughly assessed prior to being selected for group exercise

D. All exercises used in group teaching should be within the experience of the therapist in-charge of the group

Q 479. A patient diagnosed with shoulder pain of unknown etiology is referred by his physician for magnetic resonance imaging. Results of the test reveal a partial tear of the infraspinatus muscle. Which muscle group would you expect to be the most seriously affected by the injury?
[BD Chaurasia, Human Anatomy/Exercise Therapy/ 4th Ed./Pg. 146]

A. Shoulder lateral rotators   B. Shoulder medial rotators

C. Shoulder abductors   D. Shoulder adductors

Q 480. A 30-year-old man has pain under his metatarsal heads and pes cavus on both feet without any neurological abnormality. The X-ray appearance of LS spine may show:
[Essential Orthopaedics/Maheshwari/3rd Ed./Pg. 210]

A. Spondylolisthesis   B. Spina bifida occulta

C. Sacralization   D. Osteoarthritis of facet joints

Q 481. HLA-B27 is associated with:
[Essential Orthopaedics/Maheshwari/3rd Ed./Pg. 248]

A. Rheumatic arthritis   B. Ankylosing spondylitis

C. Rheumatic arthritis   D. Gouty arthritis

Q 482. Bamboo spine is seen in:
[Essential Orthopaedics/Maheshwari/3rd Ed./Pg. 248]

A. Tuberculosis   B. Rheumatoid arthritis

C. Ochronosis   D. Ankylosing spondylosis

Q 483. On chest X-ray the SILHOUTTE sign presents as:
[Refer to text]

A. The two separate structures adjacent to each other are not identified because of lack of difference in bone densities

B. Paralysis of diaphragm over shadows the lung

C. Enlargement of cardiac field in the transverse direction

D. A sharp contrast between two adjacent

Physiotherapy Gynae

Q 484. Exercises explained in the last month of pregnancy are all except:
[Therapeutic Exercise/Kisner/5th Ed./Pg. 816]

A. Contracting pelvic floor muscles

B. Contracting abdominal muscles

Answer	468 C	469 D	470 A	471 D	472 D	473 A	474 E	475 B	476 C	477 D	478 A	479 A
	480 B	481 B	482 D	483 A								

C. Straight single leg raising with extended knee
D. Straight both leg raising with extended knee

Q 485. Which of the following exercise would be inappropriate for a woman who gave birth via cesarean section two days ago?
[Therapeutic Exercise/Kisner/5th Ed./Pg. 819]
A. Pelvic tilts
B. Walking
C. Deep breathing
D. Partial sit-ups

Q 486. Which of the following conditions would be considered an absolute contraindication to exercise?
[Therapeutic Exercise/Kisner/5th Ed./Pg. 811]
A. Multiple gestation
B. Maternal diabetes
C. Phlebitis
D. Anemia

Q 487. A therapist develops exercise guidelines for a pregnant woman. Which of the following guideline is not accurate?
[Therapeutic Exercise/Kisner/5th Ed./Pg. 804]
A. Deep flexion and extension of joints should be avoided
B. Heart rate should be measured at times of peak activity
C. Duration of exercise should be influenced by perceived exertion
D. Fluid intake should be limited before and after exercise

Q 488. A therapist designs an exercise program for a woman that is pregnant. The physician referral identifies diastasis recti as a secondary diagnosis. Diastasis recti is:
[Therapeutic Exercise/Kisner/5th Ed./Pg. 804]
A. An incision made at the opening of the vagina to increases the diameter
B. When the embryo develops in the fallopian tube
C. A separation of the rectus abdominis muscle
D. When the placenta pulls away from the uterine wall

Q 489. Pelvic floor tension myalgia occurs in:
[Refer to text]
A. Adolescent boys
B. Adolescent girls
C. Adult females
D. None of these

Q 490. A woman's pulmonary and cardiovascular systems are altered physiologically during pregnancy. Which of the following would a physical therapist expect to observe when examining a pregnant woman?
[Therapeutic Exercise/Kisner/5th Ed./Pg. 800]
A. Decreased oxygen reserve ad decreased stroke volume
B. Increased oxygen reserve and increased stroke volume
C. Decreased oxygen reserve and increased cardiac output
D. Decreased stroke volume and decreased cardiac output

Q 491. A woman in her third trimester of pregnancy is referred to physical therapy with acute low back pain. During a postural examination the therapist identifies several significant findings. Which of the following postural findings is not commonly associated with pregnancy?
[Therapeutic Exercise/Kisner/5th Ed./Pg. 801]
A. Decrease in cervical lordosis
B. Increase in lumbar lordosis
C. Hyperextension of the knees
D. Protraction of the shoulder girdle

Suspension

Q 492. In axial suspension the fixed points lies:
[Concise Exercise Therapy/Roshan Lal Meena/1st Ed./Pg. 155]
A. Vertically above the joint requiring mobilization
B. Vertically above the joint proximal to the joint requiring mobilization
C. Vertically above the joint distal to the joint requiring mobilization
D. None of the above

Goniometry

Q 493. A therapist performs goniometric measurements for elbow flexion with a patient in supine. In order to isolate elbow flexion the therapist should stabilize the:
[Norkin's Goniometry/3rd Ed./Pg. 100]
A. Distal end of the humerus
B. Proximal end of the humerus
C. Distal end of the ulna
D. Proximal end of the radius

Q 494. When measuring elbow flexion, the stationary arm of the goniometer should be aligned along the:
[Norkin's Goniometry/3rd Ed./Pg. 101]
A. Humerus
B. Radius
C. Ulna
D. Fifth metacarpal

Q 495. A physical therapist obtains a goniometric measurement with a patient in supine. The stationary arm of the goniometer is positioned at the midaxillary line of the trunk. The movable arm is positioned along the lateral midline of the humerus using the lateral epicondyle as a reference. This positioning of the goniometer can be used to measure:
[Refer to text]
A. Shoulder flexion
B. Medial and lateral rotation of the shoulder
C. Shoulder extension
D. Elbow extension

Q 496 A therapist performs a range of motion screening on a 14-year-old female. The therapist instructs the patient to stand on her tiptoes. The therapist uses this command to examine:
[Daniel/7th Ed./Pg. 228]
A. Dorsiflexion and toe extension
B. Dorsiflexion and toe flexion
C. Plantar flexion and toe extension
D. Plantar flexion and toe flexion

Q 497. Forearm supination is measured with the moving arm of the goniometer placed on the _______ side of the wrist?
[Norkin's Goniometry/3rd Ed./Pg. 9]
A. Dorsal
B. Lateral
C. Medial
D. Volar

Q 498. When measuring hip abduction the stationary arm of the goniometer should be positioned _________?
[Norkin/3rd Ed./Pg. 198]
A. Between the anterior superior iliac spines
B. Parallel to the anterior aspect of the femur

Answer   484 D   485 D   486 C   487 D   488 C   489 B   490 C   491 A   492 A   493 A   494 A   495 A
496 C   497 D

C. Along the midline of the tibia
D. Along a line from the crest of the ilium, femur, and greater trochanter

Q 499. A therapist completes an upper extremity goniometric examination. The therapist records right elbow range of motion as 15-0-150 degrees. The total available range of motion for this patient is _______ degrees?

[Norkin/3rd Ed./Pg. 31]

A. 135
B. 150
C. 165
D. 180

Q 500. There are a variety of systems used to record goniometric measurements. Using the 0 to 180 system the anatomical position is used as the starting position for all movements except:

[Norkin's Goniometry/3rd Ed./Pg. 102,104]

A. Ankle inversion and eversion
B. Forearm pronation and supination
C. Shoulder flexion and extension
D. Wrist flexion and extension

Q 501. A therapist performs goniometric measurements at the carpometacarpal joint. If the therapist elects to measure carpometacarpal abduction, the stationary arm of the goniometer should be aligned with the:

[Norkin's Goniometry/3rd Ed./Pg. 164]

A. Lateral midline of the second metacarpal
B. Lateral midline of the first metacarpal
C. Palmar midline of the radius
D. Palmar midline of the first metacarpal

Q 502. A therapist performs goniometric measurements on a 38-year-old female rehabilitating from an acromioplasty. The therapist attempts on stabilize the scapula while measuring glenohumeral abduction. Failure to stabilize the scapula will led to:

[Norkin's Goniometry/3rd Ed./Pg. 78]

A. Downward rotation and elevation of the scapula
B. Downward rotation and depression of the scapula
C. Upward rotation and elevation of the scapula
D. Upward rotation and depression of the scapula

Taping

Q 503. A physical therapist traps the ankle of a young athlete with a history of recurrent inversion ankle sprains. The therapist elects to use the closed basket weave strapping technique. Which of the following is not accurate when using this technique?

[Elesiver/Jayant Joshi/ 1st Ed./Pg. 550]

A. One and one-half inch adhesive tape is traditionally used
B. Stirrups should be applied pulling the foot into inversion
C. The foot should remain in dorsiflexion during strapping to provide additional support use figure-eight with or without heel locks

Q 504. When measurement ulnar deviation of the wrist, the moveable arm of the goniometer should be aligned with the:

[Norkin's Goniometry/ 3rd Ed./Pg. 126]

A. Shaft of the second proximal phalanx
B. Shaft of the third proximal phalanx
C. Shaft of the second metacarpal
D. Shaft of the third metacarpal

Q 505. The open basket weave taping technique is commonly used as a form of treatment for an acute ankle sprain. Which of the following does not accurately describe the benefits of the open basketweave taping technique?

A. Allows freedom of movement in dorsiflexion
B. Allows freedom of movement in plantar flexion
C. Provides room for additional edema
D. Promotes proximal joint stability

Relaxation

Q 506. Sensory stimulation of either muscle contraction or relaxation was introduction by:

[Neurology/Cash's/4th Ed./ Pg. 200-201]

A. Bobath
B. Fay
C. Knott
D. Rood

Answer 498 A 499 C 500 B 501 A 502 D 503 B 504 C 505 C 506 B

2

CHAPTER

Electrotherapy

Objective Questions with Answers

General Electrotherapy

Q 1. The earth pin of the plug socket is larger as:
[Electrotherapy/Clayton/9th Ed./Pg. 48]
A. It allows one-way entry of the socket
B. It allows the earth pin to enter first and come out last
C. Both A, B
D. None of the above

Q 2. The fuse in a power circuit should break:
[Electrotherapy/Clayton/9th Ed./Pg. 46]
A. The neutral wire   B. The live wire
C. Both live and neutral wire   D. None of the above

Q 3. The switches in the apparatus should break:
[Electrotherapy Simplified/Nanda/1st Ed./Pg. 85]
A. The neutral wire   B. The live wire
C. Both live and neutral wire   D. None of the above

Q 4. The wire in a fuse should have:
[Electrotherapy Simplified/Nanda/1st Ed./Pg. 85]
A. Very high melting point   B. Very low melting point
C. High thermal tolerance   D. None of the above

Q 5. The earth pin should be connected to:
[Electrotherapy/Clayton/9th Ed./Pg. 48]
A. The wire with black or blue color
B. The wire with yellow or green color
C. The wire with red or brown color
D. None of the above

Q 6. Rectification of a circuit is achieved using:
[Electrotherapy Simplified/Nanda/1st Ed./Pg. 51-57]
A. Diode valve   B. Rheostat
C. Transformer   D. Capacitor

Q 7. The device used to regulate current is:
[Electrotherapy/Clayton/9th Ed./Pg. 39]
A. Semiconductor   B. Triode valve
C. Rheostat   D. Capacitor

Q 8. The amount of heat produced during treatment with an electric current increases if:
[Electrotherapy/Clayton/9th Ed./Pg. 117]
A. Skin impedance is high
B. The treatment time is of a short interval
C. The total current is not high
D. None of the above

Q 9. Which of the following is a true sentence:
[Electrotherapy Simplified/Nanda/1st Ed./Pg. 90]
A. After a severe shock there is paralysis of the respiratory muscles
B. Hot drinks should be avoided following a shock
C. After a severe shock there is rise in blood pressure
D. Shocks are more severe with direct currents

Q 10. The device used to regulate current by altering the resistance or the potential of the circuit is:
[Electrotherapy/Clayton/9th Ed./Pg. 39]
A. Condenser   B. Diode
C. Rheostat   D. Semiconductor

Q 11. Thermionic valve is a device that allows electrons to flow in:
[Electrotherapy/Clayton/9th Ed./Pg. 36]
A. Reverse direction   B. Both directions
C. One direction   D. All directions

Q 12. The device that measures electrical resistance is:
[Electrotherapy/Clayton/9th Ed./Pg. 36]
A. Ohmmeter   B. Potentiometer
C. Voltmeter   D. Transformer

Q 13. As the temperature of the conductor increases, the resistance to flow of electron:
[Electrotherapy Simplified/Nanda/1st Ed./Pg. 24]
A. Doubles   B. Decreases
C. Remains the same   D. Increases

Q 14. EMF of any cell can be measured by:
[Electrotherapy/Clayton/9th Ed./Pg. 81]

Answer   1 C   2 C   3 C   4 B   5 B   6 A   7 C   8 A   9 B   10 C   11 C   12 A
          13 B

A. Wheatstone bridge B. Potentiometer
C. Voltmeter D. Ammeter

Q 15. The instrument used to measure current intensity is:
[Electrotherapy Simplified/Nanda/1st Ed./Pg. 73]
A. Wheatstone bridge B. Potentiometer
C. Voltmeter D. Ammeter

Q 16. At the neuromuscular junction the chemical released is:
[Electrotherapy Simplified/Nanda/1st Ed./Pg. 111]
A. Calcium B. Prostaglandin
C. Acetylcholine D. Adrenaline

Q 17. The myelinated nerve fibers usually have diameter above:
[Neurology and Neurosurgery/Illustrated/Lindsay/
4th Ed./Pg. 428]
A. 2 µm B. 5 µm
C. 7 µm D. 3 µm

Q 18. Wallerian degeneration is completed by:
[Neurology and Neurosurgery/Illustrated/Lindsay/
4th Ed./Pg. 428]
A. 20 days B. 14 days
C. 7 days D. 1 month

Q 19. The mean dielectric constant value of body tissue is:
[Electrotherapy/Clayton/9th Ed./Pg. 117]
A. 50 B. 70
C. 80 D. None of the above

Q 20. In a step-up transformer:
[Electrotherapy Simplified/Nanda/1st Ed./Pg. 44]
A. The number of turns of wire in primary coil is more than the secondary
B. Number of turns in primary and secondary is same
C. The number of turns of wire in secondary coil is more than primary
D. None of the above

Q 21. Lenz's law deals with:
[Electrotherapy Simplified/Nanda/1st Ed./Pg. 70]
A. Inductance of the conductor
B. Rate of change of magnetic field
C. Direction of current flow
D. Direction of the induced EMF

Q 22. Joule's law expresses the relation between:
[Electrotherapy/Clayton/9th Ed./Pg. 14]
A. Current, voltage and time
B. Current, resistance and time
C. Current, Power and resistance
D. Current, EMF and time

Q 23. High inductance can be incorporated into a conducting coil by:
[Electrotherapy/Clayton/9th Ed./Pg. 21]
A. Using many turns of wire
B. Placing the turns closer
C. Winding the coil into a soft iron core
D. All of the above

Q 24. The dielectric constant of which of following is right?
[Electrotherapy/Clayton/9th Ed./Pg. 117]
A. Fatty tissue B. Skin
C. Bones D. Muscles

Q 25. Average pH of water in the therapeutic pool:
[Physical Agent in Rehabilitation/Cameron/2nd Ed./Pg. 180]
A. pH 3.75 B. pH 5.75
C. pH 7.75 D. pH 9.75

Q 26. Ideal temperature of therapeutic pool is:
[Physical Agent in Rehabilitation/Cameron/2nd Ed./Pg. 294]
A. 30.5 – 35.5°C
B. 35.5 – 40.5°C
C. 40.5 – 45.5°C
D. 26.5 – 30.5°C

Therapeutic Current

Q 27. When two opposite phases are contained in a single pulse, the wave form is termed as:
[Physical Rehabilitation O'Sullivan/4th Ed./Pg. 233]
A. Monophasic B. Biphasic
C. Asymmetric D. Symmetric

Q 28. The resting membrane potential of the skeletal muscle cell is:
[Physical Agent in Rehabilitation/Cameron/2nd Ed./Pg. 227]
A. – 60 m B. – 70 mV
C. – 90 mV D. None of the above

Q 29. The resting nerve is positive outside due to concentration of:
[Physical Agent in Rehabilitation/Cameron/2nd Ed./Pg. 227]
A. Sodium and calcium ions B. Potassium ions
C. Sodium ions D. Calcium ions

Q 30. The rate of conduction of impulses through the AA fiber is:
[Physical Agent in Rehabilitation/Cameron/2nd Ed./Pg. 229]
A. 15 m/s B. 5 m/s
C. 1 m/s D. 2 m/s

Q 31. A current that produces greater muscular hypertrophy with gain in strength is:
[Electrotherapy Simplified/Nanda/1st Ed./Pg. 267]
A. Direct current B. Faradic current
C. Russian current D. Diadynamic current

Q 32. The low frequency currents have a frequency of:
[Electrotherapy Simplified/Nanda/1st Ed./Pg. 100]
A. 50 Hz B. 100–150 Hz
C. 1–1000 Hz D. None of the above

Q 33. The circuit used to produce faradic type current is:
[Electrotherapy/Clayton/9th Ed./Pg. 56]
A. Multivibrator circuit B. Surge circuit
C. Voltage halving circuit D. Anode circuit

Q 34. The original faradic current was:
[Electrotherapy/Clayton/9th Ed./Pg. 55]
A. An unevenly alternating current
B. A constant direct current

Answer	14 B	15 D	16 C	17 A	18 B	19 C	20 C	21 D	22 B	23 D	24 D	25 C
	26 B	27 B	28 C	29 A	30 A	31 C	32 C	33 A				

C. An interrupted direct current
D. An evenly alternating current

Q 35. The minimum resistance of skin is around:
[Electrotherapy/Clayton/9th Ed./Pg. 107]
A. 1000 μ
B. 3200 μ
C. 5000 μ
D. None of the above

Q 36. When direct current is passed through the cathode, it increases the excitability of the nerve. This is termed as:
[Physical Agent in Rehabilitation/Cameron/2nd Ed./Pg. 29]
A. Anelectronus
B. Catelectronus
C. Depolarization
D. Repolarization

Q 37. The state of decreased excitability of a nerve near the anode is termed as:
[Refer to text]
A. Anelectronus
B. Catelectronus
C. Depolarization
D. Repolarization

Q 38. The smallest current that produces a muscle contraction when the stimulus is of infinite duration is:
[Electrotherapy/Clayton/9th Ed./Pg. 95]
A. Chronaxie
B. Rheobase
C. Microcurrent
D. Pulse duration

Q 39. The shape of the curve in strength duration curve indicates:
[Electrotherapy/Clayton/9th Ed./Pg. 92]
A. The site of lesion
B. Onset
C. Proportion of denervation
D. All of above

Q 40. The types of muscle fibers mostly activated by electrical stimulation are:
[Physical Agent in Rehabilitation/Cameron/2nd Ed./Pg. 231]
A. Type-I fibers
B. Type-II a, fibers
C. Type-II b, fibers
D. None of the above

Q 41. The resting nerve is:
[Physical Agent in Rehabilitation/Cameron/2nd Ed./Pg. 227]
A. Negative inside and positive outside
B. Negative outside and positive inside
C. Positive inside and positive outside
D. Negative inside and negative outside

Q 42. When a healthy innervated muscle is stimulated with an electrical current, we stimulate the:
[Physical Agent in Rehabilitation/Cameron/2nd Ed./Pg. 61]
A. The neurolemma of the axon
B. The sarcolemma of the muscle
C. The neuromuscular junction
D. All of the above

Q 43. The resting membrane potential of a nerve cell is:
[Physical Agent in Rehabilitation/Cameron/2nd Ed./Pg. 60]
A. – 70 mV
B. – 50 mV
C. – 120 mV
D. 1 mV

Q 44. Selective impulses are used for stimulation of:
[Physical Agent in Rehabilitation/Cameron/2nd Ed./Pg. 83]
A. Innervated muscles
B. Denervated muscles
C. Muscle strengthening
D. None of the above

Q 45. Conventional TENS is:
[Electrotherapy Simplified/Nanda/1st Ed./Pg. 189]
A. High intensity, low frequency stimulation
B. Low intensity, low frequency stimulation
C. High intensity, high frequency stimulation
D. High frequency, low intensity stimulation

Q 46. Which one of the following has an anesthetic effect?
[Electrotherapy Explained/Low and Reed/3rd Ed./Pg. 36]
A. High Voltage Pulsed Current
B. Continuous galvanic current
C. Diadynamic current
D. Russian currents

Q 47. The constant current stimulator is:
A. More accurate
B. More comfortable
C. Accurate as well as comfortable
D. None of the above

Q 48. Which of the statement is a false?
[Electrotherapy Explained/Low and Reed/3rd Ed./Pg. 62]
A. Edema due to disruption of blood vessels is alleviated with HVPC
B. Polarity is the predominant current characteristic to be considered in wound healing
C. HVPC can be used for muscle re-education
D. HVPC has a single monophasic wave form

Q 49. To stretch adherent scar, the ion selected for iontophoresis is:
[Electrotherapy Simplified/Nanda/1st Ed./Pg. 169]
A. Magnesium
B. Copper
C. Chloride
D. Zinc

Q 50. Which of the ions delivered through iontophoresis can be used in the treatment of calcific deposits?
[Electrotherapy Simplified/Nanda/1st Ed./Pg. 166]
A. Zinc
B. Hyaluronidase
C. Chloride
D. Acetate

Q 51. The quantity of ions introduced across the body surface by iontophoresis is directly proportional to:
[Electrotherapy Simplified/Nanda/1st Ed./Pg. 171]
A. Current intensity
B. Current density
C. Duration of current
D. Concentration of ions in solution

Q 52. Which of the following statements regarding diadynamic current is false?
[Electrotherapy Simplified/Nanda/1st Ed./Pg. 105]
A. It is sine wave at a frequency of 100 Hz
B. It is either full wave or half wave rectified
C. It is a biphasic pulsed current
D. It is a unidirectional current flow with long pulse duration

---

Answer	34 A	35 B	36 C	37 A	38 B	39 C	40 B	41 A	42 A	43 A	44 B	45 D
	46 B	47 A	48 D	49 C	50 D	51 B	52 C					

Q 53. The term Russian current applies to stimulators:
[Electrotherapy Simplified/Nanda/1st Ed./Pg. 266]
A. Which produces an asymmetric monophasic pulse from
B. Which have a ramp-up and ramp down mode
C. Which modulate a continuous sine wave
D. Which produces sine waves with full wave rectification

Q 54. Which of the following statements regarding effects of direct current is false?
[Electrotherapy Explained/Low and Reed/3rd Ed./Pg. 41]
A. It causes excitation of peripheral nerves
B. It cause alteration in protein synthesis
C. It causes smooth muscle contraction
D. It causes change in thermal and chemical balance of tissues

Q 55. In monopolar technique the dispersive electrode:
[Electrotherapy Simplified/Nanda/1st Ed./Pg. 3926]
A. Minimizes current density B. Maximizes current density
C. Increases the resistance   D. Increases the intensity

Q 56. A complete interference pattern is a feature of:
[Electrotherapy/Clayton/9th Ed./Pg. 98]
A. Normal muscle in volition
B. Denervated muscle
C. Partially innervated muscle
D. None of the above

Q 57. The reaction seen under the cathode when a direct current is passed through it is:
[Electrotherapy/Clayton/9th Ed./Pg. 36]
A. Acidic reaction
B. Neutral reaction
C. Alkaline reaction
D. No reaction

Q 58. The medium frequency currents have a frequency of:
[Electrotherapy Simplified/Nanda/1st Ed./Pg. 106]
A. 1–1000 Hz
B. Above 10,000 Hz
C. Above 1000 Hz and below 10,000 Hz
D. None of the above

Q 59. Which of the following statements regarding interferential current therapy is true?
[Electrotherapy Simplified/Nanda/1st Ed./Pg. 258]
A. Bipolar method does not provide endogenous interferential current
B. In quadripolar technique the current at the electrode skin interference is modulated
C. In quadripolar approach the stimulus is stronger on the skin
D. Bipolar method is difficult and time consuming

Q 60. In cases of diffuse area of pathology, the IFT mode selected is:
[Electrotherapy Simplified/Nanda/1st Ed./Pg. 259]
A. Scanning mode
B. Frequency sweep mode
C. Quadripolar mode
D. None of the above

Q 61. In order to produce muscle contraction the frequency of interferential current selected is:
[Electrotherapy Simplified/Nanda/1st Ed./Pg. 257]
A. 1–10 Hz   B. 1–100 Hz
C. 80–150 Hz   D. None of the above

Q 62. High frequency currents have a frequency of:
[Electrotherapy Simplified/Nanda/1st Ed./Pg. 108]
A. Above 10,000 Hz   B. Below 10,000 Hz
C. 500 Hz   D. None of the above

Q 63. The modality of choice for the treatment of postnatal perineal pain would be:
[Electrotherapy Simplified/Nanda/1st Ed./Pg. 46]
A. Ultraviolet radiation
B. Microwave diathermy
C. Pulsed electromagnetic energy
D. None of the above

Q 64. The unknown resistance of a circuit can be known by:
[Electrotherapy Simplified/Nanda/1st Ed./Pg. 69]
A. Potentiometer   B. Wheatstone bridge
C. Ammeter   D. None

Q 65. A patient sustains a deep laceration on the right anterior thigh after stumbling and falling in a modality cart. The therapist's most immediate response should be to:
[Physical Agent in Rehabilitation/Cameron/2nd Ed./Pg. 32]
A. Apply direct pressure over the wound
B. Apply heat
C. Apply ice
D. Fill out an incident report

Q 66. Thermal conductivity of which of the following is least?
[Physical Agent in Rehabilitation/Cameron/2nd Ed./Pg. 35]
A. Muscle   B. Skin
C. Ligaments   D. Fat

Q 67. Cold reduces pain as it is:
[Physical Agent in Rehabilitation/Cameron/2nd Ed./Pg. 40]
A. Reduce transmission of neural impulses
B. Act as counter irritant
C. Releases opioids
D. All of the above

Q 68. PUVA therapy is not used for:
[Electrotherapy/Clayton/9th Ed./Pg. 189]
A. Alopecia   B. Pressure sores
C. Plantar warts   D. All of the above

Q 69. TENS is a:
[Electrotherapy Simplified/Nanda/1st Ed./Pg. 103]
A. Low frequency type of current
B. Microcurrent
C. High frequency type of current
D. Medium frequency type of current

Q 70. The dielectric constant of tissues with high water content:
[Refer to text]

Answer	53 C	54 C	55 A	56 A	57 C	58 C	59 B	60 A	61 B	62 A	63 C	64 B
	65 A	66 D	67 B	68 B	69 A							

A. is less than the fatty tissue
B. is less than the skin
C. is less than the bony tissue
D. is more than the tissue with low water content

Q 71. The dielectric constant of water is:
A. 0.81
B. 81.1
C. 18.1
D. 1.08

Q 72. Most useful modality for rehabilitation in cervical spine injury with quadriplegia is:
A. CPM upper limb
B. CPM lower limb
C. Tilt table
D. Wax bath

Q 73. A capacitor is a device for:
[Electrotherapy/Clayton/9th Ed./Pg. 32]
A. Storing an electrical charge
B. Stepping up voltage
C. Producing magnetic field
D. None of the above

Q 74. Contraindications for hydrotherapy pool treatment is:
[Cameron, Saunder/2nd Ed./Pg. 294]
A. Bowel incontinence
B. Fits and seizures
C. Open wounds
D. all of above

Q 75. Which of the following situations would be contraindicated when using transcutaneous electrical nerve stimulation?
[Electrotherapy Simplified/Nanda/1st Ed./Pg. 196-197]
A. Use over an arthritic joint
B. Use during labor and delivery
C. Use over a pregnant uterus
D. Use to diminish phantom limb sensation.

Q 76. A therapist applies an electrical stimulation unit to a patient rehabilitating from an Achilles tendon rupture. Which of the following types of current has the lowest total average current?
[Electrotherapy Simplified/Nanda/1st Ed./Pg. 200-201]
A. Low volt
B. High volt
C. Russian
D. Interferential

Q 77. A therapist explains to a patient the benefits of using electrical stimulation for muscle reduction. The patient appears to understand the therapist's explanation, however seems extremely fright and asks the therapist not to use electrical device. The most appropriate therapist action is:
[Electrotherapy/Clayton/9th Ed./Pg. 68]
A. Reassure the patient that the electrical stimulation will not be harmful
B. Use only small amounts of current
C. Select another appropriate treatment technique
d. Discharge the patient from physical therapy

Q 78. A physical therapist treats a patient using transcutaneous electrical nerve stimulation. Which condition would not be considered a contraindication for TENS?
[Electrotherapy Simplified/Nanda 1st Ed./Pg. 198]
A. Placement over the carotid sinus
B. Placement over a pregnant uterus
C. Use on a patient with a cardiac pacemaker
D. Use during labor and delivery

Heating Modalities

Q 79. Energy required to change the state of a substance is:
[Electrotherapy/Clayton/9th Ed./Pg. 5]
A. Kinetic energy
B. Potential energy
C. Latent heat
D. Chemical energy

Q 80. The property of a device that enables it to store electrical energy by means of an electromagnetic field:
[Electrotherapy/Clayton/9th Ed./Pg. 18]
A. Conductance
B. Capacitance
C. Inductance
D. Impedance

Q 81. A choke coil is used in a circuit:
[Electrotherapy/Clayton/9th Ed./Pg. 242]
A. To supply uniform current flow
B. To allow the flow of low frequency, and prevent the flow of high frequency currents
C. Both A and B
D. None of the above

Q 82. Transmission of heat due to convection primarily takes place in:
[Electrotherapy/Clayton/9th Ed./Pg. 6]
A. Solids
B. Fluids
C. Metals
D. Atoms

Q 83. The law that tells about the direct relationship of the metabolic rate to increase in tissue temperature is:
[Electrotherapy/Clayton/19th Ed./Pg. 6]
A. Joule's law
B. Van't Hoff's law
C. Grotthus low
D. Eddy's law

Q 84. Skin resistance can be decreased by:
[Electrotherapy Simplified/Nanda/1st Ed./Pg. 24]
A. Warming
B. Cooling
C. Drying
D. Use of law voltage current

Q 85. The statement that is true for inductothermy is:
[Electrotherapy Clayton/9th Ed./Pg. 130]
A. It effects more of tissues with high impedance
B. It produce greater tissue temperature than capacitor field method
C. It is applied by the disc electrodes
D. None of the above

Q 86. In tissue heating by SWD, complex permittivity is dependent upon:
[Electrotherapy Simplified/Nanda/1st Ed./Pg. 322]
A. Frequency
B. Intensity
C. Duration of application
D. None of the above

Answer	70 D	71 D	72 C	73 A	74 D	75 C	76 D	77 C	78 D	79 C	80 C	81 C
	82 B	83 B	84 A	85 B	86 A							

Q 87. A magnaplode stands for:
[Electrotherapy Simplified/Nanda/1st Ed./Pg. 343]
A. Flat helix
B. Drum electrode
C. Pad electrode
D. disc electrode

Q 88. For thermal effect to be produced by PSWD, the mean power exceeds:
[Electrotherapy Simplified/Nanda/1st Ed./Pg. 364]
A. 3 W
B. 5 W
C. 10 W
D. None of the above

Q 89. Strong superficial heating relieves pain by:
[Electrotherapy Simplified/Nanda/1st Ed./Pg. 274]
A. Counter irritation
B. Increased blood supply
C. Muscle relaxation
D. Increased metabolic rate

Q 90. The term decimeter wave applies:
[Electrotherapy/Clayton/9th Ed./Pg. 157]
A. Infrared
B. Shortwave
C. Microwaves
D. None of the above

Q 91. The term diathermy means:
[Physical Agent in Rehabilitation Cameron/2nd Ed./Pg. 388]
A. Superficial heating
B. Deep heating
C. Through and through heating
D. None of the above

Q 92. The cable method in SWD is called:
[Electrotherapy Simplified/Nanda/1st Ed./Pg. 342]
A. Pulsed SWD
B. Cross fire method
C. Inductothermy
D. Contraplanar method

Q 93. The position of SWD electrodes when treating a structure of high impedance should be such that:
[Electrotherapy Simplified/Nanda/ 1st Ed./Pg. 336]
A. The tissue remain at right angles to the electric field
B. The tissues remain parallel to the electric field
C. One electrode nearer to the skin than other
D. Both the electrodes nearer the skin

Both the Electrodes Nearer the Skin

Q 94. Which of the following fields predominate when SWD is applied by the cable method to a material of high impedance?
[Electrotherapy/Clayton/9th Ed./Pg. 130-131]
A. Electromagnetic field
B. Electric field
C. Magnetic field
D. None of the above

Q 95. The commonly used therapeutic frequency of SWD is:
[Electrotherapy/Clayton/9th Ed./Pg. 114]
A. 29.17 MHz
B. 27.12 MHz
C. 30.12 MHz
D. 20.19 MHz

Q 96. Whenever deeply placed structures are to be treated with the capacitor field method, which of the following technique would be used?
[Electrotherapy/Clayton/9th Ed./Pg. 126]
A. Coplanar
B. Crossfire
C. Contraplanar
D. Cable

Q 97. While applying SWD by the inductive method to treat structures of high impedance the part of the cable used by:
[Electrotherapy Simplified/Nanda/1st Ed./Pg. 134]
A. Middle of the cable
B. The spiral coil
C. Both ends and middle of the cable
D. Ends of the cable

Q 98. What would be ideal during positioning of the SWD electrodes relative to the tissue:
[Electrotherapy/Clayton/9th/Pg. 124]
A. Placing at an angle to each other
B. Placing parallel to each other
C. Placing parallel to the skin
D. None of the above

Q 99. The electrode spacing material used in SWD should be:
[Electrotherapy/Clayton/9th Ed./Pg. 121]
A. Of high dielectric constant
B. Of low dielectric constant
C. A good conductor
D. None of the above

Q 100. For a given treatment area what should be the appropriate size of the SWD electrodes?
[Electrotherapy Simplified/Nanda/1st Ed./Pg. 1331]
A. Smaller than of the part to be treated
B. Little larger than the part to be treated
C. One electrode larger than the other
D. Equal to the area to be treated

Q 101. The amount of heat delivered to the body by moist hot pack is more than PWB, because:
[Electrotherapy Simplified/Nanda/1st Ed./Pg. 221]
A. The specific heat of water is more than wax
B. The specific heat of wax is more than convection
C. Moist heat produces heat in body by convection
D. None of the above

Q 102. The number of layers of towel between the moist pack and skin should have at least:
[Electrotherapy Simplified/Nanda/1st Ed./Pg. 285]
A. 4 layers
B. 16 layers
C. 8 layers
D. 6 layers

Q 103. The proportion of solid wax to mineral oil in Paraffin wax treatments should be:
[Electrotherapy Simplified/Nanda/1st Ed./Pg. 276]
A. 7:1
B. 5:1
C. 4:1
D. None of the above

Answer	87 A	88 B	89 A	90 C	91 C	92 C	93 A	94 B	95 B	96 C	97 D	98 C
	99 B	100 B	101 A	102 D	103 A							

Q 104. In Paraffin wax treatments there should be at least:
[Electrotherapy Simplified/Nanda/1st Ed./Pg. 278]
A. 203 mm, thickness of wax on the part
B. 5 mm, thickness of wax on the part
C. 6 mm, thickness of wax on the part
D. 9 mm, thickness of wax on the part

Q 105. Which one of the following regarding dry and moist heat treatment is true?
[Physical Agent in Rehabilitation/Cameron/2nd Ed./ Pg. 168/174]
A. Dry heat causes strong superficial heating whereas moist heat causes deep heating
B. Moist heat causes strong superficial heating whereas dry heat causes deep heating
C. Both cause strong deep heating
D. None of the above

Q 106. The temperature of fluidotherapy unit should be:
[Physical Agent in Rehabilitation/Cameron/2nd Ed./Pg. 173]
A. Above 45°C
B. Between 38 – 45°C
C. Below 38°C
D. None of the above

Q 107. Therapeutically eddy current is used to:
[Electrotherapy Simplified/Nanda/1st Ed./Pg. 42]
A. Produce heat
B. Produce nerve stimulation
C. Apply drugs in iontophoresis
D. None of the above

Q 108. Fluidotherapy refers to:
[Physical Agent in Rehabilitation/Cameron/2nd Ed./Pg. 173]
A. Dry heat modality
B. Fluid immersion therapy
C. Application of analgesic fluid
D. Application of radiation through fluid

Q 109. The contraplanar, capacitor field method of shortwave diathermy is used for treatment of:
[Electrotherapy Clayton/9th Ed./Pg. 126]
A. Superficial lesions of the skin
B. Subcutaneous injuries
C. Deeply placed structures
D. Superficial muscles of spine

Q 110. When different sized electrodes are used for application of SWD by coplanar method:
[Electrotherapy Simplified/Clayton/9th Ed./Pg. 121]
A. The heating effect will not be there
B. Very deep effect will be achieved
C. Concentration of heat will be achieved
D. Superficial heating under the small electrodes will occur

Q 111. In contrast bath he period of immersion in hot and cold bath is as:
[Physical Agent in Rehabilitation/Cameron/Pg. 291]
A. Hot water – 30 seconds, cold water – 10 seconds
B. Hot water – 10 seconds, cold water – 30 seconds
C. Hot water – 3 – 4 minutes, cold water – 1 minute
D. Hot water – 1 minutes, cold water – 3 – 4 minutes

Q 112. The choice of modality to treat painful joints of hand of a rheumatoid arthritic patient is:
[Electrotherapy Simplified/Nanda/1st Ed./Pg. 1280]
A. Hot packs
B. Infrared rays
C. Microwave diathermy
D. Paraffin wax bath

Q 113. The thermal conductivity in which of the following tissues is higher?
[Physical Agent in Rehabilitation/Cameron/2nd Ed./Pg. 135]
A. Muscles
B. Skin
C. Ligaments
D. Fat

Q 114. Heliotherapy is treatment by:
[Electrotherapy Simplified/Nanda/Heliotherapy 1st Ed.]
A. Natural sunlight
B. Russian current
C. Didynamic current
D. Mud packs

Q 115. A 55-year-old female diagnosed with a right hip intertrochanteric fracture is eight weeks status post-open reduction and internal fixation with a plate and pinning. The patient has pain with active hip flexion and abduction. Acceptable modalities for this patient would include all of the following except:
[Physical Agent in Rehabilitation/Cameron/2nd Ed./Pg. 394]
A. Hot packs
B. Whirlpool
C. Pulsed ultrasound
D. Shortwave diathermy

Q 116. A therapist examines a morbidly obese patient in physical therapy. The therapist would like to incorporate modalities into the patient's care plan, but is concerned about excessively elevating the patient's tissue temperature. Which modality would potentially be the most hazardous?
[Physical Agent in Rehabilitation/Caneroon/2nd Ed./Pg. 395-397]
A. Diathermy
B. Hot packs
C. Paraffin
D. Pulsed ultrasound

Q 117. An 18-year-old male six weeks status post-open reduction of a Colle's fracture is referred to physical therapy. Examination reveals mild swelling on the dorsum of the hand and limited flexion of the metacarpophalangeal joints in all digits. The most appropriate heating agent for the patent is:
[Electrotherapy Simplified/Nanda/1st Ed./Pg. 281]
A. Paraffin
B. Hot packs
C. Vapocoolant sprays
D. Ultrasound

Q 118. A patient rehabilitating from a lower extremity injury is referred to physical therapy for hydrotherapy treatments. The therapist would like the patient to fully extend the involved lower extremity while in the hydrotherapy tank. Which type of whirlpool would not allow the patient to extend the involved lower extremity?
[Physical Agent in Rehabilitation/Cameron/2nd Ed./Pg. 286, 289]
A. Hubbard tank
B. Highboy tank
C. Lowboy tank
D. Walk tank

Q 119. Whirlpool treatments are commonly used in physical therapy to stimulate circulation promote muscle relaxation, and provide pain relief. Which statement regarding hydrotherapy is not true?
[Physical Agent in Rehabilitation/Cameron/2nd Ed./Pg. 287]

Answer   104 A   105 A   106 B   107 A   108 A   109 C   110 C   111 C   112 D   113 A   114 A   115 D
116 A   117 A   118 B

A. 41 – 46 degrees Celsius is an acceptable range for water temperature
B. The region to be treated should be thoroughly inspected prior to beginning treatment
C. The tank and turbine should be cleaned after each treatment
D. The agitation force should be adjusted initially at a minimum level and increased as desired

Q 120. All of the following are used frequently by a physical therapist to treat temporomandibular joint disorders except:
[Electrotherapy Simplified/Nanda/1st Ed./Pg. 363]
A. Postural training
B. Diathermy
C. Electrical stimulation
D. Ultrasound

Q 121. A patient ambulates outside rehabilitation hospital as part of a therapy session. The therapist monitors the patient closely during the session due to extreme heat and humidity. What is the primary mode of beat loss during exercise?
[Physical Agent in Rehabilitation/Cameron/2nd Ed./Pg. 137]
A. Conduction
B. Convection
C. Evaporation
D. Radiation

Q 122. An example of a heating agent which can cause temperature elevation in tissues to depths of three centimeters or more includes:
[Electrotherapy Simplified/Nanda/1st Ed./Pg. 391-392]
A. Paraffin
B. Moist heating packs
C. Whirlpool
D. Ultrasound

Q 123. Shortwave diathermy is used for all of the following except:
[Electrotherapy Simplified/Nanda/1st Ed./Pg. 328]
A. Back pain
B. Hemophiliac joint
C. Osteoarthritis
D. Sprain

Ultrasound

Q 124. Which one of the following is true regarding production of ultrasound?
[Physical Agent in Rehabilitation/Cameron/2nd Ed./ Pg. 193]
A. Ultrasound is produced by electromagnetic induction
B. Ultrasound is produced by piezo- electric effect
C. Ultrasound is produced by reverse piezoelectric effect
D. None of the above

Q 125. The depth of near field of an ultrasonic beam can be calculated by:
[Physical Agent in Rehabilitation/Cameron/2nd Ed./Pg. 140]
A. $1/r^2$
B. $2/r^2$
C. r^2/lc
D. r^2

Q 126. The half value depth of 1 MHz ultrasound is:
[Electrotherapy Simplified/Nanda/1st Ed./Pg. 388]
A. 1 cm
B. 3 cm
C. 5.6 cm
D. 6.5 cm

Q 127. The following statements regarding coupling medium used with ultrasound are true except:
[Physical Agent in Rehabilitation/Cameron/2nd Ed./Pg. 207]
A. Transmission of ultrasound by aquasonic gel is 40%
B. A gel is an ideal coupling medium
C. It helps in the transmission of ultrasound
D. To eliminate air between transducer head and the patient

Q 128. As an ultrasonic beam travels through tissues, the energy contained with in it decreases with the distance traversed. This phenomenon is known as:
[Physical Agent in Rehabilitation/Cameron/2nd Ed./Pg. 191]
A. Absorption
B. Attenuation
C. Conduction
D. Reflection

Q 129. When an ultrasonic beam travels in a medium in which its velocity is law into one in which its velocity is high, it is?
[Physical Agent in Rehabilitation/Cameron/2nd Ed./Pg. 191]
A. Reflected
B. Refracted away from the normal
C. Refracted towards the normal
D. Not transmitted

Q 130. The vibrating source required to produce ultrasound is achieved using:
[Electrotherapy Simplified/Nanda/1st Ed./Pg. 377]
[Clayton/9th Ed./Pg. 165]
A. Sodium citrate
B. Barium titanate
C. Silver nitrate
D. Chromium oxide

Q 131. The percentage of transmission of a aquasonic gel is:
[Electrotherapy Clayton/9th Ed./Pg. 171]
A. 59%
B. 19%
C. 67%
D. 72%

Q 132. A patient with a cardiac pacemaker suffers from shoulder pain and stiffness. Which of the following modality would be indicated?
[Physical Agent in Rehabilitation/Cameron/2nd Ed./Pg. 423]
A. TENS
B. IFT
C. Ultrasound
D. None of the above

Q 133. The ratio of spatial peak intensity to spatial average intensity is:
[Physical Agent in Rehabilitation/Cameron/2nd Ed./Pg. 188]
A. Far field
B. Near field
C. Effective radiation area
D. Beam nonuniformity ratio

Q 134. A duty cycle of 20 percent is equivalent to a m:s ratio of
[Physical Agent in Rehabilitation/Cameron/2nd Ed./Pg. 185]
A. 1:7
B. 1:4
C. 1:8
D. 2:5

Q 135. When an ultrasonic beam is applied to a cell membrane, it causes unidirectional flow of tissue components. This is termed as:
[Physical Agent in Rehabilitation/Cameron/2nd Ed./Pg. 191]
A. Cavitation
B. Attenuation
C. Adsorption
D. Acoustic streaming

Q 136. The resistance to passage of sound is called as:
[Physical Agent in Rehabilitation/Cameron/2nd Ed./Pg. 192]

Answer											
119 A	120 B	121 C	122 D	123 B	124 C	125 C	126 D	127 A	128 B	129 B	130 B
131 D	132 C	133 D	134 B	135 D							

A. Cavitation
B. Attenuation
C. Phonation
D. Acoustic impedance

Q 137. The unit of ultrasound is:
[Physical Agent in Rehabilitation/Cameron/2nd Ed./Pg. 208]
A. Watts
B. Watts/cm²
C. Volts/sqinch
D. Newton

Q 138. The frequency of therapeutic ultrasound is:
[Physical Agent in Rehabilitation/Cameron/2nd Ed./Pg. 186]
A. 1 MHz – 3 MHz
B. 0.75 MHz – 3.3 MHz
C. 0.5 MHz – 1 MHz
D. None

Q 139. The amount of US reflected at the bone periosteum interface is:
[Electrotherapy Simplified/Nanda/1st Ed./Pg. 380]
A. 30%
B. 20%
C. 70%
D. 100%

Q 140. The absorption coefficient of muscle for ultrasound absorption is:
[Electrotherapy Simplified/Nanda/1st Ed./Pg. 383]
A. Double of fat
B. Same as fat
C. Half of fat
D. None of the above

Q 141. Phonophoresis occurs due to:
[Physical Agent in Rehabilitation Cameron/2nd Ed./Pg. 193]
A. Acoustic streaming
B. Unstable cavitation
C. Attenuation
D. Reflection

Q 142. The frequency of infrasonic waves lie between:
[Electrotherapy Simplified/Nanda/1st Ed./Pg. 1375]
A. Below 20 Hz
B. 1-5 KHz
C. 10-20 KHz
D. 1-3 MHz

Q 143. The cavitation effect of ultrasound application to body is:
[Physical Agent in Rehabilitation/Cameron/2nd. Ed./Pg. 192 and Clayton/9th Ed./Pg. 173]
A. Micromassage
B. Rise in local temperature
C. Analgesic effect on nerves
D. Gas bubbles in tissues

Q 144. To treat open wounds by ultrasonic the following gel is used as couplant medium:
[Physical Agent in Rehabilitation/Cameron/2nd Ed./Pg. 198]
A. Cobadex cream
B. Geliperm sterile pack
C. Emla gel
D. Xylocaine ointment

Q 145. A frequency of 3 MHz ultrasonic waves have a half value depth of penetration equal to:
[Electrotherapy Simplified/Nanda/1st Ed./Pg. 380]
A. 3 mm
B. 0.3 cm
C. 100 mm
D. 25 mm

Q 146. Ultrasound may be safely employed over:
[Electrotherapy Clayton/9th Ed./Pg. 176]
A. Tumor
B. Growing epiphysis
C. Abdomen in pregnancy
D. Metal implants

Q 147. Using the water bag technique for application of ultrasonic therapy:
[Electrotherapy Simplified/Nanda/1st Ed./Pg. 414]
A. Couplant is not used
B. Couplant is contained inside the water bag
C. Couplant is applied over the upper surface of the bag on which transducer head is used
D. Couplant is applied on both the sides of water bag

Q 148. Treatment of choice for supraspinatus tendinitis is which of the following?
[Electrotherapy Simplified/Nanda/1st Ed./Pg. 403]
A. Short wave diathermy
B. Ultrasonic therapy
C. LASER
D. CPM

Q 149. In acute fracture what type of ultrasound should be used?
[Physical Agent in Rehabilitation/Cameron/2nd Ed./Pg. 200]
A. Low intensity pulsed
B. High intensity pulsed
C. Low intensity continuous
D. High intensity pulsed

High intensity pulsed

Q 150. A physical therapist elects to use ultrasound on a patient diagnosed with a second degree lateral ankle sprain. The therapist uses the underwater technique due to the uneven joint surface and the patient's extreme sensitivity to pressure. Which description of ultrasound using the underwater techniques is true?
[Physical Agent in Rehabilitation/Cameron/2nd Ed./Pg. 198]
A. The transducer should be place directly on the skin
B. A commercial gel is appropriate for a coupling medium
C. the transducer should be held one-half to one inch from the skin and moved throughout the entire section
D. The patient should move the transducer once it is immersed in the water

Q 151. Which therapeutic modality would be a relative contraindication in a pediatric patient with juvenile rheumatoid arthritis?
[Electrotherapy Simplified/Nanda/1st Ed./Pg. 415-442]
A. Superficial heat
B. Ultrasound
C. Transcutaneous electrical nerve stimulation
D. Ice

Q 152. A 28-year-old male referred to physical therapy by his primary physician complains of recurrent ankle pain. As part of the treatment program the therapist uses ultrasound ever the peroneus longus and brevis tendons. The most appropriate location for ultrasound applications is:
A. Inferior to the sustentaculum tali
B. Over the sinus tarsi
C. Posterior to the lateral malleolus
D. Anterior to the lateral malleolus

Q 153. Iontophoresis and phonophoresis are commonly used to deliver a specified medication through the skin to underlying tissues. Which route of administration does iontophoresis and phonophoresis utilize?
[Electrotherapy Simplified/Nanda/1st Ed./Pg. 417]
A. Inhalation
B. Sublingual
C. Topical
D. Transdermal

Answer	136 D	137 B	138 A	139 C	140 A	141 A	142 A	143 A	144 B	145 B	146 D	147 C
	148 B	149 A	150 C	151 B	152 C	153 D						

Q 154. A therapist prepares to treat a patient with continuous ultrasound. Which general rule best determines the length of treatment when using ultrasound?

[Electrotherapy Simplified/Nanda/1st Ed./Pg. 407]

A. 2 minutes for every area that is 2–3 times the size of the transducer face
B. 5 minutes for every area that is 2–3 time the size of the transducer face
C. 5 minutes is the maximum treatment time regardless of the treatment area
D. 10 minutes is the maximum treatment time regardless of the treatment area

Q 155. All of the following modalities would be indicated in the treatment of a pregnant woman except:

[Physical Agent in Rehabilitation/Cameron/2nd Ed./Pg. 206]

A. Vapocoolant sprays in the treatment of muscle spasms
B. Transcutaneous electrical nerve stimulation used for pain relief during labor
C. Phonophoresis in the treatment of lateral epicondylitis
D. Continuous ultrasound over an area of diminished circulation

Q 156. A therapist observes random changes in the intensity of an ultrasound generator during patient treatment. The most appropriate response is to:

[Electrotherapy Clayton/9th Ed./Pg. 165-176]

A. Ignore the changes in the intensity since they are normal when using ultrasound
B. Continue to use the machine at intensity levels less than 1.0 w/cm^2
C. Closely monitor the machine during use
D. Discontinue use the machine and contract a service technician

Q 157. Tissues of high collagen content are affected to a greater extent by ultrasound energy. Which tissue would you expect to absorb the most ultrasound energy?

[Physical Agent in Rehabilitation/Cameron/2nd Ed./Pg. 191]

A. Bone
B. Muscle
C. Tendon
D. Skin

Q 158. Biophysical effects of ultrasound include thermal and nonthermal effects. The amount of heat absorbed using ultrasound is least dependent upon:

[Electrotherapy Simplified/Nanda/1st Ed./Pg. 409]

A. The intensity
B. The duration of exposure
C. The choice of coupling agent
D. The size of the area sonated

Q 159. A recreational tennis player is diagnosed with lateral epicondylitis. All of the following are considered appropriate forms of treatment for acute lateral epicondylitis except:

[Physical Agent in Rehabilitation/Cameron/2nd Ed./Pg. 195]

A. Modification of tennis grip and string tension
B. Phonophoresis
C. Curvilinear brace applied just below the bed in the elbow
D. Curvilinear brace applied just below the bend in the elbow
E. Progressive resistive emphasizing the wrist extensors

Q 160. A therapist uses ultrasound to elevate the tissue temperature at the insertion of the supra of the supraspinatus. What would be the most appropriate patient for the ultrasound application?

[Physical Agent in Rehabilitation/Cameron/2nd Ed./Pg. 199-200]

A. Patient in supine with the arm abducted and externally rotated
B. Patient in supine with the arm adducted and medially rotated
C. Patient in supine with the arm abducted and medially rotated
D. Patient in supine with the arm adducted and externally rotated

Q 161. A patient with degenerative joint disease is referred to physical therapy with right shoulder pain. During the initial examination the therapist identifies significant muscle guarding and spasm throughout the right shoulder. If the therapist elects to treat the patient using ultrasound, which patient position would be the most appropriate?

[Electrotherapy Simplified/Nanda/1st Ed./Pg. 412]

A. Supine with the upper extremity slightly flexed and adducted
B. Supine with the arm resting against the abdomen
C. Supine with the glenohumeral joint in the resting position
D. A position where the patient is comfortable and relaxed

Infrared and UVR

Q 162. The angle of incidence for the electromagnetic rays to have maximum absorption should be:

[Electrotherapy Clayton/9th Ed./Pg. 194]

A. 0^0
B. 90^0
C. 180^0
D. None of the above

Q 163. The most susceptible peripheral nerve fibers to be affected by cold application are:

[Electrotherapy Clayton/19th Ed./Pg. 201]

A. B
B. C
C. A™
D. D

Q 164. In the electromagnetic spectrum infrared occupy a place between:

[Physical Agent in Rehabilitation/Cameron/2nd Ed./Pg. 372]

A. 400 nm – 750 nm
B. 10 nm – 400 nm
C. 200 nm – 350 nm
D. 750 nm – 400,000 nm

Q 165. The depth of penetration of luminous infrared is:

[Electrotherapy/Clayton/9th Ed. Ed./Pg. 36]

A. 15 mm
B. 3 cm
C. 2 mm
D. 5 – 10 mm

Q 166. Which one statement regarding infrared generators are true?

[Electrotherapy Simplified/Nanda/1st Ed./Pg. 423]

A. The luminous lamp longer for warming up than nonluminous lamp
B. The nonluminous lamp takes longer for warming-up than luminous lamp

---

Answer   154 B   155 D   156 D   157 A   158 C   159 D   160 C   161 D   162 B   163 B   164 D   165 D
166 B

C. Nonluminous generators produce visible radiation and IR
D. None of the above

Q 167. Which of the statements for luminous IR is false?
[Electrotherapy Simplified/Nanda/1st Ed./Pg. 423]
A. Luminous IR is considered in acute conditions
B. Luminous IR penetrates deeper than nonluminous
C. Luminous IR is produced along with visible radiation
D. None of the above

Q 168. The law that states about the absorption of electromagnetic waves in the tissue to have an effect is:
[Electrotherapy Clayton/9th Ed./Pg. 26]
A. Joule's law　　　　B. Grotthus law
C. Snell's law　　　　D. None of the above

Q 169. The latent period for the appearance of a third degree erythema is:
[Electrotherapy Clayton/9th Ed./Pg. 186]
A. 10 – 12 hours
B. 1 – 4 hours
C. 8 – 10 hours
D. None of the above

Q 170. Treatment of psoriasis with Leeds regimen includes all except:
[Electrotherapy Clayton/9th Ed./Pg. 189]
A. Local application of coal tar
B. Test reaction to UVR in the sensitized condition
C. E2 dose is given to the patient.
D. A Theraktin tunnel or an air cooled lamp can be used

Q 171. Which of the following statements regarding Theraktin tunnel is false?
[Electrotherapy Clayton/9th Ed./Pg. 184]
A. It is an easier way to give general irradiation with UVR
B. It emits only UVB rays
C. A suberythemal dose is given
D. Dosage I progressively increased by 12.5%

Q 172. In UVR lamp the heat produced in the burner changes the quartz to:
[Electrotherapy Clayton/9th Ed./Pg. 182]
A. Silicone　　　　B. Boron
C. Tridymite　　　　D. Silicon oxide

Q 173. Which of the following would be a choice in order to irradiate a sinus with UVR?
[Electrotherapy Clayton/9th Ed./Pg. 183]
A. Air cooled lamp
B. Theraktin tunnel
C. Kromayer with an applicator
D. Fluorescent tube

Q 174. UVR reacts with oxygen in air to produce:
[Electrotherapy Clayton/9th Ed./Pg. 182]
A. Neon　　　　B. Argon
C. Ozone　　　　D. Helium

Q 175. Erythema obtained due to application of UVR is due to:
[Electrotherapy Clayton/9th Ed./Pg. 180]
A. Release of chemical substances
B. Arterial dilatation
C. Venous dilation
D. Damage to RBC

Q 176. The wavelength of UVA is:
[Electrotherapy Clayton/9th Ed./Pg. 180]
A. 280 nm – 315 nm
B. 260 nm – 280 nm
C. 315 nm – 400 nm
D. 220 nm – 260 nm

Q 177. Which of the following statement regarding UVR is false?
[Electrotherapy Clayton/9th Ed./Pg. 188]
A. Carcinogenesis is a danger due to long exposure to UVR
B. Short UVR can be used for sterilization
C. UVB damages granulation tissue
D. Minimal erythemal dose is given for treatment of acne

Q 178. In the quartz applicator, ultraviolet is transmitted by:
[Electrotherapy Simplified/Nanda/1st Ed./Pg. 459]
A. Refraction　　　　B. Total internal reflection
C. Diffusion　　　　D. None of the above

Q 179. The epidermal transit time is:
[Electrotherapy Simplified/Nanda/1st Ed./Pg. 465]
A. 14 days　　　　B. 5 days
C. 28 to 70 days　　　　D. None of the above

Q 180. For the treatment of psoriasis:
[Electrotherapy Clayton/9th Ed./Pg. 189]
A. E1 dose is used
B. Suberythemal dose is used
C. Suberythemal or E1 dose is used
D. None of the above

Q 181. The life of fluorescent tubes are limited to:
[Electrotherapy Simplified/Nanda/1st Ed./Pg. 460]
A. 1000 hours　　　　B. 500 hours
C. < 500 hours　　　　D. None of the above

Q 182. The phosphor coating in fluorescent tubes:
[Electrotherapy Clayton/9th Ed./Pg. 184]
A. Absorbs the long ultraviolet rays
B. Allows both short and long ultraviolet rays to pass
C. Allows short ultraviolet to pass
D. Allows long ultraviolet rays to pass

Q 183. The length of fluorescent tube is:
[Electrotherapy Clayton/9th Ed./Pg. 120]
A. 20 cm　　　　B. 50 cm
C. 100 cm　　　　D. 120 cm

Q 184. In PUVA treatments, application of UVR is done:
[Electrotherapy Clayton/9th Ed./Pg. 196]
A. 2 hours before ingestion of psoralen
B. 2 hours after ingestion of psoralen
C. After application of coal tar
D. None of the above

Answer	167 A	168 B	169 B	170 C	171 B	172 C	173 C	174 C	175 A	176 C	177 D	178 B
	179 C	180 C	181 A	182 D	183 D	184 B						

Q 185. UVA can penetrate up to:
[Electrotherapy Clayton/9th Ed./Pg. 85]
A. Superficial epidermis
B. Superficial fascia
C. Deep epidermis
D. Capillary layers of dermis

Q 186. Due to thickening of epidermis, an E3 dose should increase by:
[Electrotherapy Simplified/Nanda/1st Ed./Pg. 476]
A. 75%
B. 50%
C. 25%
D. None of the above

Q 187. In psoriasis, the epidermal transit time is reduced to:
[Electrotherapy Simplified/Nanda/1st Ed./Pg. 467]
A. 7 days
B. 5 days
C. 28 days
D. None of the above

Q 188. After taking the photoactive drug, the patient should take eye protection measures for:
[Electrotherapy Simplified/Nanda/1st Ed./Pg. 147]
A. 2 hours
B. 6 hours
C. 12 hours
D. None of the above

Q 189. The unit of UVR intensity is:
[Electrotherapy Clayton/9th Ed./Pg. 196]
A. J/cm^2
B. Watt
C. mW/cm^2
D. None of the above

Q 190. For the treatment of open wound, UVR is applied at:
[Clayton/9th Ed./Pg. 190]
A. E4 dose
B. E2 dose
C. E1 dose
D. E0 dose

Q 191. Which type of UVR is ionizing and germicidal:
[Electrotherapy Simplified/Nanda/1st Ed./Pg. 454]
A. UVA
B. UVB
C. UVC
D. None of the above

Q 192. The type of UVR filtered by the ozone layer is:
[Electrotherapy Simplified/Nanda/1st Ed./Pg. 454]
A. UVA
B. UVC
C. UVB
D. None of the above

Q 193. The term vacuum UV refers to:
[Electrotherapy Simplified/Nanda/1st Ed./Pg. 454]
A. UVR with wavelength between 100–200 nm
B. UVR with wavelength between 50 and 100 nm
C. UVR with wavelength of 50 nm
D. None of the above

Q 194. The Alpine sun lamp is positioned at a distance of:
[Electrotherapy Simplified/Nanda/1st Ed./Pg. 458]
A. 20 cm
B. 100 cm
C. 45050 cm
D. None of the above

Q 195. The depth of penetration of UVC is approximately:
[Electrotherapy Simplified/Nanda/1st Ed./Pg. 462]
A. 70 – 80 μm
B. 20 – 30 μm
C. 40 – 50 μm
D. None of the above

Q 196. Maintenance of erythema due to UVB is because of:
[Electrotherapy Simplified/Nanda/ 1st Ed./Pg. 462]

A. Calcium oxide
B. Oxygen
C. Nitric oxide
D. None of the above

Q 197. Thickening of skin following UVR is due to:
A. Stimulation of fibroblasts
B. Stimulation of keratinocytes
C. Stimulation of sebaceous glands
D. None of the above

Q 198. The protective thickening of the skin due to UVR is gradually lost in:
[Electrotherapy Simplified/Nanda/1st Ed./Pg. 465]
A. 2 – 3 weeks
B. 4 – 6 weeks
C. 3 – 4 weeks
D. None of the above

Q 199. Vitamin D is produced by the effect of:
[Electrotherapy Simplified/Nanda/1st Ed./Pg. 465]
A. UVB
B. UVA
C. UVC
D. None of the above

Q 200. Skin cancer due to UVR is due to:
[Electrotherapy Simplified/Nanda/1st Ed./Pg. 465]
A. Thickening of epidermis
B. Production of erythema
C. Immunosuppressive effects
D. None of the above

Q 201. Due to carcinogenesis, short UVR should not be applied for:
[Electrotherapy Simplified/Nanda/1st Ed./Pg. 466]
A. More than 3 weeks
B. More than 8 weeks
C. More than 4 weeks
D. None of the above

Q 202. The filter used for filtering short UVR is:
[Electrotherapy Clayton/9th Ed./Pg. 183]
A. Cellophane or blue uviol
B. Litmus paper
C. Wire mesh filter
D. None of the above

Q 203. The wavelength of nonluminous infrared rays lies from:
[Electrotherapy Simplified/Nanda/1st Ed./Pg. 422]
A. 350 nm to 400 nm
B. 770 nm to 1500 nm
C. 70 nm to 110 nm
D. 7.7 nm to 15 nm

Q 204. PUVA therapy is used for:
[Electrotherapy Clayton/9th Ed./Pg. 184]
A. Alopecia
B. Psoriasis
C. Pressure sores
D. Plantar warts

Q 205. To counter the effect of an overdose of UVR traditionally:
[Electrotherapy Clayton/9th Ed./Pg. 152]
A. Application of infrared ray is used
B. Application of us therapy is used
C. Cryotherapy is given
D. IFT application given

Q 206. Infected wounds are treated by application of the following dose of UVR:
[Electrotherapy Clayton/9th Ed./Pg. 189-190]
A. Suberythemal dose
B. Half of E1 dose
C. E4 dose
D. E1 dose

Answer	185 D	186 A	187 A	188 C	189 C	190 A	191 C	192 B	193 A	194 C	195 C	196 C
	197 B	198 B	199 A	200 A	201 C	202 A	203 B	204 B	205 A	206 C		

Q 207. According to cosine law for maximal absorption of UVR it must strike the surface at:
[Electrotherapy Clayton/9th Ed./Pg. 27]
A. An acute angle
B. Right angle
C. An obtuse angle
D. 45 degree angle

Q 208. A therapist prepares to treat a patient using ultraviolet light by determining the patient's minimal erythemal dose. The most common location for testing is:
[Electrotherapy Simplified/Nanda/1st Ed./Pg. 145]
A. On the posterior aspect of the upper arm
B. On the anterior aspect of the forearm
C. On the anterior aspect of the thigh
D. On the area to be treated

Q 209. A therapist revises the results of ultraviolet testing. Which grade of erythemal dose best describe the time required for mold reddening of the skin?
[Electrotherapy Clayton/9th Ed./Pg. 186]
A. Suberythemal dose
B. Minimal erythemal dose
C. Second degree erythema
D. Third degree erythema

Microwave

Q 210. The frequency of microwaves are:
[Electrotherapy Clayton/2nd Ed./Pg. 372]
A. 300 MHz – 300 GHz
B. 10 MHz – 100 MHz
C. 200 MHz
D. None of the above

Q 211. Which of following modality has maximum frequency?
[Electrotherapy Clayton/9th Ed./Pg. 159]
A. Ultrasound waves
B. MWD waves
C. SWD waves
D. Infrared radiation waves

Q 212. Microwaves are more absorbed in tissues with:
[Electrotherapy Clayton/9th Ed./Pg. 159]
A. More fat content
B. More water content
C. More osseous in nature
D. None of the above

Q 213. The very high frequency of microwaves can be produced by:
[Physical Agent in Rehabilitation/Cameron/2nd Ed./Pg. 392]
A. Repetitively charging and discharging of condenser
B. Thermionic valve
C. Magnetron
D. Transistor

Q 214. The depth of penetration of microwave diathermy is:
[Electrotherapy Simplified/Nanda/1st Ed./Pg. 364]
A. 0.5 cm
B. 3.0 cm
C. 1.3 cm
D. 9.0 cm

Q 215. Microwave diathermy is contraindicated in all of the following except:
[Electrotherapy Simplified/Nanda/1st Ed./Pg. 374]
A. Infections
B. Pregnancy
C. Tumorous conditions
D. Sprain

Laser

Q 216. The depth of penetration of He-Ne laser is:
[Electrotherapy Clayton/AITBS/9th Ed./Pg. 154]
A. 6 mm
B. 2 – 4 mm
C. 1 – 2 mm
D. None of the above

Q 217. Which one of the statement for laser therapy is true?
[Electrotherapy Clayton/9th Ed./Pg. 154]
A. The penetration depth of IR laser < He-Ne laser
B. The penetration depth of IR laser > He-Ne laser
C. Laser produces heat
D. Laser produces nerve stimulation

Q 218. First generation laser refers to:
A. IR laser
B. He-Ne laser
C. Diode based units
D. None of the above

Q 219. The term population inversion refers to:
A. A state where elections in the metastable level > ground level
B. A state where electrons in the ground level > metastable level
C. A state of electron jump
D. None of the above

Q 220. The effect of laser in nerve conduction is to:
A. Increase rate of conduction
B. Decrease rate of conduction
C. May increase rate decrease conduction
D. None of the above

Q 221. In physiotherapy the class of laser used is:
[Electrotherapy Simplified/Nanda/1st Ed./Pg. 437]
A. Class-1
B. Class-4
C. Class-2
D. Class-3

Q 222. Laser promotes wound healing by:
[Electrotherapy Simplified/Nanda/1st Ed./Pg. 442]
A. Cell proliferation
B. Increase in RNA production
C. Increase in collagen formation
D. All of the above

Q 223. Laser beam is characterized by:
[Electrotherapy Simplified/Nanda/1st Ed./Pg. 433-434]
A. Monochromaticity
B. Coherence
C. Collimation
D. All of the above

Q 224. What is the wavelength of radiation emitted by He-Ne laser?
[Physical Agent in Rehabilitation/Cameron/2nd Ed./Pg. 383]
A. 833 nm
B. 694.3 nm
C. 633 nm
D. None of the above

Q 225. The rate at which laser energy produced or absorbed is measured in:
[Physical Agent in Rehabilitation/Cameron/2nd Ed./Pg. 384]
A. Joules
B. J/s
C. J/m^2
D. J/cm^2

Q 226. When treating a large wound, the method of application of laser selected is:
[Physical Agent in Rehabilitation/Cameron/2nd Ed./Pg. 386]
A. Grid method
B. Scanning method
C. Grid or scanning method
D. None of the above

Answer	207 B	208 B	209 B	210 A	211 B	212 B	213 C	214 B	215 D	216 C	217 B	218 B
	219 A	220 A	221 D	222 D	223 D	224 C	225 D	226 C				

Q 227. Laser acronym is used for:
[Physical Agent in Rehabilitation/Cameron/2nd Ed./Pg. 383]
A. Low amplitude stimulated electrical response
B. Light amplification by stimulated emission of radiation
C. Light amplitude of strong electrical rays
D. Light amplification by stimulated echogenic response

Q 228. Helium neon laser has penetration of up to:
[Physical Agent in Rehabilitation/Cameron/2nd Ed./Pg. 383]
A. 6 mm B. 7 mm
C. 8 mm D. 9 mm

Q 229. Cold lasers are used in treatment of:
[Physical Agent in Rehabilitation/Cameron/2nd Ed./Pg. 385]
A. Fractures B. Soft tissues injuries
C. Cartilaginous injuries D. Others

Cryotherapy

Q 230. Which of the following statement is false?
[Electrotherapy Simplified/Nanda/1st Ed./Pg. 295-296]
A. Motor conduction velocity of nerves decreases with cooling
B. Cooling reduces the metabolic rate of tissues
C. Motor skills are enhanced as a result of cooling
D. Cooling diminishes muscle strength

Q 231. The alternating vasodilatation and vasoconstriction during the application of cold is:
[Electrotherapy Clayton/9th Ed./Pg. 200]
A. Joules effect B. Turners effect
C. Lewis hunting reaction D. Hunters effect

Q 232. When ice is applied to the body the initial reaction is:
[Electrotherapy Clayton/9th Ed./Pg. 200]
A. Vasoconstriction B. Vasodilatation
C. Increase in blood pressure D. Fall in blood pressure

Q 233. When vasodilatation is not desired, the duration of cryotherapy should be:
[Electrotherapy Simplified/Nanda/1st Ed./Pg. 287]
A. 30 minutes
B. More than 15 minutes
C. Less than 15 minutes
D. None of the above

Q 234. The pattern of heat to cold application in contrast bath is:
[Electrotherapy Simplified/Nanda/1st Ed./Pg. 221]
A. 3 minutes of hot bath followed by 1 minute of cold bath
B. 4 minutes of hot bath followed by 1 minutes of cold
C. 3 minutes of hot bath followed by 2 minutes of cold bath
D. None of the above

Q 235. Optimal temperature for the cold pack therapy is between:
[Physical Agent in Rehabilitation/Cameron/2nd Ed./Pg. 48]
A. 10 to 15 °C B. – 10 to 15 °C
C. 5 to 10 °C D. – 5 to 0 °C

Q 236. For immediate management of soft tissue injury acronym RICE stands for:
[Physical Agent in Rehabilitation/Cameron/2nd Ed./Pg. 426]
A. Rubbing, instant heat, clean and elevation
B. Reassurance, immunization, cold and electrical stimulation
C. Rest, ice, compression and elevation
D. Resisted, isometric contracted by electric stimulation

Q 237. To reduce spasticity following modality is more suitable:
[Physical Agent in Rehabilitation/Cameron/2nd Ed./Pg. 180]
A. Cryotherapy B. Ultrasonic
C. TENS D. Hot packs

Q 238. A physical therapist immerses a patient's edematous ankle in cold water. When a body part comes in direct contact with a cold agent the energy is transferred through:
[Electrotherapy Clayton/9th Ed./Pg. 5]
A. Conduction B. Convection
C. Evaporation D. Radiation

Q 239. Which objective would not be accomplished using cold packs on an involved lower extremity?
[Physical Agent in Rehabilitation/Cameron/2nd Ed./Pg. 135]
A. Decrease nerve conduction velocity
B. Increase vasodilation
C. Decrease metabolism
D. Temporarily reduce spasticity

Q 240. A therapist tests a small area of skin for hypersensitivity prior to using a cold immersion bath. The patient begins to demonstrate evidence of cold intolerance within 60 seconds after cold application. The most appropriate response is to:
[Physical Agent in Rehabilitation/Cameron/2nd Ed./Pg. 144]
A. Limit cold exposure to ten minutes or less
B. Select an alternative cryotherapeutic agent
C. Continue with the cold immersion bath
D. Discontinue cold application and document you findings

Traction

Q 241. The traction used to immobilize a symptomatic spinal area:
[Physical Agent in Rehabilitation/Cameron/2nd Ed./Pg. 310]
A. Intermittent traction B. Static traction
C. Continuous traction D. None of the above

Q 242. In cervical spine, posterior vertebral separation occurs at a flexion angel of:
[Electrotherapy Simplified/Nanda/1st Ed./Pg. 486]
A. 5° B. 15°
C. 20 – 30° D. None of the above

Q 243. To apply tractive force to upper cervical spine:
[Electrotherapy Simplified/Nanda/1st Ed./Pg. 486]
A. The spine should be kept in extension
B. The spine should be kept neutral
C. The spine should be kept in flexion
D. None of the above

Q 244. In prone lying the lumbar spine is:
[Physical Agent in Rehabilitation/Cameron/2nd Ed./Pg. 310]
A. Flexed
B. Partially extended

Answer	227 B	228 A	229 A	230 C	231 C	232 A	233 C	234 A	235 A	236 C	237 A	238 A
	239 B	240 D	241 C	242 C	243 A	244 B						

C. Neither flexed nor extended
D. None of the above

Q 245. Which of the following is a contraindication for cervical traction?
[Physical Agent in Rehabilitation/Cameron/2nd Ed./Pg. 305]
A. Cervical spondylosis   B. Rheumatoid arthritis
C. Muscle spasm   D. None of the above

Q 246. Which one of the following professionals advocated the use traction first?
A. Mackenzie   B. Mennel
C. Cyriax   D. None of the above

Q 247. Continuous traction is applied with:
[Physical Agent in Rehabilitation/Cameron/2nd Ed./Pg. 318-319]
A. Small weights for long periods of time
B. Small weights for short periods of time
C. Heavier weights for long periods of time
D. Heavier weights for short periods of time

Q 248. A physical therapist receives a referral for lumbar traction on a 61 year old female diagnosed with chronic lumbar pain. During the history the patient states that she sustained a compression fracture at the L4 level six weeks ago. The most appropriate action is:
[Electrotherapy Simplified/Nanda/1st Ed./Pg. 485]
A. Initiate lumbar traction in a prone position only
B. Initiate lumbar traction since the compression fracture was six weeks age
C. Contact the physician and discuss your concerns
D. Inform the physician that the referral showed poor judgment

Q 249. A therapist designs a plan of care for a patient with left hemiparesis. Which treatment option would not assist with the facilitation of motor return and control?
[Physical Agent in Rehabilitation/Cameron/2nd Ed./Pg. 308]
A. Biofeedback
B. Icing
C. Functional electrical stimulation
D. Back's traction

Q 250. The tractive force applied for the lumber spine in PIVD is:
[Physical Agent in Rehabilitation/Cameron/2nd Ed./Pg. 324]
A. 50% of body weight   B. 25% of body weight
C. 75% of body weight   D. None of the above

Q 251. The tractive force applied for cervical spine in PIVD is:
[Physical Agent in Rehabilitation/Cameron/2nd Ed./Pg. 324]
A. 50% of body weight   B. 25% of body weight
C. 5–7 kg   D. None of the above

Q 252. For joint distraction the tractive force required in cervical spine is:
[Physical Agent in Rehabilitation/Cameron/2nd Ed./Pg. 324]
A. 7% of body weight   B. 25% of body weight
C. 5 – 7 kg   D. None of the above

Q 253. Which of the following is a contraindication for lumbar traction?
[Physical Agent in Rehabilitation/Cameron/2nd Ed./Pg. 324]

A. Cord signs   B. PIVD
C. Muscle spasm   D. None of the above

Electrostatics

Q 254. The law that gives reciprocal relationship between the distance and intensity from the source to surface is:
[Electrotherapy Clayton/9th Ed./Pg. 243]
A. Grotthus law   B. Inverse square law
C. Cosine law   D. None of the above

Q 255. The reflector that makes the rays to emerge parallel from its surface, thereby having uniform irradiations a:
[Electrotherapy Simplified/Nanda/9th Ed./Pg. 423]
A. Spherical reflector   B. Parabolic reflector
C. Plane mirror   D. None of the above

Q 256. The ability of a conductor to have electric current induced is known as:
[Electrotherapy Clayton/9th Ed./Pg. 21,115]
A. Resistance   B. Impedance
C. Inductance   D. Conductance

Q 257. The capacitance of a condenser is:
[Electrotherapy Clayton/9th Ed./Pg. 37]
A. The ratio of the charge to its potential
B. Product of its charge to potential
C. Ratio of its potential to the charge
D. Product of charge and potential

Q 258. Dielectric constant of dry air is:
[Electrotherapy Simplified/Nanda/1st Ed./Pg. 15]
A. 2   B. 1
C. 5   D. 10

Q 259. In a condenser the spacing material should have:
[Electrotherapy Simplified/Nanda/1st Ed./Pg. 5]
A. High dielectric constant   B. Low dielectric constant
C. Both A, B   D. None of the above

Q 260. Thoracic outlet syndrome is usually diagnosed by:
A. Nerve conduction velocity tests and EMG
B. MRI and CT
C. Arteriograms and ultrasound
D. Careful clinical examination

Electrodiagnosis

Q 261. Statement is true:
[Electrotherapy/Clayton/9th Ed./Pg. 60]
A. Rheobase is the duration of impulse that produces a muscle contraction
B. In an UMN lesion there is an altered response to electrical stimulation
C. A current which rises or falls suddenly is more effective in stimulating an innervated muscle
D. Strength—duration curve indicates the site of lesion

Q 262. A normal pulse ratio value should be:
[Electrotherapy Simplified/Nanda/1st Ed./Pg. 223]

Answer	245 B	246 C	247 A	248 C	249 D	250 B	251 C	252 A	253 A	254 B	255 B	256 C
	257 A	258 B	259 B	260 B	261 C							

A. Above 2.2
B. 2.2 and less
C. Below 3.2
D. None of the above

Q 263. Insertional activity is found in:
[Physical Rehabilitation O'Sullivan/4th Ed./Pg. 222]
A. Denervated muscle
B. Innervated muscle
C. Both A and B
D. None of the above

Q 264. An EMG potential is called polyphasic if:
[Physical Rehabilitation O'Sullivan/4th Ed./Pg. 223]
A. It has two phases
B. It has four phases
C. It has more than four phases
D. None of the above

Q 265. S-D curve was used to investigate human nerve injuries by:
[Physical Rehabilitation O'Sullivan/4th Ed./Pg. 212]
A. Adrian
B. Erb
C. Duchenne
D. None of the above

Q 266. The normal values of motor NCV in the upper limb are:
[Electrotherapy Simplified/Nanda/1st Ed./Pg. 226]
A. Less than 40 m/s
B. 45 – 70 m/s
C. 70 – 80 m/s
D. None of the above

Q 267. Abnormal dorsal root function in radiculopathies shows:
[Electrotherapy Simplified/Nanda/1st Ed./Pg. 227]
A. Increased H-reflex latency
B. Decreased H-reflex latency
C. Normal H-reflex latency
D. None of the above

Q 268. Which of the following EMG picture is true in the diagnosis of myopathy?
[Physical Rehabilitation O'Sullivan/4th Ed./Pg. 223]
A. Spontaneous activity and partial interference pattern of decreased amplitude and duration on volition
B. Spontaneous activity with short duration low amplitude polyphasic potential on volition
C. High frequency respective discharge with alternate increased and decreased in amplitude
D. None of the above

Q 269. In the event of cardiac arrest, the right step to follow immediately is:
[Tidy/Wright Bristol/4th Ed./Pg. 425]
A. Apply external cardiac massage and mouth to mouth breathing
B. Inform the head of the department
C. Call for the doctor
D. None of the above

Q 270. In addition to therapeutic intervention, the therapist should also do:
[Refer to text]
A. Documentation
B. Counselling
C. Both A and B
D. None of the above

Q 271. The optimal pH level of water in therapeutic pool is maintained at:
[Refer to text]
A. 5.7 pH
B. 1.75 pH
C. 7.5 pH
D. 0.75 pH

Answer   262 B   263 B   264 C   265 A   266 B   267 B   268 B   269 A   270 C   271 C

3

CHAPTER

Biomechanics

Objective Questions with Answers

General Biomechanics

Q 1. The specific gravity of the human body is:

[Mcardle/4th Ed./Pg. 551]

A. 1.995
B. 0.095
C. 0.95
D. 9.05

Q 2. Normally in the standing position the center of gravity lies:

[Joint Structure and Function/Norkin/Pg. 10]

A. 5 cm anterior to second sacral vertebra
B. 5 cm posterior to second sacral vertebra
C. Around umbilicus
D. 5 cm anterior to second lumbar vertebra

Q 3. Vector is a physical force that has:

[Joint Structure and Function/Norkin/Pg. 7]

A. Magnitude
B. Direction
C. Magnitude and direction both
D. Fixed point of application of force

Q 4. In the second order lever the arrangement is:

[Joint Structure and Function/Norkin/Pg. 28]

A. Weight in middle, fulcrum and effort point are either end
B. Fulcrum is in middle, weight and effort point are on either end
C. Effort point is in middle, weight and fulcrum are on either end
D. None of the above

Q 5. The body's center of gravity in an adult normally has up and down movements of:

[Joint Structure and Function/Norkin/Pg. 449]

A. 1.5 inch
B. 2.5 inch
C. 3.5 inch
D. 4.5 inch

Q 6. A therapist examines joint play movement by placing the joint in is resting position. This position is best described as:

[Joint Structure and Function/Norkin/3rd Ed./Pg. 77]

A. Maximal congruency between the articular surfaces and the joint capsule
B. Minimal congruency between the articular surfaces and the joint capsule
C. Passive separation of the joint surfaces is limited
D. Parallel to the joint treatment plane.

Q 7. If a plumb line is positioned laterally to a patient so it runs along the line of gravity, where should the line fall with respect to the midline of the knee?

[Joint Structure and Function/Norkin/3rd Ed./Pg. 412]

A. Anterior
B. Posterior
C. Directly through the knee joint
D. Posterior and medial

Q 8. A physical therapist instructs a patient to move her lower teeth forward in relation to the upper teeth. This motion is termed:

[Orthopedic Physical Assessment/Magee/3rd Ed./Pg. 164]

A. Protrusion
B. Retrusion
C. Lateral deviation
D. Occlusal position

Q 9. Tests for the length of the hamstrings typically involve stabilization of the uninvolved leg while raising the leg to be tested. It is important to stabilize the uninvolved leg because it:

[Orthopedic Physical Assessment/David J. Magee/5th Ed./Pg. 698]

A. Prevents excessive posterior pelvic tilt and excessive flexion of the lumbar spine
B. Prevents excessive posterior pelvic tilt and excessive extension of the lumbar spine
C. Prevents excessive anterior pelvic tilt and excessive flexion of the lumbar spine
D. Prevents excessive anterior pelvic tilt and excessive extension of the lumbar spine

Q 10. A physical therapist consistently falls behind with his documentation due to an excessive patient load. The most appropriate action is:

[Refer to text]

Answer   1 C   2 A   3 C   4 A   5 B   6 B   7 A   8 A   9 A

A. Discuss the situation with other staff physical therapists
B. Ignore the situation and attempt to complete the documentation in a timely fashion
C. Discuss the situation with the immediate supervisor
D. Discuss the situation with the director of rehabilitation

Q 11. Which of the following muscles are stance phase muscles?
[Joint Structure and Function/Norkin/3rd Ed./Pg. 440]
A. Quadriceps
B. Hamstring muscles
C. Tibialis anterior
D. Peroneus longus
E. Soleus gastrocnemius

Q 12. The most important factor in fracture healing is:
[Essential Orthopedics/Maheshwari/3rd Ed./Pg. 9]
A. Good alignment
B. Organization of blood clot
C. Accurate reduction and 100% opposition of fractured fragments
D. Immobilization
E. Adequate calcium intake

Muscle Biomechanics

Q 13. The resting membrane potential of skeletal muscle fiber is:
[Textbook of Physiology/AK Jain/3rd Ed./Pg. 167]
A. $-90\,mV$
B. $-0.9\,mV$
C. $-0.09\,mV$
D. $-0.009\,mV$

Q 14. Conduction of nerve impulses is faster in myelinated nerves because of:
[Textbook of Physiology/AK Jain/3rd Ed./Pg. 167]
A. Uninterrupted flow of impulse
B. Saltatory conduction
C. Circular current flow
D. Quick reversal of current flow

Q 15. Cardiac muscles ability to regenerate is:
[Textbook of Physiology/AK Jain/3rd Ed./Pg. 189]
A. Partial
B. None
C. Full and complete
D. Variable

Q 16. Presence of muscle fibrillation indicates which of the following?
[Neurology and Neurosurgery/Illustrated/Lindsay/Pg. 57]
A. Hyperexcitability of motor unit
B. High neural discharge rate
C. Loss of muscle innervation
D. Upper motor neuron defect

Q 17. Which type of contraction occurs when the force of the muscles is less than the resistance?
[Principles of Exercise Therapy/Gardiner/4th Ed./Pg. 22]
A. Concentric
B. Eccentric
C. Isometric
D. Isokinetic

Q 18. The cross-section of muscle is equal to:
[Approximately/Macardle/4th Ed./Pg. 321]
A. Length × width
B. Length × ½ thickness
C. 2 (thickness) ÷ 2 (width)
D. Width × thickness

Q 19. During rest the flow of blood to muscle is:
[Approximately/Macardle/4th Ed./Pg. 316]
A. $3-4\,mL/100\,gm/min$
B. $3-4\,mL/100\,gm/sec$
C. $3-4\,mL/10\,gm/30\,sec$
D. $3-4\,mL/1000\,gm/min$

Q 20. One of the function of basal ganglia is to:
[Human Anatomy/BDC/Vol. 3/4th Ed./Pg. 316]
A. Increase the muscle tone
B. Produce small jerky movements
C. Inhibit stretch reflex
D. Control auditory function

Q 21. A patient who recently sustained a gastrocnemius strain asks a therapist what factors may have contributed to the muscle strain. Which statement does not accurately describe contributing factors to a muscle strain?
[Therapeutic Exercise/Kisner/5th Ed./Pg. 776]
A. The muscle may have been poorly prepared due to inadequate warm up
B. The muscle may have been weakened by a previous injury
C. The muscle may have been exposed to heat which would cause the muscle to be less contractile than normal
D. The muscle may previously have been extensively injured with resultant scar tissue formation

Biomechanics of Spine

Q 22. Action of latissimus dorsi muscle is:
[Joint Structure and Function/Norkin/3rd Ed./Pg. 222]
A. Supraspinatus, infraspinatus, teres major and latissimus dorsi
B. Infraspinatus, subscapularis, latissimus dorsi and pectoralis major
C. Teres minor, subscapularis, latissimus dorsi and pectoralis major
D. Teres minor, infraspinatus, supraspinatus subscapularis

Q 23. A 23-year-old suffered from spinal-cord injury while rock climbing and is independent in transfers with assistive devices most likely spinal cord level involved is:
[Physical Rehabilitation/Sullivan/5th Ed./Pg. 963]
A. C5
B. C6
C. C7
D. T1

Q 24. A patient with a T6 spinal cord injury prepares for discharge from a rehabilitation center following 15 weeks of intensive therapy. Which of the following does not accurately describe the patient's expected functional ability at the conclusion of rehabilitation?
[Physical Rehabilitation/Sullivan/5th Ed./Pg. 976]
A. Independent in light housekeeping and meal preparation
B. Independent bowel and bladder care with appropriate equipment
C. Independent self-feeding
D. Independent ambulation with forearm crutches and bilateral knee-ankle-food orthoses

Answer	10 C	11 A	12 C	13 A	14 B	15 B	16 C	17 B	18 D	19 A	20 A	21 C
	22 A	23 D	24 D									

Q 25. A patient exhibits pain and sensory loss in the posterior leg, calf, and dorsal foot. Extension of the hallux is poor, however the Achilles reflex is normal. What spinal level would you expect to be involved?
[Orthopedic Physical Assessment/Magee/3rd Ed./Pg. 369]
A. L4   B. L5
C. S1   D. S2

Q 26. A 26-year-old male involved in a motorcycle accident sustains a T10 vertebral fracture. The patient's physician attempts to restrict forward thoracic flexion by using an externally applied device. Which of the following would be the most appropriate selection?
[Physical Rehabilitation/Sullivan/5th Ed./Pg. 956]
A. Minerva cervical-thoracic orthosis
B. Philadelphia collar
C. Sternal-occipital-mandibular immobilizer
D. Thoracolumbar-sacral orthosis

Q 27. A sensory examination reveals light touch impairment to the buttock, thigh, and posterior leg the corresponding dermatome should be recorded as:
[Orthopedic Physical Assessment/Magee/3rd Ed./Pg. 382]
A. L1   B. L2
C. L4   D. S1

Q 28. A therapist orders a wheelchair for a patient with T8-T9 paraplegia. Which wheelchair option is not usually necessary for a patient with paraplegia?
[Physical Rehabilitation/Sullivan/5th Ed./Pg. 1307]
A. Detachable Leg Rests   B. Pneumatic Tires
C. Removable Arms   D. Wheel Rim Projections

Q 29. A therapist works on range of motion of the lower extremities with a patient rehabilitating from spinal cord injury. Independent range of motion of the lower extremities is a realistic goal for which spinal cord level?
[Physical Rehabilitation/Sullivan/5th Ed./Pg. 965]
A. C2   B. C4
C. C5   D. C7

Q 30. A therapist examines a patient with a C5 spinal cord injury. A realistic goal for the patient is:
[Physical Rehabilitation/Sullivan/5th Ed./Pg. 963]
A. Independent sliding board transfer
B. Forward raise in wheelchair using loops for pressure relief
C. Independent rolling from prone to supine and supine to prone
D. Independent scooting

Q 31. The following description best describes a patient with a spinal cord injury at the _____ level? Biceps, deltoids, and rotator cuff musculature are intact. Independent transfers with a sliding board may be possible.
[Human Anatomy/Vol. 1/BDC/4th Ed./Pg. 85]
A. C2   B. C4
C. C6   D. C8

Q 32. A realistic long-term goal for a patient with T10 paraplegia is:
[Physical Rehabilitation/Sullivan/5th Ed./Pg. 964]

A. The patient is able to ambulate with bilateral knee-ankle-foot orthoses using forearm crutches and a four-point gait pattern
B. The patient is able to ambulate with bilateral ankle-foot orthoses using forearm crutches and a three-point gait pattern
C. The patient is able to ambulate with bilateral knee-ankle-foot orthoses using forearm crutches and a swing-to gait pattern
D. The patient is able to ambulate independently in the parallel bars with bilateral ankle-foot orthoses and a swing-to gait pattern

Q 33. A therapist orders a wheelchair for a patient with C4 tetraplegia. Which power wheelchair option would be inappropriate for the patient?
[Physical Rehabilitation/Sullivan/5th Ed./Pg. 961]
A. Full length arm supports   B. Reclining frame
C. Hand controls   D. Elevating leg rests

Q 34. A respiratory examination is performed on a patient with tetraplegia with the following results: the patient attains seventy percent of standard vital capacity, he is able to verbalize eight syllables per breath, and is able to mobilize and clear secretions from his longs. Which level of injury does this best describe?
[Physical Rehabilitation / Sullivan / 5th Ed./Pg. 963]
A. C2 – C3   B. C4 – C5
C. C7 – C8   D. T2 – T3

Q 35. A therapist utilizes resistive testing as part of an initial examination. To assess the C5 myotome the therapist should resist:
[Orthopedic Physical Assessment/Magee/3rd Ed./Pg. 104]
A. Wrist radial deviation   B. Elbow extension
C. Shoulder abduction   D. Thumb extension

Q 36. A therapist develops a chart detailing expected functional outcomes for a variety of spinal cord injuries. Which is the highest spinal level at which independent transfers with sliding board would be feasible?
[Physical Rehabilitation/Sullivan/5th Ed./Pg. 962]
A. C4   B. C6
C. T1   D. T3

Q 37. A patient with complete C5 tetraplegia works on a forward raise for pressure relief with his therapist. The patient utilizes loops that are attached to the back of the wheelchair to assist with successful with the forward raise:
[Physical Rehabilitation/Sullivan/5th Ed./Pg. 962]
A. Brachioradialis, brachialis
B. Rhomboids, levator scapulae
C. Biceps, deltoids
D. Triceps, flexor digitorum

Q 38. A therapist treats a patient with complete C6 tetraplegia. Which of the following would not be an expected functional outcome for the patient?
[Physical Rehabilitation/Sullivan/ 5th Ed./Pg. 964]
A. Independent transfers with a sliding board
B. Independent bowel and balder care

Answer
| 25 B | 26 D | 27 D | 28 D | 29 D | 30 B | 31 C | 32 C | 33 C | 34 C | 35 C | 36 B |
| 37 C | 38 B | | | | | | | | | | |

C. Independent manual wheelchair propulsion
D. Independent self-feeding

Q 39. Which statement best describes the realistic functional status of a patient with C4 tetraplegia after completing rehabilitation?
[Physical Rehabilitation/Sullivan/5th Ed./Pg. 961]
A. Able to ambulate independently
B. Independent in all activities of daily living
C. Able to propel a manual wheelchair independently
D. Able to operate a power wheelchair

Q 40. A patient reports pain radiating down her posterior leg into the foot. She also exhibits weakness in plantar flexion and an absent Achilles reflex. Which spinal level would you expect to be involved?
[Orthopedic Physical Assessment/Magee/5th Ed./Pg. 550]
A. L2
B. L3
C. L5
D. S2

Q 41. A therapist completes a sensory examination on a patient diagnosed with an incomplete spinal cord injury. To assess the C5 dermatome the therapist should examine the:
[Orthopedic Physical Assessment / Magee/5th Ed./Pg. 183]
A. Neck
B. Superior portion of the chest above the axilla
C. Thumb and index finger
D. Deltoid area of the lateral arm

Q 42. A therapist orders a wheelchair for a patient in a rehabilitation hospital. Which of the following patients would be most in need of a wheelchair with handrim projections?
[Physical Rehabilitation/Sullivan/5th Ed./Pg. 962]
A. A patient with a C3 spinal cord injury
B. A patient with a C5 spinal cord injury
C. A patient with hemiparesis
D. A patient with a cauda equina lesion

Q 43. A therapist an in-service to the rehabilitation staff on the anatomy of the spine. As part of the presentation the therapist discusses the role of each of the ligaments of the spine. Which ligament of the spine acts to prevent hyperextension?
[Joint Structure and Function/Norkin/3rd Ed./Pg. 122]
A. Ligamentum flavum
B. Interspinous ligaments
C. Anterior longitudinal ligament
D. Posterior longitudinal ligament

Q 44. A patient is positioned in supine with the hips flexed to 90 degrees and knees extended. As the patient slowly lowers her extended legs toward the horizontal, there is an increase in lordosis of the low back. This finding is indicative of weakness of the:
[Human Anatomy/BDC/4th/Pg. 200]
A. Hip flexors
B. Back extensors
C. Hip extensors
D. Abdominals

Q 45. A therapist examines a patient with a C6 spinal cord injury. Which muscle would not be innervated based on the patient's level of injury?
[Physical Rehabilitation/Sullivan/5th Ed./Pg. 962]
A. Biceps
B. Deltoids
C. Triceps
D. Diaphragm

Q 46. At what level is it realistic for a patient with a spinal cord injury to functionally ambulate?
[Physical Rehabilitation/Sullivan/5th Ed./Pg. 964]
A. C7
B. T1
C. T6
D. L1

Q 47. Median nerve injury above elbow leads to:
[Orthopedic Physical Assessment/Magee/5th Ed./Pg. 650]
A. Ape thumb
B. Trigger finger
C. Wrist drop
D. Claw hand

Q 48. Cartilage is quite vascular in:
[Essential of Orthopedicss/Jayant Joshi/Reprint 2006/Pg. 406]
A. Embryonic life
B. Early childhood
C. Early adulthood
D. Old age

Q 49. Osteophytes developing at the joint at Luscka characteristically compress spinal nerves at:
[Essential Orthopedics/Maheshwari/3rd Ed./Pg. 229]
A. Intervertebral foramen
B. Anterior part of body
C. Posterior part of body
D. Paradural areas

Q 50. Minimum intradiscal pressure in vertebral column is seen when a person is:
[Orthopedic Physical Assessment/Magee/5th Ed./Pg. 523]
A. Standing
B. Sitting
C. Lying flat
D. Lying on one side

Q 51. Dislocation of the vertebrae is uncommon in thoracic region because:
[Refer to text]
A. The articular processes are interlocked
B. The vertebral body is long
C. Anterior longitudinal ligament is strong
D. Spinous process is long and pointed

Biomechanics of U/L

Q 52. The rotator cuff of the glenohumeral joint is formed by the tendons of:
[Joint Structure and Function/Norkin/Pg. 220]
A. Supraspinatus, infraspinatus, teres major and latissimus dorsi
B. Infraspinatus, subscapularis, latissimus dorsi and pectoralis major
C. Teres minor, subscapularis, latissimus dorsi and pectoralis major
D. Teres minor, infraspinatus, supraspinatus and subscapularis

Q 53. Deltoid muscle is supplied by:
[Human Anatomy BDC/Pg. 76]
A. Suprascapular nerve C 4, 5, 6
B. Radial nerve C 7, 8
C. Musculocutaneous nerve C 5, 6
D. Axillary nerve C 5,6

Q 54. The ROM of abduction at thumb (CMC) is
[David/7th Ed./Pg. 168]

Answer										
39 D	40 D	41 D	42 B	43 C	44 D	45 C	46 D	47 A	48 A	49 A	50 C
51 B	52 D	53 D								

A. 50°
B. 90°
C. 225°
D. 15°

Q 55. Loss of active extension of metacarpophalangeal joint occurs in the injury of which of the following nerves?
[Essential of Orthopedicss of Applied Physiotherapy/ Jayant Joshi/Pg. 262]
A. Median
B. Ulnar
C. Posterior interosseous
D. Musculocutaneous

Q 56. Wrist drop occurs in radial nerve injury of all levels except:
[Essential of Orthopedicss/Maheshwari/Pg. 53]
A. Axilla
B. Radial groove
C. Proximal to elbow
D. Distal to elbow

Q 57. All the following are correct about clavicle except:
[Human Anatomy/BDC/Pg. 7]
A. Only long bone in body to ossify in membrane
B. Only long bone in body which connects limb to axial skeleton
C. Only long bone in body to ossify in intrauterine life
D. Only long bone in body to ossify by endochondral ossification

Q 58. Crazy bone or crazy nerve contusion is associated with:
[Human Anatomy/BDC/4th Ed./Pg. 111]
A. Ulnar nerve at elbow level
B. Axillary nerve at shoulder level
C. Radial nerve at spiral groove in humerus
D. Median nerve in carpal tunnel

Q 59. Brachioradialis muscle is paralyzed in radial nerve injuries of all the following levels except:
[Human Anatomy/BDC/Vol. 1/4th Ed/Pg. 96]
A. Axilla
B. Middle of the arm
C. Proximal to elbow
D. Distal to elbow

Q 60. Ulnar nerve injury at elbow would involve all of the following except:
[Human Anatomy/BDC/Vol. 1/4th ed./Pg. 104]
A. Flexor Carpi Ulnaris
B. Hypothenar Muscles
C. Flexor Digitorum Profundus
D. Interossei

Q 61. A patient sustains an injury to the dorsal scapular nerve. Which muscle not innervated by this nerve can elevate the scapula?
[BDC/Vol. 1/4th Ed./Pg. 61]
A. Latissimus dorsi
B. Levator scapulae
C. Rhomboid minor
D. Trapezius

Q 62. While palpating the wrist and hand, it should become apparent that the hamate articulates with the ________ metacarpal?
[Musculoskeletal System/Neumann/Pg. 179]
A. First
B. Second
C. Third
D. Fourth

Q 63. A therapist reviews the medical record of a patient with a peripheral nerve injury. The most common site for an ulnar never is the:
[Musculoskeletal System/Neuman/Pg. 156]
A. Brachial plexus
B. Medial epicondyle of the humerus
C. Superficial surface of the flexor retinaculum
D. Distal wrist crease.

Q 64. A physical therapist reviews a physician's examination of a patient that will be seen in therapy later in the day. The examination identifies excessive medial displacement of the elbow during ligamentous testing. Which ligament is typically involved in medial instability of the elbow?
[Orthopedic Physical Assessment/Magee/3rd Ed./Pg. 266]
A. Anular
B. Radial collateral
C. Ulnar collateral
D. Volar radioulnar

Q 65. A therapist measures a patient for a wheelchair. Which measurement is used to determine armrest height in a wheelchair?
[Physical Rehabilitation/Sullivan/5th Ed/Pg. 1306]
A. Seat to anterior superior iliac spine
B. Seat to olecranon distance
C. Femur to radial head distance
D. Elbow to acromion distance

Q 66. A physical therapist instructs a patient to reach behind her head and touch the superior medial angle of the opposite scapula. Which shoulder motions are necessary in order to follow this command?
[Orthopedic Physical Assessment/ David J. Magee/5th Ed./Pg. 255]
A. Flexion and lateral rotation
B. Flexion and medial rotation
C. Abduction and lateral rotation
D. Abduction and medial rotation

Q 67. If the radial nerve is severed above the origin of the triceps muscle, what motion of the elbow joint in impossible?
[Vol. 1/BDC/Vol. 1/4th Ed./Pg. 96]
A. Flexion
B. Extension
C. Pronation
D. Supination

Q 68. A therapist begins to suspect neurological involvement after completing an upper quarter screening examination. Which anatomic are would be most appropriate to gather information on the C8 dermatome?
[Orthopedic Physical Assessment/Maggi/5th Ed./Pg. 159]
A. Thumb and index finger
B. Radial border of the hand
C. Middle three fingers
D. Ulnar border of the hand

Q 69. A therapist examines the elbow of a patient rehabilitating from a radial head fracture. Which of the following most accurately describes the close packed position of the radiohumeral joint?
[Orthopedic Physical Assessment/Magee/5th Ed./Pg. 362]

Answer	54 A	55 C	56 D	57 D	58 A	59 D	60 C	61 D	62 D	63 B	64 C	65 B
	66 C	67 B	68 D									

A. 45 degrees flexion, 10 degrees supination
B. 60 degrees flexion, 20 degrees supination
C. 90 degrees flexion, 5 degrees supination
D. 120 degrees flexion, 10 degrees supination

Q 70. A therapist completes a goniometric assessment of a patient's wrist. Assuming normal range of motion, which of the following motions would you expect to have the greatest available range?
[Joint Structure and Function/Norkin/3rd Ed./Pg. 253]
A. Extension
B. Flexion
C. Radial deviation
D. Ulnar deviation

Q 71. A therapist measures passive forearm pronation and concludes the results are within normal limits. Which measurement would be classified as within normal limits?
[Joint Structure and Function/Norkin/3rd Ed./Pg. 234]
A. 65 degrees
B. 85 degrees
C. 105 degrees
D. 125 degrees

Q 72. A patient status post stroke presents with a hypotonic left upper extremity. While performing sitting activities the position of choice for the left upper extremity is:
[Physical Rehabilitation/Sullivan/5th Ed./Pg. 751]
A. In the patient's lap
B. In a sling
C. Weight bearing through the upper extremity with the elbow extended
D. Weight bearing through the upper extremity with the elbow and wrist flexed

Q 73. A therapist practices assessing joint end-feel. The therapist would most accurately classify normal elbow extension end-feel as:
[Physical Rehabilitation/Sullivan/5th Ed./Pg. 175]
A. Firm
B. Hard
C. Soft
D. Empty

Q 74. A forearm laceration causes damage to the median nerve. Which muscle not innervated by the media nerve can flex the wrist?
[BDC/Vol. 1/4th Ed./Pg. 102]
A. Flexor carpi radialis
B. Flexor carpi ulnaris
C. Flexor digitorum superficialis
D. Flexor longus

Q 75. A patient sustained a knife would which severed the distal lateral cord of the brachial plexus EMG testing reveals no damage to the median nerve. The injury will likely result in impairment of:
[BDC/Vol. 1/4th Ed./Pg. 53]
A. Elbow Flexion and Forearm Supination
B. Elbow Extension and Forearm Pronation
C. Shoulder Flexion and Abduction
D. Shoulder Lateral Rotation

Q 76. If the axillary nerve was severed, what muscle could laterally rotate the humerus?
[BDC/Vol. 1/4th Ed./Pg. 52]
A. Teres major
B. Subscapularis
C. Infraspinatus
D. Teres minor

Q 77. A physical therapist palpates the muscle bellies of the wrist extensors. The therapist follows the muscles proximally to their common origin. This bony landmark is termed the:
[BDC/Vol. 1/4th Ed./Pg. 131]
A. Lateral epicondyle
B. Medial epicondyle
C. Radial head
D. Olecranon

Q 78. A therapist attempts to palpate the lunate by moving his finger immediately distal to lister's tubercle. Which wrist motion with allow the therapist to facilitate palpation of the lunate?
[Joint Structure Function/Norkin/3rd Ed./Pg. 252]
A. Extension
B. Flexion
C. Radial deviation
D. Ulnar deviation

Q 79. A therapist palpates the bony structures of the wrist and hand. Which of the following structures would not be identified in the distal row of carpals?
[Joint Structure Function/Norkin/3rd Ed./Pg. 252]
A. Capitate
B. Hamate
C. Triquetrum
D. Trapezoid

Q 80. A therapist examines a patient with limited range of motion at the glenohumeral joint. Which of the following is considered a capsular pattern of the glenohumeral joint?
[Orthopedic Physical Assessment/Magee/ 5th Ed./Pg. 253]
A. Greatest limitation in flexion flowed by medial rotation
B. Greatest limitation in lateral rotation, followed by abduction
C. Greatest limitation in medial rotation, followed by abduction
D. Greatest limitation in extension and lateral rotation

Q 81. A therapist measures a patient's shoulder medial rotation with patient positioned in supine with glenohumeral joint in 90 degrees of abduction and the elbow in 90 degrees of flexion. The therapist records the patient's shoulder medial rotation is 0–70 degrees and classifies the end-feel as firm. Which portion of the joint capsule is primarily responsible for the firm end-feel?
[Cynthia Norkin/3rd Ed./Pg. 207]
A. Anterior joint capsule
B. Posterior joint capsule
C. Inferior joint capsule
D. Superior joint capsule

Q 82. A physical therapist examines a patient with a dorsal scapular nerve injury. Which muscles would you expect to be most affected by this condition?
[BDC/Vol. 1/Pg. 52]
A. Serratus anterior, pectoralis minor
B. Levator scapulae, rhomboids
C. Latissimus dorsi, teres major
D. Supraspinatus, infraspinatus

Q 83. The lesion in Klumpke's paralysis is at:
[BDC/Vol.1/Pg. 53]
A. Cervical plexus
B. Lower brachial
C. Upper brachial
D. Sacral plexus

Q 84. Muscles involved in Volkman's ischemic contracture:
[Essential of Orthopedics and Applied Physiotherapy/Jayant Joshi/Reprint 2009/ Elsevier/Pg. 99]
A. Flexor pollicis longus
B. Flexor profundus
C. Flexor sublimis
D. All of the above

Answer	69 C	70 B	71 B	72 C	73 B	74 B	75 A	76 C	77 A	78 B	79 D	80 B
	81 B	82 B	83 B	84 D								

Q 85. True flexors of the elbow joint are:
[FA David/Norkin/Joint Structure and Function/3rd Ed./Pg. 242]
A. Biceps
B. Brachialis
C. Brachioradialis
D. Teres minor

Q 86. Joint least affected by neuropathy:
[Essential of Orthopedics and Applied Physiotherapy/Jayant Joshi/Reprint 2009/Pg. 489]
A. Shoulder
B. Hip
C. Wrist
D. Elbow

Q 87. Dorsum of the middle finger is supplied by:
[BDC/Vol. 1/Pg. 66]
A. Radial nerve
B. Median Nerve
C. Ulnar nerve
D. A and B

Q 88. Sensory supply of the tip of the ring fingers:
[BDC/Vol. 1/Pg. 66]
A. Radial nerve
B. Median nerve
C. Ulnar nerve
D. Posterior interosseous nerve

Q 89. Which nerve repair has worst prognosis:
[Essential of Orthopedicss and Applied Physiotherapy/Jayant Joshi/Reprint 2009/Pg. 266]
A. Ulnar
B. Radial
C. Median
D. Lateral popliteal

Q 90. Medial meniscus is more vulnerable to injury because of:
[Essential orthopedics/Maheshwari/3rd Ed./Pg. 129]
A. Its fixity to tibial collateral ligament
B. Its semicircular shape
C. Action of adductor magnus
D. Its attachment to fibrous capsule

Q 91. Median nerve injury above elbow leads to:
[BDC/Vol. 1/Pg. 110]
A. Ape thumb
B. Trigger finger
C. Wrist drop
D. Claw hand

Q 92. Sprengel's deformity of scapula is:
[Orthopedic Physical Assessment/Magee/5th Ed./Pg. 544]
A. Undescended/elevated scapula
B. Undescended neck of scapula
C. Exostosis scapula
D. None of the above

Q 93. Most commonly injured nerve in anterior dislocation of shoulder is:
[Jayant Joshi/Reprint 2009/Pg. 80/]
A. Nerve of Bell
B. Axillary nerve
C. Radial nerve
D. Median nerve

Q 94. Injury of median nerve at wrist is best detected by:
[BDC/Vol. 1/Pg. 116]
A. Action of abductor pollicis brevis
B. Action of flexor pollicis brevis
C. Loss of sensation of radial half of palm
D. Loss of sensation of tip of ring finger

Q 95. All are components of rotator cuff except:
[Jayant Joshi/Reprint 2009/Pg. 473]
A. Supraspinatus
B. Infraspinatus
C. Subscapularis
D. Teres major

Q 96. Brachialis is supplied by:
[BDC/Vol. 1/Pg. 85]
A. Radial and Ulnar nerve
B. Median and Musculocutaneous nerve
C. Radial and Musculocutaneous nerve
D. Radial and median nerve

Q 97. Nerve which responds best to repair is:
[Jayant Joshi/Reprint 2009/Pg. 262]
A. Median
B. Ulnar
C. Sciatic
D. Radial

Q 98. Luxatio erecta:
[Essential Orthopedics/Maheshwari/3rd Ed./Pg. 74]
A. Tear of the glenoidal labium
B. Inferior dislocation of shoulder
C. Anterior dislocation of shoulder
D. Defect in the humeral head

Q 99. Bankhart's lesion involves:
[Essential Orthopedics/Maheshwari/3rd Ed./Pg 74]
A. Anterior aspect of the head of humerus
B. Anterior aspect of glenoid labrum
C. Posterior aspect of glenoid labrum
D. Posterior aspect of the head of humerus

Q 100. Extension of the metacarpophalangeal joint is lost in injury to:
[Jayant Joshi/Reprint 2009/Pg. 262]
A. Radial nerve
B. Ulnar nerve
C. Median nerve
D. Posterior interosseous nerve

Q 101. Clumsiness of the hand in case of leprosy is due to involvement of:
[Essential Orthopedics/Maheshwari/3rd Ed./Pg. 168]
A. Interosseous muscle
B. Abductor pollicis longus
C. Extensor carpi ulnaris
D. Flexor carpi radialis

Biomechanics of L/L

Q 102. To determine real leg length measurement is taken from:
[Essential Orthopedics/] Maheshwari/3rd Ed./Pg. 309]
A. ASIS to lateral malleolus on the same side
B. ASIS to the great toe on the same side
C. ASIS to the heel on the same side
D. ASIS to the medial malleolus of the leg

Q 103. Tightness of tensor fascia latae causes:
[Joint Structure and Function/Norkin/3rd Ed./Pg. 311]
A. Adduction of the hip
B. Extension of the hip
C. Knocking (genu valgum) of the knee
D. Plantar flexion of the ankle

Q 104. The ligaments of the hip are very weak:
[Joint Structure and Function/Norkin/3rd Ed./Pg. 298]

Answer	85 A	86 C	87 D	88 B	89 A	90 A	91 A	92 A	93 B	94 A	95 D	96 C
	97 D	98 B	99 B	100 D	101 A	102 D	103 C					

A. On anterior side
B. On posterior side
C. On lateral side
D. On anterolateral side

C. Flexion of hip and knee on same side, i.e. left side
D. Plantar flexion of right ankle to increase the leg length

Q 105. Normal angle between vertical lines of femur and tibia is:
[Joint Structure and Function/Norkin/Pg. 450]
A. 7 Degrees
B. 12 Degrees
C. 1.5 Degrees
D. 0.5 Degrees

Q 106. Management of CDH by splintage is done with the hip placed in:
[Essential Orthopedics/Maheshwari/Pg. 203]
A. Flexion and abduction
B. Extension and abduction
C. Flexion and adduction
D. Extension and adduction

Q 107. Piriformis muscle is inserted at:
[Joint Structure and Function/Norkin/3rd Ed./Pg. 312]
A. Trochanteric fossa
B. Pectineal line
C. Greater trochanter
D. Quadrate tubercle

Q 108. Loss of active dorsiflexion of ankle occurs in the injury of which of the following nerves?
[Essential of Orthopedics/Jayant Joshi/Pg. 262]
A. Sciatic
B. Obturator
C. Femoral
D. Radial

Q 109. Loss of active knee extension occurs in the injury of which of the following nerves?
[Essentials of Orthopedics/Jayant Joshi/Pg. 262]
A. Sciatic
B. Obturator
C. Femoral
D. Radial

Q 110. All of the following are components of quadriceps muscle except:
[Joint Structure and Function/Norkin/Pg. 349]
A. Vastus medialis
B. Vastus lateralis
C. Vastus intermedius
D. Rectus femoris

Q 111. The most powerful muscle of body is:
[Joint Structure and Function/Norkin/Pg. 347]
A. Quadriceps
B. Gluteus maximus
C. Gastrocsoleus
D. Deltoid

Q 112. Inversion of foot occurs at:
[Joint Structure and Function/Norkin/Pg. 376]
A. Ankle joint
B. Subtalar joint
C. Talonavicular joint
D. Tibiofibular joint

Q 113. All is correct about the true measurement of the limb except:
[Essential Orthopedics/Maheshwari/Pg. 309]
A. Length is measured after marking the bony points anterior superior iliac spine and medial malleolus
B. The pelvis should be made square
C. Length is measured keeping the limb in identical position
D. Measurement is taken from xiphisternum to medial malleolus

Q 114. Due to paralysis or marked weakness of gluteus medius muscle the positive Trendelenburg's sign results into:
[Orthopedic Physical Assessment/Magee/3rd Ed./Pg. 690]
A. Dropping of pelvis on opposite side, i.e. left side
B. Dropping of pelvis on same side, i.e. right side

Q 115. Hip joint is weakest in which of the following attitudes?
[Kinesiology of Musculoskeletal System/Neuman/Pg. 400]
A. Neutral position
B. Flexion, adduction and external rotation
C. Flexion, adduction and internal rotation
D. None of the above

Q 116. The main dorsiflexor of foot is:
[Kinesiology of Musculoskeletal System/Neuman/Pg. 510]
A. Tibialis anterior
B. Extensor digitorum longus
C. Extensor digitorum brevis
D. Extensor hallucis longus

Q 117. In adduction deformity of hip. Anterior ASIS move in which direction.
[Orthopedic Physical Assessment/Magee/3rd Ed./Pg. 463]
A. ASIS of affected hip move proximal
B. ASIS of affected hip move distal
C. ASIS of normal hip move proximal
D. ASIS of normal hip move distal

Q 118. Which of the following maneuver will bring the raised ASIS to normal level?
[Orthopedic Physical Assessment/Maggi/3rd Ed./Pg. 452]
A. Adduction of Normal Hip
B. Abduction of Normal Hip
C. Adduction of Diseased Hip
D. Abduction of Diseased Hip

Q 119. Tuber joint angle in normal adult is:
[Essential Orthopedics/Maheshwari/3rd Ed./Pg. 140]
A. 10 degrees
B. 30 degrees
C. 60 degrees
D. 90 degrees

Q 120. Tuber joint angle is important in which of the following fractures?
[Essential Orthopedics/Maheshwari/3rd Ed./Pg. 140]
A. Femoral neck
B. Trochanter
C. Calcaneum
D. Navicular

Q 121. The nodule of trigger point is palpable at which of the following sites?
A. Proximal interphalangeal joint
B. Neck of metatarsal
C. Terminal interphalangeal joint
D. Middle phalanx

Q 122. A therapist examines a patient seated in a wheelchair. After completing the examination the therapist determines the wheelchair has inadequate seat width. Which of the following is the most likely consequences?
[Physical Rehabilitation/Sullivan/5th Ed./Pg. 1323]
A. Excessive pressure under the distal thigh
B. Excessive pressure under the ischial tuberosities
C. Excessive pressure in the popliteal fossa
D. Excessive pressure on the greater trochanters

Answer	104 B	105 A	106 A	107 C	108 A	109 C	110 D	111 C	112 B	113 D	114 A	115 C
	116 A	117 A	118 A	119 B	120 C	121 B	122 D					

Q 123. The Q angle is utilized as a measure to determine the amount of lateral force on the patella. Which three bony landmarks are used to measure the Q angle?

[Kinesiology of Musculoskeletal System/Neuman/Pg. 461]

A. Anterior superior iliac spine, superior border of the patella, tibial tubercle
B. Anterior superior iliac spine, midpoint of the patella, tibial tubercle
C. Anterior superior iliac inferior border of the patella, midpoint of the patella tendon
D. Greater trochanter midpoint of the patella, superior border of the patella tendon

Q 124. A patient positioned in supine on a mat table is instructed to flex her right hip and knee to her chest and hold it. This evaluative technique can be used to assess the length of the:

[Essential Orthopedics/David J Maheshwari/3rd Ed./Pg. 482]

A. Hamstrings on the left   B. Hamstrings on the right
C. Hip flexors on the left   D. Hip flexors on the right

Q 125. A patient is instructed to lie supine with his knees bent to 90 degrees over the edges of a treatment table. The patient is then asked to bring his right knee to his chest. By examining the angle of the left knee, the therapist can obtain information on the length of the ___muscle?

[Orthopedic Physical Assessment/Magee/3rd Ed./Pg. 482]

A. Biceps femoris   B. Rectus femoris
C. Sartorius   D. Tensor fasciae latae

Q 126. A physical therapist examines a patient's hip range of motion. Which pattern of limitation is typically considered to be a capsular pattern?

[Orthopedic Physical Assessment/ Magee/3rd Ed./Pg. 460]

A. Limitation of flexion, abduction, and medial rotation
B. Limitation of flexion, adduction, and lateral rotation
C. Limitation of extension, adduction, and medial rotation
D. Limitation of extension abduction and Lateral rotation

Q 127. A therapist treats a patient with emphysema. As part of the treatment session the therapist teaches the patient to perform diaphragmatic breathing exercise. The primary goal for diaphragmatic breathing to:

[CBS/BDC/Vol. 2/4th Ed./Pg. 311]

A. Decrease Tidal Ventilation
B. Increase Respiration Rate
C. Decrease Accessory Muscle Use
D. Decrease oxygenation

Q 128. A therapist attempts to reduce a child's genu recurvatum using an ankle-foot orthosis. Which ankle setting would be the most effective to achieve the therapist's objective?

[Kinesiology of Musculoskeletal/System/Neuman/ 1st Ed./Pg. 473]

A. 5-10 degrees of dorsiflexion
B. Neutral
C. 5-10 degrees of plantar flexion
D. 15-20 degrees of plantar flexion

Q 129. A therapist places patient's hip in the resting position prior to assessing joint play. Which of the following would be considered the resting position of the hip?

[Orthopedic Physical Assessment/David J Magee/3rd Ed./Pg. 460]

A. 10 degrees flexion, 15 degrees abduction, slight medial rotation
B. 30 degrees flexion, 30 degrees abduction slight lateral rotation
C. 30 degrees flexion, 30 degrees adduction, 20 degrees lateral rotation
D. 10 degrees extension, 20 degrees adduction, 20 degrees medial rotation

Q 130. A therapist attempts to palpate the peroneus longus and brevis tendons on a patient diagnosed with chronic ankle instability. The facilitate palpation of these structures the therapist should:

[BDC/Vol. 2/4th Ed/Pg. 106]

A. Ask the patient to invert and dorsiflex his foot
B. Ask the patient to evert and plantarflex his foot
C. Ask the patient to invert and plantarflex his foot
D. Ask the patient to evert and dorsiflex his foot

Q 131. An elderly patient with a minor right ankle inversion sprain is learning to use a straight cane. Which of the following instructions would be the most appropriate?

[Neuman/1st Ed./Pg. 422]

A. Hold the cane in the right hand, step left, then step right
B. Hold the cane in the left hand, step left, the step right
C. Hold the cane in the right hand, step right, then step left
D. Hold the cane in the left hand step right, then step left

Q 132. The length of a patient's hamstrings is tested in supine using a straight leg raise. While raising the tested lower extremity the therapist attempts to stabilize the contralateral limb. If the patient has tight hip flexions which result in an excessive anterior pelvic tilt what can the physical therapist conclude about the patient's measured hamstrings length?

[Orthopedic Physical Assessment/Magee/3rd Ed./Pg. 389]

A. Actual length is greater than measured length
B. Actual length is less than measured length
C. Short hip flexors do not influence apparent hamstrings length
D. The apparent length measured is the actual length

Q 133. If a leg length measurement is 28. inches when taken in a supine position and 30.2 inches when taken in a standing position, the leg length difference is probably due to:

[Essential Orthopedics/Maheshwari/3rd Ed./Pg. 309]

A. Poor standing posture
B. Pelvic asymmetry
C. An actual leg length difference
D. Not enough information is given to form a conclusion

Q 134. A physical therapist observes a patient ambulating with a Trendelenburg gait pattern. This deviation is often caused by weakness of the:

[Joint Structure and Function/Norkin/3rd Ed./Pg. 317]

A. Gluteus maximus   B. Gluteus medius
C. Gluteus minimus   D. Piriformis

Answer   123 B   124 C   125 B   126 A   127 C   128 C   129 B   130 B   131 D   132 A   133 D   134 B

Q 135. A high school basketball player is treated in physical therapy after spraining her ankle. Palpation reveals an extremely painful area extending from the anterior portion of the lateral malleolus to the lateral aspect of the talar neck. The ligament most likely associated with the discomfort is the:

[Essentials of Orthopedics/Jayant Joshi/Reprint 2009/ Pg. 556]

A. Deltoid
B. Calcaneofibular
C. Posterior talofibular
D. Anterior talofibular

Q 136. A physical therapist observes that a patient's medial longitudinal arch is extremely depressed. Which ligament helps to maintain the medial longitudinal arch?

[Joint Structure and Function/Norkin/3rd Ed./Pg. 399]

A. Talonavicular
B. Anterior talofibular
C. Calcaneonavicular
D. Posterior talofibular

Q 137. A patient rehabilitating from greater trochanteric bursitis completes active range of motion exercises. Which of the following best describes the arthrokinematics associated with hip flexion?

[Joint Structure and Function/Norkin/3rd Ed./Pg. 301]

A. Superior glide of the femoral head
B. Anterior glide of the femoral head
C. Inferior glide of the femoral head in the acetabulum
D. Posterior and inferior glide of the femoral head in the acetabulum

Q 138. A physical therapist observes a patient performing active hip abduction in supine. The patient is limited by 10 degrees in abduction, but appears to be moving through the full range of motion. What compensatory measures might the patient use to seemingly increase hip abduction:

[Joint Structure and Function/Norkin/3rd Ed./Pg. 317]

A. Hip flexion and lateral rotation
B. Hip flexion and medial rotation
C. Hip hyperextension and lateral rotation
D. Hip hyperextension and medial rotation

Q 139. A patient with a fractured right tibia who is partial weight bearing is referred to physical therapy for fitting and instruction with an assistive device. During the examination the physical therapist identifies poor lower extremity strength and coordination. Which assistive device would be most appropriate for the patient?

[Physical Rehabilitation/Sullivan/5th Ed./Pg. 549]

A. Axillary crutches
B. Cane
C. Lofstrand crutches
D. Walker

Q 140. A therapist observes the gait of a patient status post right CVA with a metal upright ankle-foot orthosis. The therapist notes left knee instability with left stance. The ankle-foot orthosis most likely has:

[Physical Rehabilitation/Sullivan/5th Ed./Pg. 1236]

A. A long foot plate
B. Inadequate knee lock
C. Inadequate dorsiflexion stop
D. Inadequate plantar flexion stop

Q 141. A physical therapist observes a patient dragging his toe during the swing phase of gait. All of the following are possible causes except:

[Joint Structure and Function/Norkin/3rd Ed./Pg. 478]

A. Weakness of dorsiflexors
B. Spasticity of plantar flexors
C. Weakness of plantar flexors
D. Inadequate knee flexion

Q 142. A patient performs bridging in supine a part of an exercise program. The therapist increases the difficulty by applying agonistic reversals as the patient maintains the bridge position. The application of atomistic reversals promotes eccentric control of the:

[Physical Rehabilitation/Sullivan/5th Ed./Pg. 601]

A. Hip Extensions, Hamstrings
B. Hip Flexion Quadriceps
C. Hip Extensors, Adductors
D. Adductor Hamstrings

Q 143. A patient lies supine with one knee over the edge of a treatment table and the other held against his chest. The therapist notes that the knee over the edge of the treatment table is flexed to 45 degrees. A probable cause of this position of the knee includes tightness of the:

[Therapeutic Exercise/Kisner/5th Ed./Pg. 674]

A. Iliopsoas
B. Rectus Femoris
C. Tensor Fascia Latae
D. Vastus Medialis

Q 144. The most common type of contracture in a patient with a transfemoral amputation is:

[Essential of Orthopedics/Jayant Joshi/Reprint 2009/Pg. 236]

A. Hip Flexion
B. Hip Extension
C. Hip Adduction
D. Knee Flexion

Q 145. A therapist attempts to determine if a patient has muscular weakness in the gastrocnemius or soleus by observing the patient's gait. Which objective finding would not be consistent with weakness in this area?

[Joint Structure and Function/Norkin/3rd Ed./Pg. 464]

A. Inability to dorsiflex the ankle during midswing phase
B. Inability to perform a calf raise against resistance
C. Inability to walk on toes decreased toe off
D. Decreased toe off

Q 146. A patient is limited in passive ankle dorsiflexion when the knee is extended, but is not limited, when the knee is flexed. The most logical explanation is:

[Joint Structure and Function/Norkin/3rd Ed./Pg. 347]

A. The gastrocnemius is responsible for the limitation
B. The soleus is responsible for the limitation
C. The popliteus is responsible for the limitation
D. The gastrocnemius and soleus are both responsible for the limitation

Q 147. A therapist classifies a patient's end-feel as soft after completing a specific passive movement. Which of the following joint motions would typically produce a soft end-feel?

[Physical Rehabilitation/Sullivan/5th Ed./Pg. 175]

Answer   135 D   136 C   137 D   138 A   139 D   140 C   141 C   142 A   143 B   144 A   145 A   146 A

A. Hip flexion with the knee extended
B. Knee flexion
C. Elbow extension
D. Forearm supination

Q 148. A physical therapist positions a patient's hip in the resting position. This position for the hip is:
[Orthopedic Physical Assessment/Magee/5th Ed./Pg. 659]
A. 30 degrees of hip flexion, 30 degrees of abduction, and 5 degrees of lateral rotation
B. 60 degrees of hip flexion, 30 degrees of abduction, and 15 degrees of lateral rotation
C. 90 degrees of hip flexion, 15 degrees of abduction, and 5 degrees of lateral rotation
D. 120 degrees of hip flexion, 15 degrees of abduction, and 15 degrees of lateral rotation

Q 149. A physical therapist positions a patient in prone to measure passive knee flexion. Range of motion may be limited in this position due to:
[Joint Structure and Function/Norkin/3rd Ed./Pg. 97]
A. Active insufficiency of the knee extensors
B. Active insufficiency of the knee flexors
C. Passive insufficiency of the knee extensors
D. Passive insufficiency of the knee flexors

Q 150. Which of the following is correct in medial meniscus tear?
[Essential Orthopedics/Jayant Joshi/Reprint 2009/Pg. 537]
A. Rotation of femur on tibia
B. Meniscus do not heal
C. Locking and unlocking episodes
D. Meniscus should be excised
E. All of the above are correct

Q 151. Most common dislocation of the hip is:
[Essential Orthopedics/Jayant Joshi/Reprint 2009/Pg. 151]
A. Posterior
B. Anterior
C. Central
D. None

Q 152. Spontaneous rupture of the Achilles' tendon in an 18-year-old male is most likely to be due to excess
[Refer to text]
A. Tendon strength
B. Bone strength
C. Muscle strength
D. Musculotendinous junction strength

Q 153. The tension resistance of normal fascia per square inch, such as the fascia lata, has been determined to be:
A. 550 pounds
B. 1,000 pounds
C. 2,000 pounds
D. 5,000 pounds
E. 7,000 pounds

Q 154. Maximal shortening of lower limb is with:
[Essential Orthopedics/Maheshwari/3rd Ed./Pg. 111]
A. Posterior dislocation
B. Central dislocation
C. Fracture neck of femur
D. Trochanteric fracture

Q 155. Most common recurrent dislocation is seen with:
[Essential Orthopedics/Maheshwari/3rd Ed./Pg. 74]
A. Shoulder
B. Patella
C. Elbow
D. Hip

Q 156. Most common ligament injured in ankle sprain:
Essential Orthopedics/Jayant Joshi/Reprint 2009/Pg. 556]
A. Anterior talofibular
B. Posterior talofibular
C. Deltoid
D. Spring ligament

Q 157. Medial meniscus is more injury, because:
[Orthopedic Physical Assessment/Magee/5th Ed./Pg. 790]
A. It is semilunar in shape
B. Medial portion is thicker
C. Medial collateral ligament is attached to it
D. Avascular

Posture

Q 158. Normal stride length is about:
[Joint Structure and Function/Norkin/Pg. 445]
A. 35 to 41 cm
B. 41 to 47 cm
C. 15 to 20 cm
D. 70 to 82 cm

Q 159. A physical therapist instructs a woman with left unilateral lower extremity weakness to descend stairs. The most appropriate position for the therapist to guard the patient is:
[Physical Rehabilitation/Sullivan/5th Ed./Pg. 556]
A. In front of the patient toward the left side
B. In front of the patient toward the right side
C. Behind the patient toward the left side
D. Behind the patient toward the right side

Q 160. A therapist completes a postural examination on a patient with low back ....deformity is often associated with weak abdominal muscles?
[Physical Rehabilitation/David J Magee/5th Ed./Pg. 531]
A. Increased lordosis
B. Decreased lordosis
C. Increased posterior pelvic tilt
D. Increased kyphosis

Q 161. Studies using intradiscal pressures in the lumbar spine have given physical therapists valuable information on the importance of body position. Which body position would you expect to place the most pressure on the lumbar spine:
[Physical Rehabilitation/David J Magee/5th Ed./Pg. 523]
A. Standing in the anatomical position
B. Standing with 45 degrees of hip flexion
C. Sitting in a chair
D. Sitting in a chair with reduced lumbar lordosis

Q 162. A physical therapist guards a patient during stair training. The most appropriate position for the therapist as the patient descends the stairs is:
[Physical Rehabilitation/Sullivan/5th Ed./Pg. 556]
A. Beside the patient on the involved side
B. Beside the patient on the uninvolved side
C. Behind the patient on the uninvolved side
D. In front of the patient on the involved side

Q 163. A physical therapist palpates along the lateral portion of the hamstring musculature to its tendinous attachment on the fibular head. The hamstring muscle should be identified as the:
[BDC/Vol. 2/4th Ed./Pg. 90]

Answer	147 B	148 A	149 C	150 E	151 A	152 B	153 E	154 A	155 A	156 A	157 A	158 D
	159 A	160 A	161 D	162 D								

A. Biceps femoris   B. Gracilis
C. Sartorius   D. Semitendinosus

Q 164. A physical therapist observes the standing posture of a patient from a lateral view. If the patient has normal anatomical alignment, a plumb line would fall:
[Joint Structure and Function/Norkin/3rd Ed./Pg. 412]
A. Posterior to the lobe of the ear
B. Anterior to the greater trochanter of the femur
C. Slightly anterior to a midline through the knee
D. Slightly posterior to the lateral malleolus

Q 165. A patient presents with orthostatic hypotension. The most appropriate treatment technique to assist the patient with standing is:
[Physical Rehabilitation/Sullivan/5th Ed./Pg. 111]
A. Standing in parallel bars for increasing time intervals
B. Using a standing table
C. Standing in a pool
D. Tilt table with progressive vertical positioning

Q 166. A therapist places a patient's knee in the resting position. This position is best described as:
[Orthopedic Physical Assessment/Magee/5th Ed./Pg. 727]
A. 5 degrees flexion   B. 15 degrees flexion
C. 25 degrees flexion   D. Complete extension

Gait and Locomotion

Q 167. The stance phase compromises of the following percentage of gait cycle during normal walking:
[Joint Structure and Function/Norkin Pg. 438]
A. 60%   B. 50%
C. 75%   D. 25%

Q 168. Weakness of hip flexors leads to:
[Kinesiology of Musculoskeletal System/Donald. A Neumann/ 1st Ed./Pg. 548]
A. Abducted gait   B. Lurching gait
C. Trendelenburg's gait   D. Circumduction gait

Q 169. In high steppage gait there is paralysis of:
[Kinesiology of Musculoskeletal System/Donald. A Neumann/ 1st Ed./Pg. 693]
A. Dorsiflexors of ankle   B. Plantar flexors of ankle
C. Extensors of knee joint D. Flexors of hip joint

Q 170. Average axial rotation of the lower extremity during walking is:
[Neumann/Pg. 542]
A. 8 degrees   B. 16 degrees
C. 24 degrees   D. 32 degrees

Q 171. A therapist completes a gait analysis of a patient rehabilitating from a motor vehicle accident. Which descriptive term is not associated with the stance phase of the gait cycle?
[Joint Structure and Function/Norkin/3rd Ed./Pg. 443]
A. Heel strike   B. Deceleration
C. Loading response   D. Midstance

Q 172. What muscle controls with position of the ankle joint at heel strike?
[Joint Structure and Function/Norkin/3rd Ed./Pg. 459]
A. Eccentric contraction of the anterior tibialis
B. Eccentric contraction of the gastrocnemius-soleus
C. Concentric contraction of the anterior tibialis
D. Concentric contraction of the gastrocnemius-soleus

Q 173. A 47-year-old male uses a straight cane during gait activities. The patient is two weeks status postoperative left total hip replacement using a posterolateral approach and is full weight bearing. Which of the following would not be considered good advice when making a 180 degree turn?
[Essential Orthopedics/Jayant Joshi/Reprint 2004/Pg. 208]
A. Move in a slow and cautions manner
B. Turn towards your affected side
C. Maintain an adequate base of support
D. Keep the cane in front of you

Q 174. A therapist examines a 25 year old male rehabilitating from a tibial plateau fracture. The physician orders indicate the patient is non-weight bearing on the involved lower extremity. The most appropriate gait pattern for the patient is:
[Hoppen field/Pg. 351]
A. Two-point   B. Three-point
C. Four-point   D. Swing-to

Q 175. A therapist instructs a patient ambulating with axillary crutches to move cautiously and deliberately on any potentially hazardous surface. Which gait pattern would allow the patient maximum security?
[Physical Rehabilitation/Sullivan/5th Ed./Pg. 549]
A. Swing-to   B. Swing-though
C. Three-point   D. Four-point

Q 176. A therapist measures a patient for a straight cane prior to beginning ambulation activities. Which gross measurement method would provide the best estimate of cane length?
[Roshan Meena concise/Exercise therapy/Pg. 77]
A. Measuring from the head of the fibula straight to the floor and multiplying by two
B. Measuring from the iliac crest straight to the floor
C. Measuring from the grate trochanter straight to the floor
D. Dividing the patient's height by two and adding three inches

Q 177. A physician instructs a therapist to begin gait training with a patient one day status post cemented total hip replacement. Assuming the patient has not had any significant problems postoperatively, which weight bearing status would be the most appropriate to begin the treatment session?
[Essential Orthopedics/Jayant Joshi/Reprint 2004/Pg. 209]
A. Nonweight bearing
B. Partial weight bearing
C. Weight bearing as tolerated
D. Full weight bearing

Q 178. A therapist observes a patient walking at various speeds. Which of the following does not occur as the speed of ambulation increases?
[Joint Structure and Function/Norkin/3rd Ed./Pg. 446]

Answer

163 A	164 C	165 D	166 C	167 A	168 D	169 A	170 A	171 B	172 A	173 B	174 B
175 D	176 C	177 A								

A. Stride length increases
B. Angle of toe out increases
C. Width of the base of support decreases
D. Cadence increases

Q 179. A physical therapist notes during a gait examination that a patient plantar flexes from neutral to 15 degrees as the lower extremity moves from initial contact to then of the loading response. This is indicative of:
[Joint Structure and Function/Norkin/3rd Ed./Pg. 440]
A. Early terminal stance
B. Decreased ankle motion
C. Normal gait pattern
D. Late terminal stance

Q 180. A patient positioned in kneeling works on weight shifting activities. Which stage of control is demonstrated with this activity?
[Physical Rehabilitation/Sullivan/5th Ed./Pg. 528]
A. Mobility
B. Stability
C. Controlled mobility
D. Skill

Q 181. A therapist attempts to identify an appropriate gait pattern for a patient with bilateral lower extremity involvement due to muscle weakness. The patient presents with balance and coordination deficits. The most appropriate gait pattern using axillary crutches is:
[Physical Rehabilitation/Sullivan/5th Ed./Pg. 548]
A. Swing-to
B. Swing-through
C. Four-point
D. Two-point

Q 182. Which of the following factors is of least importance when selecting an assistive device?
[Physical Rehabilitation/Sullivan/5th Ed./Pg. 541]
A. The patient's level of understanding
B. The patient's height and weight
C. The patient's upper and lower extremity strength
D. The patient's level of coordination

Q 183. A patient with a transfemoral amputation is referred to physical therapy for gait training. During the initial examination the therapist identifies lateral trunk bending towards the affected side during the stance phase of gait. A possible cause of this deviation is:
[Essential Orthopedics/Jayant Joshi/Reprint 2004/Pg. 248]
A. The prosthesis is too long
B. The prosthesis is too short
C. The socket diameter is too small
D. There is an increased amount of edema in the residual limb

Q 184. A physical therapist observes a patient ambulating with a normal gait pattern. The therapist notices that approximately _____ percent of the normal gait cycle is spent in the stance phase?
[Joint Structure and Function/Norkin/3rd Ed./Pg. 438]
A. 20
B. 40
C. 60
D. 80

Q 185. A patient who is partial weight bearing on the left ambulates with a walker. The patient advances the walker followed by a step with the left and then a step with the right. This gait pattern is termed:
[Physical Rehabilitation/Sullivan/5th Ed./Pg. 549]
A. Two-point
B. Three-point
C. Four-point
D. Swing-to

Q 186. A physical therapist treats a patient with a fractured left hip. The patient is weight bearing as tolerated and uses a large base quad cane for gait activities. Correct use of the quad cane would include:
[Physical Rehabilitation/Sullivan/5th Ed./Pg. 543]
A. Using the quad cane on the left with the longer legs positioned away from the patient
B. Using the quad cane on the right with the longer legs positioned away from the patient
C. Using the quad cane on the left with the longer legs positioned toward the patient
D. Using the quad cane on the right with the longer legs positioned toward the patient

Q 187. Which type of gait pattern would be most appropriate for a patient who exhibits unilateral lower extremity weakness?
[Physical Rehabilitation/Sullivan/5th Ed./Pg. 549]
A. Four-point
B. Two-point
C. Three-point
D. Swing-through

Q 188. A patient requires a walker for gait training. When fitting the walker for the patient the elbow should be place in:
[Physical Rehabilitation/Sullivan/5th Ed./Pg. 547]
A. 10 – 20 degrees of flexion
B. 20 – 30 degrees of flexion
C. 40 – 50 degrees of flexion
D. Complete Extension

Q 189. Weakness in the _______ would make it extremely difficult to ambulate on crutches?
[Joint Structure and Function/Norkin/3rd Ed./Pg. 440]
A. Medial deltoid
B. Erector spinae
C. Latissimus dorsi
D. Rhomboids

Q 190. A therapist instructs a patient diagnosed with multiple sclerosis to ambulate using two canes. Which gait pattern would be the most appropriate when using two canes?
[Physical Rehabilitation/Sullivan/5th Ed./Pg. 803]
A. Swing-to
B. Swing-through
C. Three-point gait
D. Four-point gait

Q 191. A physical therapist instructs a patient diagnosed with Parkinson's disease in ambulation activities. Which of the following would be helpful to improve the quality of the patient's gait:
[Physical Rehabilitation/Sullivan/5th Ed./Pg. 879]
A. Decrease stride length
B. Increase trunk rotation
C. Increase forward head posture
D. Decrease base of support

Q 192. A therapist observes the gait of a patient of post pneumonia. The therapist notices that the patient walks on his heels. Possible causes of this deviation include all of the following except:
[Joint Structure and Function/Norkin/3rd Ed./Pg. 478]

Answer 178 B 179 C 180 C 181 C 182 B 183 B 184 C 185 B 186 B 187 C 188 B 189 C
190 D 191 B

A. Weakness of the gastrocnemius muscle
B. Tightness of the dorsiflexor muscle
C. Decreased strength in the dorsiflexors
D. Pes calcaneus deformity

Q 193. A patient with latissimus dorsi and lower trapezius weakness would have the most difficulty performing which of the following activities?
[Physical Rehabilitation/Sullivan/5th Ed./Pg. 545]
A. Four-point gait with Lofstrand crutches
B. Modified two-point gait with a straight cane
C. Swing-through gait with axillary crutches
D. Wheelchair propulsions

Q 194. A student physical therapist is treating a 65 year old mildly obese patient. The patient is status post total hip replacement and is cleared for 25 pounds of weight bearing through the involved lower extremity. Appropriate assistive devices for gait training would include all of the following except:
[Essential Orthopedics/Jayant Joshi/Reprint 2009/Pg. 208]
A. Parallel Bars   B. Walker
C. Axillary Crutches   D. Straight Cane

Q 195. A physical therapist is required to train a 71-year-old patient to ascend and descend a flight of stairs. The patient presents with a fractured left tibia and is weight bearing as tolerated. There is moderate weakness in the involved lower extremity secondary to the fracture. The most appropriate instruction are:
[Physical Rehabilitation/Sullivan/5th Ed./Pg. 556]
A. "One step at a time, right foot first to ascend and to ascend and to descend the stairs."
B. "One step at a time, right foot first to ascend the stairs and left foot first to descend the stairs."
C. "Step over step slowly."
D. "One step at a time left foot first to ascend and to descend the stairs."

Q 196. A patient with an ankle foot orthosis demonstrates genu recurvatum during the stance phase of gait. Which action would be the most appropriate action to decrease the recurvatum?
[Joint Structure and Function/Norkin/3rd Ed./Pg. 473]
A. Increase the plantar flexion stop
B. Increase the dorsiflexion stop
C. Allow full range of motion at the ankle
D. Ankle joint position does not affect recurvatum

Q 197. A physical therapist observes excessive knee flexion from heel strike to midstance while observing patient with a transtibial amputation during gait training. A possible cause for this deviation is:
[Essential Orthopedics/Jayant Joshi/Reprint 2009/Pg. 249]
A. The foot is set in neutral
B. The socket is set posterior in relation to the foot
C. The prosthesis is too short
D. The socket is aligned in excessive flexion

Q 198. Which assistive device allows for a two-point, three-point, and four-point gait pattern?
[Physical Rehabilitation/Sullivan/5th Ed./Pg 548]

A. Straight cane   B. Walker
C. Quad cane   D. Axillary crutches

Q 199. A therapist orders a wheelchair for a patient with C5 tetraplegia. Which type of wheelchair would be the most appropriate for this patient?
[Physical Rehabilitation/Sullivan/5th Ed./Pg. 962]
A. Electric wheelchair
B. Manual wheelchair with handrim projections
C. Manual wheelchair with friction surface handrims
D. Manual wheelchair with standard handrims

Q 200. A 54 year old male rehabilitating from a fractured ankle is referred to physical therapy for gait training. The patient is in a short leg cast and is not permitted to bear weight through the involved lower extremity. Which gait pattern is the most appropriate for the patient?
[Physical Rehabilitation/Sullivan/5th Ed./Pg. 803]
A. Three-point gait using axillary crutches
B. Three-point swing-through using a walker
C. Three-point swing-to using a walker
D. Four-point alternating gait using axillary crutches

Q 201. A patient is referred to physical therapy for gait training following an extended illness. The patient has poor balance, but is able to move her legs alternately. Which of the following gait patterns would be the most stable?
[Physical Rehabilitation/Sullivan/5th Ed./Pg. 803]
A. Two-point   B. Three-point
C. Four-Point   D. Swing-through

Q 202. A therapist views a videotape which compares and contrasts the normal gait of toddlers and adults. Which of the following statements is not accurate when comparing the gait of these two groups?
[Joint Structure and Function/Norkin/3rd Ed./Pg. 472]
A. Toddlers walk with a wider base of support
B. Toddlers walk with an increased single leg support time
C. Toddlers walk with a higher cadence
D. Toddlers walk with a shorter step length

Q 203. A physical therapist observes a patient during gait training. The patient has normal strength and equal leg length. As the patient passes midstance he slightly vaults and has early toe off. The most likely cause of this deviation is:
[Joint Structure and Function/Norkin/3rd Ed./Pg. 478]
A. Patient has excessive forefoot pronation
B. Patient has limited hamstrings length
C. Patient has limited plantar flexion
D. Patient has limited dorsiflexion

Q 204. A physical therapist might select a metal upright ankle-foot orthosis instead of a plastic ankle-foot orthosis if the patient exhibits:
[Physical Rehabilitation/Sullivan/5th Ed./Pg. 1217]
A. Mild sensory loss   B. Significant fluctuating edema
C. Cosmetic concerns   D. Mediolateral ankle instability

Q 205. Which of the following muscles are stance phase muscles?
[Joint Structure and Function/Norkin/3rd Ed./Pg. 440]

Answer   192 C   193 B   194 D   195 B   196 A   197 D   198 D   199 B   200 A   201 C   202 B   203 D
204 B

A. Quadriceps
B. Hamstring muscles
C. Tibialis anterior
D. Peroneus longus
E. Soleus-gastrocnemius

Physiology

Q 206. The principle of diet planning for an individual comprises that out of the total calories requirement the carbohydrates should provide:

[Mcardle/4th Ed./Pg. 84]

A. 15% of the total calories required
B. 50% of the total calories required
C. 80% of the total calories required
D. 79% of the total calories required

Q 207. Coughing is usually considered a reflex controlled by afferent stimulation of the:

[Textbook of Physiology/AK Jain/Pg. 472]

A. Trigeminal nerve
B. Vagus nerve
C. Phrenic nerve
D. Glossopharyngeal nerve

Q 208. The normal A-VpO$_2$ difference is

[Textbook of Physiology/AK Jain/Pg. 460]

A. 5 mm Hg
B. 95 mm Hg
C. 9.5 mm Hg
D. 55 mm Hg

Q 209. The normal breath holding time in a normal young individual is:

[Textbook of Physiology/AK Jain/Pg. 481]

A. 2.5 mins
B. 22 secs
C. 45 – 55 secs
D. 10 secs

Q 210. With each 1*F rise in body temperature heart rate increases by about:

[Textbook of Physiology/AK Jain/Pg. 351]

A. 2 beats per minute
B. 3 beats per minute
C. 4 beats per minute
D. 10 beats per minute

Q 211. A 16-year-old male engaged in light work needs an average Kcal/day of:

[Mcardle/4th Ed./Pg. 86]

A. 2,000 Kcal/day
B. 10,000 Kcal/day
C. 3,500 Kcal/day
D. 1,500 Kcal/day

Q 212. In deep inspiration the central tendon of diaphragm is drawn downwards by:

[Mcardle/4th Ed.Pg. 86]

A. 2.7 cm
B. 1.5 cm
C. 7 cm
D. 1.7 cm

Q 213. The normal residual volume of air in lungs is

[Textbook of Physiology/AK Jain/Pg. 436]

A. 120 mL
B. 210 mL
C. 500 mL
D. 1200 mL

Q 214. The duration of normal cardiac cycle is:

[Textbook of Physiology/AK Jain/Pg. 297]

A. 2 sec
B. 1.2 sec
C. 0.8 sec
D. 1.8 sec

Q 215. In ECG "QRS" complex represents

[Textbook of Physiology/AK Jain/3rd Ed./Pg. 304]

A. Atrial depolarization
B. Atrial repolarization and closure of semilunar valves
C. Ventricular repolarization and opening of semilunar valves
D. Ventricular depolarization and it precedes ventricular systole

Q 216. The speed of conduction of impulse in a nerve fiber depends upon:

[Textbook of Physiology/AK Jain/3rd Ed./Pg. 1490]

A. The diameter
B. The strength of current
C. The muscles it supplies
D. Absence of myelin sheath

Q 217. In neuropraxia the conduction of impulse in a nerve is blocked due to:

[Essential Orthopedics/Maheshwari/Pg. 50]

A. Segmental demyelination
B. Wallerian degeneration
C. Division of nerve trunk
D. Neuroma

Q 218. The head of femur receives blood supply from:

[Human Anatomy/BD Chaurasia/Vol. 2/4th Ed./Pg. 56]

A. Medial and lateral femoral artery
B. Medial and lateral circumflex artery
C. Medial and lateral iliac artery
D. Medial and lateral gluteal artery

Q 219. Rhesus (Rh) factor is positive in:

[Textbook of Physiology/AK Jain/for PT and OT/4th Ed./Pg. 61]

A. 15% people
B. 26% people
C. 28% people
D. 85% people

Q 220. An athlete engaged in intense training can have expenditure of energy up-to:

[Mcardle/4th Ed./Pg. 769]

A. 1,800 Kcal per day
B. 3,000 Kcal per day
C. 5,000 Kcal per day
D. 10,000 Kcal per day

Q 221. Average chest expansion of an normal healthy Indian adult is:

[Mcardle/4th Ed./Pg. 220]

A. 3 cm
B. 5 cm
C. 7 cm
D. 9 cm

Q 222. The average rate of nerve regeneration after nerve repair is:

[Essential Orthopedics/Maheshwari/3rd Ed./Pg. 59]

A. 1 mm per day
B. 1 cm per day
C. 2 mm per day
D. 2 cm per day

Q 223. A therapist completes a fitness screening for a 34-year-old male prior to prescribing an aerobic exercise program. Which number is most representative of the patient's age predicted maximal heart rate?

[Mcardle/4th Ed./Pg. 266]

A. 168
B. 174
C. 180
D. 196

Q 224. A therapist commonly uses ice to decrease inflammation following arthroscopic surgery. Which type of pharmacological agent would have an antagonistic effect on joint inflammation?

[Mehta pub./J Maheshwari/3rd Ed./Pg. 257]

Answer	205 A	206 C	207 B	208 A	209 C	210 D	211 C	212 C	213 D	214 C	215 D	216 A
	217 A	218 B	219 D	220 C	221 B	222 A	223 C					

A. Anti-inflammatory steroids
B. Nonsteroidal anti-inflammatory drugs
C. Peripheral vasodilators
D. Systemic vasoconstrictors

Q 225. A therapist completes a developmental assessment of a seven month old infant. Assuming normal developmental which of the following reflexes would not be integrated?
[Sophie Levitt/4th Ed./Pg. 90]
A. Asymmetrical tonic neck reflex
B. Moro reflex
C. Landau reflex
D. Symmetrical tonic neck reflex

Q 226. Metabolic equivalents can be a useful device to compare the energy cost of various activities to the resting state. Which of the following activities would you expect to have the lowest metabolic equivalent?
[Textbook of Physiology/AK Jain/Pg. 447]
A. Ambulation with crutches B. Cycling at 10 mph
C. Sexual intercourse D. Walking at 3.0 mph

Q 227. A therapist records the vital signs of individuals at a health and wellness fair designed to promote physical therapy week. Which age group should the therapist expect to have the highest resting pulse rate?
[Joint Structure and Function/Norkin/3rd Ed./Pg. 440]
A. Infants B. Children
C. Teenagers D. Adults

Q 228. A therapist observes a patient's breathing as part of a respiratory assessment. Which muscle of respiration most active during expiration?
[Human Anatomy/Vol. 1/BDC/4th Ed./Pg. 207]
A. Diaphragm B. External intercostals
C. Internal intercostals D. Upper trapezius

Q 229. A physical therapist records the blood pressure of a ten year old child. Which measurement would be considered normal for this age group?
[Mcardle/4th Ed./Pg. 269]
A. 40 mm Hg systolic, 70 mm Hg diastolic
B. 90 mm Hg systolic, 60 mm Hg diastolic
C. 115 mm Hg systolic, 70 mm Hg diastolic
D. 130 mm Hg systolic, 85 mm Hg diastolic

Q 230. A physical therapist instructs a female athlete to complete ten minutes of stretching before beginning her treadmill program. While observing the athlete stretching her hamstring, the therapist notices repetitive bouncing and a failure to maintain the stretch for more than five seconds. Why is this type stretching considered to be inadequate?
[Therapeutic Exercise/Kisner/4th Ed./Pg. 178]
A. The athlete should maintain each stretch for at least 30 seconds
B. The athlete should stretch only after running on the treadmill
C. The athlete is activating the stretch reflex
D. The athlete should remain activity specific and does not need to stretch the hamstrings if she is running on the treadmill

Q 231. A therapist attempts to assess the dorsal pedal pulse of a patient diagnosed with peripheral vascular disease. The locate the dorsal pedal pulse the therapist should palpate:
[Human Anatomy/BDC/Vol. 2/4th Ed./Pg. 104]
A. Between the extensor hallucis longus and the extensor digitorum longus tendons on the dorsum of the foot
B. Between the flexor digitorum longus and the flexor hallucis longus tendons on the dorsum of the foot
C. Immediately posterior to the medial malleolus
D. Immediately posterior to the lateral malleolus

Q 232. A therapist determines a patient's heart rate by counting the number of QRS complexes in a six second electrocardiogram strip. Assuming the therapist identifies eight QRS complexes in the strip, the patient's heart rate should be recorded as:
[Mcardle/4th Ed./Pg. 287]
A. 40 bpm B. 60 bpm
C. 80 bpm D. 100 bpm

Q 233. A patient with an irregular heart rate is monitored using a single lead electrocardiogram during exercise. Which of the following techniques would provide the therapist with the most accurate measurement of heart rate?
[Mcardle/4th Ed./Pg. 287]
A. Count the number of QRS complexes that occur in sixty seconds
B. Count the number of R waves the occur in thirty second and multiply by two
C. Count the number of P wave that occur in fifteen seconds and multiply by four
D. Count the number of T waves that occur in six seconds and multiply by ten

Q 234. A therapist reviews the results of a patients arterial blood gases. The report indicates the following: PaO_2 = 45 mm Hg, $PaCO_2$ = 55 mm, HCO_3 = 24 mEq/L, pH = 7.20. These values are most indicative of:
[Textbook of Physiology/AK Jain/Vol. 1/3rd Ed./Pg. 478]
A. Respiratory acidosis B. Respiratory alkalosis
C. Metabolic acidosis D. Metabolic alkalosis

Q 235. Patients are often placed on diuretics to control high blood pressure and fluid retention. Which of the flowing side effects of diuretics can require immediate medical attentions?
[Textbook of Physiology/AK Jain/Vol. 1/3rd/Pg. 560]
A. Elevated cholesterol and lipoprotein levels
B. Nausea
C. Elevated white blood cell count
D. Potassium depletion

Q 236. A therapist develops an exercise program for a young boy with insulin dependent diabetes. What effect does exercise have on the patient's insulin requirements?
[Textbook of Physiology/AK Jain/Vol. 1/3rd Ed./Pg. 771]
A. Exercise may reduce a patient's insulin requirements
B. Exercise often increases a patient's insulin requirements
C. Exercise has no effect on a patient's insulin requirements
D. Exercise is contraindicated for insulin dependent diabetics

---

Answer 224 C 225 C 226 D 227 A 228 C 229 C 230 C 231 A 232 C 233 A 234 A 235 D 236 A

Q 237. A therapist determines that patient's age predicted maximal heart rate is 165 beats per minute. Which of the following would be most representative of the patient's target heart rate during cardiovascular exercise?
[Physical Rehabilitation/Sullivan/5th Ed./Pg. 598]
A. 82 – 99 beats per minute   B. 99 – 115 beats per minute
C. 99 – 132 beats per minute   D. 132 – 148 beats per minute

Q 238. A note in a patient's medical chart indicates the presence of an acid-base disturbance of metabolic origin. Which condition is not typically associated with metabolic acidosis?
[Textbook of Physiology/AK Jain/Vol. 1/3rd Ed./Pg. 478]
A. Vomiting   B. Secondary hyperventilation
C. Lethargy   D. Syncope

Q 239. A therapist revises literature which details the expected changes in endurance and physical work capacity as an individual progress from middle age to an older adult. Which or the following measurements would not be affected by this transition?
[Physical Rehabilitation/Sullivan/5th Ed./Pg. 601]
A. Resting heart rate
B. Stroke volume
C. Cardiac output
D. Blood pressure

Q 240. A physical therapist studies a normal resting electrocardiogram for one cardiac cycle. What wave or change in shape of the electrocardiogram results from atrial depolarization?
[Physical Rehabilitation/Sullivan/5th Ed./Pg. 603]
A. P wave   B. QRS complex
C. ST segment   D. T wave

Q 241. A therapist records the blood pressure of a two-year-old child in the medical record. Assuming normal values the most typical blood pressure reading is:
[Textbook of Physiology/AK Jain/Vol. 1/3rd/Pg. 35]
A. 80 systolic, 35 diastolic   B. 85 systolic, 60 diastolic
C. 105 systolic, 65 diastolic   D. 120 systolic, 80 diastolic

Biomechanics of Bone

Q 242. Skeletal muscles in a normal adult contribute:
A. 10 to 15% to the total body weight
B. 15 to 20% to the total body weight
C. 40 to 50% to the total body weight
D. 0 to 5% to the total body weight

Q 243. The frequency of post-traumatic osteonecrosis of femoral head is highest in which age group:
[Essential Orthopedic/Maheshwari/Pg. 188]
A. 1 – 10 yrs   B. 10 – 30 yrs
C. 30 – 60 yrs   D. Above 60 yrs

Q 244. The frequency of aseptic necrosis of femoral head in hip dislocations is highest in:
[Essential of Orthopedics/Maheshwari/Pg. 112]
A. Children   B. Adolescents
C. Adults   D. Old persons

Q 245. Length growth of bone is accomplished by:
[Essential of Orthopedics/Maheshwari/Pg. 8]
A. Periosteum   B. Epiphysis
C. Metaphysic   D. Epiphyseal plate

Q 246. The first bone to ossify in fetal life is:
[BDC/4th Ed./Pg. 7]
A. Skull   B. Vertebrae
C. Clavicle   D. Femur

Q 247. The most uncommon site for secondary deposits in bone is:
[Essential of Orthopedics/Maheshwari/Pg. 225]
A. Skull   B. Spine
C. Pelvis   D. Calcaneum

Q 248. The following bone is a pneumatic bone:
[BDC/Vol. 3/4th Ed./Pg. 35]
A. Patella   B. Pisiform
C. Maxilla   D. 12th pair of rib

Q 249. The best technique to demonstrate the orientation of collagen fibers within bone:
[Joint Structure and Function/Norkin/3rd Ed./Pg. 53]
A. Toluidine Blue Strain   B. H&E strain
C. Polarized light   D. Ultraviolet light

Q 250. The structure responsible for longitudinal growth is:
[Essential of Orthopedics/Maheshwari/3rd Ed./Pg. 7]
A. Epiphysis   B. Epiphyseal plate
C. Metaphysis   D. Diaphysis

Q 251. The pre-cartilaginous analog to bone arises from:
[Joint Structure and Function/Norkin/Pg. 65]
A. Ectoderm   B. Endoderm
C. Mesenchyme   D. None of the above

Q 252. Distal femoral epiphysis is seen at the age of:
[BDC/Vol. 2/4th Ed./Pg. 22]
A. Just after birth   B. 10 weeks
C. 20 weeks   D. 34 weeks

Q 253. Most common bone to fracture in body is:
[Essential of Orthopedics/Jayant Joshi/Reprint 2009/Pg. 74]
A. Radius   B. Clavicle
C. Femur   D. Vertebra
E. Pelvis

Q 254. Longitudinal bone growth is dependent on:
[Essential of Orthopedics/Maheshwari/3rd Ed./Pg. 8]
A. Metaphysis   B. Diaphysis
C. Epiphysis   D. None

Tissue Biomechanics

Q 255. Most sensitive structure in a joint is:
[Joint Structure and Function/Norkin/3rd Ed./Pg. 70]
A. Articular cartilage   B. Synovium
C. Fibrous capsule   D. Bone

Q 256. Cartilage is quite vascular in:
[Joint Structure and Function/Norkin/3rd Ed./Pg. 56]

Answer											
237 C	238 D	239 A	240 A	241 B	242 C	243 D	244 D	245 D	246 C	247 A	248 C
249 B	250 B	251 C	252 C	253 B	254 C	255 C					

A. Embryonic life
B. Early childhood
C. Early adulthood
D. Old age

Q 257. The characteristic of collagen is presence of:
[Joint Structure and Function/Norkin/3rd Ed./Pg. 56]

A. Glycine
B. Methionine
C. Hydroxyproline
D. None of the above

Q 258. The factors responsible for viscosity of synovial fluid is/are:

[Joint Structure and Function/Norkin/ 3rd Ed./Pg. 71]

A. Chondroitin sulphate
B. Hyaluronic acid
C. Heparin sulphate
D. All of the above

Q 259. Which of the following is not found normally in synovial membrane?
[Joint Structure and Function/Norkin/3rd Ed./Pg. 71]

A. Two layers of lymphatics
B. Pacinian corpuscles
C. Basement membrane
D. A fibrocollagenous layer

Q 260. In long-term therapy vitamin-D resistant rickets, the best guide to safe treatment is:
[AK Jain/Vol. 1/3rd Ed./Pg. 720]

A. Urinary phosphate excretion
B. Urinary calcium excretion
C. Serum alkaline phosphatase
D. Serum phosphate level
E. Serum calcium level

Answer   256 A   257 A   258 B   259 A   260 E

4

Orthopedics

Objective Questions with Answers

Rheumatoid Arthritis

Q 1. Treatment of rheumatoid arthritis include all except:
[Karen At Kinson, et al./Elsevier/2005,203
A. Give rest to the joint   B. Correction of deformities
C. Synovectomy   D. Exercises
E. Immunosuppressive drugs

Q 2. Following is involved in rheumatoid arthritis:
[J. Ebnezar/1st Ed./Pg. 393]

A. Synovial fluid   B. Synovial membrane
C. Cartilage   D. Subchondral bone

Q 3. The cause of rheumatoid arthritis is:
[J. Ebnezar/1st Ed./Pg. 392]

A. Familial   B. Immunological
C. Infective   D. Traumatic

Q 4. Epiphyseal wafering may be seen in:
A. Rheumatic arthritis
B. Juvenile rheumatoid arthritis
C. Osteoarthritis
D. Gouty arthritis

Q 5. Distal interphalangeal joint is not involved in:
[J. Ebnezar/1st Ed./Pg. 365]
A. Rheumatoid arthritis   B. Osteoarthritis
C. Psoriatic arthropathy   D. Multiple histiocytosis

Q 6. In rheumatic arthritis the pathology starts in:
[Essential Orthopedics/Maheshwari/3rd Ed./Pg. 345]
A. Articular cartilage   B. Synovial
C. Capsule   D.   Muscles

Q 7. Para-articular erosions are most commonly seen in:
[Essential Orthopedics/Maheshwari/3rd Ed./Pg. 246]
A. Osteoarthritis   B. Rheumatoid arthritis
C. Gout   D. Acute suppurative arthritis

Q 8. Tom Smith arthritis manifest as:
[Essential Orthopedics/Maheshwari/3rd Ed./Pg. 166]

A. Increase hip mobility and instability
B. Hip stiffness
C. a + b
D. Shortening of limb

Q 9. Disease where distal interphalangeal joint is characteristically involved:
[Essential Orthopedics/Maheshwari/3rd Ed./Pg. 251]
A. Psoriatic arthritis   B. Rheumatoid
C. SLE   D. Gout

Q 10. The rheumatoid factor immunoglobulin is against:
[Medicine/Davidson/20th Ed./Pg 1105]
A. Fab portion of immunoglobulin
B. Fc portion of immunoglobulin
C. Double strand DNA
D. Mitochondria

Q 11. In rheumatoid arthritis the part which is affected most is:
[Essential Orthopedics/Maheshwari/ Pg. 244]

A. Synovium   B. Subchondral bone
C. Cartilage   D. Tendon

Q 12. Most common cause of septic arthritis in all ages:
[Essential Orthopedics/Maheshwari/ Pg. 163]

A. *Streptococcus*   B. *Staphylococcus*
C. *Gonococcus*   D. *Pseudomonas*

Osteoarthritis

Q 13. Herbeden's nodules are seen in:
[Turek's/4th Ed./Pg. 388]
A. Osteoarthritis   B. Rheumatoid arthritis
C. Rheumatic arthritis   D. Psoriatic arthritis

Q 14. Commonest degenerative joint disease is:
[J. Ebnezar/1st Ed./Pg. 380]
A. Gout   B. Osteoporosis
C. Rheumatoid arthritis   D. Osteoarthritis

Answer   1 A   2 B   3 B   4 B   5 A   6 B   7 B   8 A   9 A   10 B   11 A   12 B
     13 A   14 D

Q 15. Osteoarthritis does not affect:
[J. Ebnezar/1st Ed./Pg. 381]
A. Knee joint
B. Hip joint
C. Interphalangeal joint
D. Metacarpophalangeal joint
E. Shoulder joint

Q 16. Which of the following is not a predisposing factor for osteoarthritis (OA):
[J. Ebnezar/1st Ed./Pg. 381]
A. Diabetes mellitus
B. Defective joint Position
C. Weight bearing joints
D. Incongruity of articular surfaces
E. Old age

Q 17. Treatment of osteoarthritis include all except:
[Essential Orthopedics/Maheshwari/3rd Ed./Pg. 253]
A. Graded muscle exercises
B. Replacement of articular surfaces
C. Correction of deformities
D. Increase the weight bearing by the affected joint
E. Rest to the joint in acute phase

Fracture

Q 18. Avascular necrosis of head of femur can occur in :
[Essential Orthopedics/Maheshwari/2005/Pg. 118]
A. Sickle cell anemia
B. Caison's disease
C. Intracapsular fracture neck
D. Trochanteric fracture

Q 19. The long flexor tendon of the thumb can be advanced for more than 1 cm for repair in Zone 1 because:
[Kinesiology of Musculoskeletal System/Neumann/1st Ed./Pg. 217]
A. Paratendinous adhesions are fewer following advancement than following free tendon graft
B. Only two annular pulleys bind the tendon to bone
C. Vascularity of the tendon is not compromised because vinculum is absent
D. The tendon is long enough to allow easy advancement

Q 20. March Fracture is:
[Essential Orthopedics/Maheshwari/2005/Pg. 203]
A. Stress fracture of neck of second metatarsal
B. Stress fracture of neck of talus
C. Compression fracture of calcaneum
D. Fracture lower end of fibula

Q 21. Commonest complication of extra capsular fracture of neck of femur is:
[Essential Orthopedics/Maheshwari/2005/Pg. 119]
A. Nonunion
B. Ischemic necrosis
C. Malunion
D. Pulmonary complications

Q 22. The best radiological view for fracture scaphoid is:
[Refer to Text]
A. AP
B. PA
C. Lateral
D. Oblique

Q 23. Commonest fracture in childhood is:
[Essential Orthopedics/Maheshwari/3rd ed/Pg. 46]
A. Femur
B. Distal humerus
C. Clavicle
D. Radius

Q 24. Fracture femur in infants is best treated by:
[J. Ebnezar/1st Ed./Pg. 129]
A. Open reduction
B. Closed reduction
A. IM nailing
B. Gallows splinting

Q 25. Treatment of fracture patella in 24-year-old young male is:
[Essential Orthopedics/Maheshwari/3rd Ed./Pg. 126]
A. Patellectomy if undisplaced
B. No treatment required
C. Internal fixation if comminuted fracture
D. POP in full extension

Q 26. Nonunion in long bones is treated by:
[Essential Orthopedics/Maheshwari/3rd Ed./Pg. 39]
A. Intramedullary nailing
B. Pop cast
C. Conservative treatment
D. Open reduction and internal fixation with bone grafting

Q 27. An oblique fracture of olecranon if displaced proximally. The treatment is:
[Essential Orthopedics/Maheshwari/3rd Ed./Pg. 88]
A. Excision and re-suturing
B. Tension band wiring
C. Resection
D. Elbow is immobilized in cast

Q 28. Bennet's fracture is fracture dislocation of base of metacarpal:
[Essential Orthopedics/Maheshwari/3rd Ed./Pg. 2]
A. 4th
B. 3rd
C. 2nd
D. 1st

Q 29. Patient when comes with fracture femur in an acute accident, the first thing to do:
[Essential Orthopedics/Maheshwari/3rd Ed/Pg. 11]
A. Secure airway and treat the shock
B. Splinting
C. Physical examination
D. X-rays

Q 30. Which fracture in children requires operative reduction?
[Essential Orthopedics/Maheshwari/3rd Ed./Pg. 48]
A. Epiphyseal separation
B. Both upper limb bones
C. Dislocation of humerus
D. Fracture humerus

Q 31. Meyer's operation is done for:
[Essential Orthopedics/Maheshwari/3rd Ed./Pg. 117]
A. Dislocation of patella
B. Fracture neck of femur
C. Dislocation of shoulder
D. fibula fracture

Q 32. Commonest complication of intracapsular Fracture neck of femur is:
[Essential Orthopedics/Maheshwari/3rd Ed./Pg. 117]
A. Osteoarthritis
B. Shortening
C. Malunion
D. Nonunion

Q 33. Battle's sign is seen in:
A. Fracture middle cranial fossa
B. Fracture base of skull
C. Fracture anterior cranial fossa
D. all of the above

Answer	15 D	16 A	17 D	18 C	19 A	20 A	21 C	22 D	23 C	24 D	25 D	26 D
	27 B	28 D	29 A	30 A	31 B	32 D	33 A					

Q 34. Which is true about Perthe's disease?
[Essential Orthopedics/Maheshwari/3rd Ed.Pg. 270]
A. Not painful
B. It manifests at puberty
C. Involves fracture of neck of femur
D. Viral etiology

Q 35. Open reduction in children is done for:
[Essential Orthopedics/Maheshwari/3rd Ed./Pg. 48]
A. Supracondylar fracture   B. Forearm both bone fracture
C. Femoral condyle fracture   D. Lateral condylar fracture

Q 36. Which Fracture in children requires open reduction?
[Essential Orthopedics/Maheshwari/3rd Ed./Pg. 47]
A. Fracture tibial epiphysis
B. Fracture shaft of femur
C. Fracture both bones forearm
D. Fracture femoral condyle

Q 37. Reduction of Bennett's fracture is difficult to keep in position due to the pull of:
[J. Ebnezar/1st Ed./Pg. 111]
A. Abductor pollicis brevis   B. Abductor pollicis longus
C. Flexor pollicis longus   D. flexor pollicis brevis

Q 38. Which one of the following statements is not correct regarding fracture of the scaphoid?
[Essential Orthopedics/Maheshwari/3rd Ed/Pg. 97]
A. It is the most commonly fractured carpal bone
B. Persistent tenderness in the anatomical snuffbox is highly suggestive of fracture
C. Immediate X ray of hand may not reveal fracture line
D. Malunion is a frequent complication

Q 39. The treatment of choice in grade 4 subcapital fractured neck of femur in a 50 year old patient:
[J. Ebnezar/1st Ed./Pg. 121]
A. Pin in situ   B. Reduction
C. Hemiarthroplasty   D. Total hip replacement

Q 40. The ideal treatment of a 3-day- old fracture neck of femur is a 50-year- old male would be:
[J. Ebnezar/1st Ed./Pg. 420]
A. Compression screw fixation
B. POP hip spica
C. Hemi replacement arthroplasty
D. Total hip replacement

Q 41. Which is not a principle of compound fracture treatment?
[J. Ebnezar/1st Ed./Pg. 36]
A. No tendon repair
B. Aggressive Antibiotic cover
C. Wound debridement
D. Immediate wound closure

Q 42. Stress fractures are known to occur in the:
[J. Ebnezar/1st Ed./Pg. 36]
A. Metatarsals   B. Tibia
C. Femur   D. Pelvis
E. Radius and ulna

Q 43. Intramedullary nailing is contraindicated in fracture shaft femur if:
[J. Ebnezar/1st Ed./Pg. 130]
A. The fracture is compound
B. The fracture is near the knee joint
C. The epiphysis have not fused
D. Any of the above is present
E. None of the above is present

Q 44. In fracture neck of femur in a 64-year-old-lady the treatment of choice is:
[Essential Orthopedics/Maheshwari/3rd Ed./Pg. 117]
A. Prosthetic replacement of head of femur
B. Conservative
C. Austin Moore's pin
D. S P nailing

Q 45. Fracture neck of femur in old persons is best treated by:
[Essential Orthopedics/Maheshwari/3rd Ed./Pg. 117]
A. Replacement arthroplasty
B. Thomas splint support
C. No treatment
D. Internal fixation with S P nail

Q 46. Treatment after removal of plaster for supracondylar fracture of humerus is:
[Essential Orthopedics/Maheshwari/3rd Ed./Pg. 83]
A. Active mobilization at elbow joint
B. Massage
C. No treatment
D. Passive movements at elbow joint

Q 47. Most common type of Supracondylar fracture is
[J. Ebnezar/1st Ed./Pg. 190]
A. Extension type   B. Flexion type
C. Abduction type   D. Adduction type

Q 48. Excision of fractured fragment is practised in all fractures except:
[J. Ebnezar/1st Ed./Pg. 151]
A. Patella   B. Olecranon
C. Head of radius   D. Lateral condyle of humerus

Q 49. The most preferred treatment of fracture of neck of femur in young person is:
[Essential Orthopedics/Maheshwari/3rd Ed./Pg. 116]
A. Hemiarthroplasty
B. Total hip replacement
C. Conservative treatment
D. Closed reduction & Internal fixation

Q 50. In treatment of hand injuries the greatest priority is:
[J. Ebnezar/1st Ed./Pg. 275]
A. Repair of tendons   B. Restoration of skin cover
C. Repair of nerves   D. Repair of blood vessels

Q 51. Oblique view is required to diagnosis fracture of:
[Essential Orthopedics/Maheshwari/3rd Ed./Pg. 97]
A. Capitate   B. Scaphoid
C. Navicular   D. Hamate

Answer	34 C	35 B	36 A	37 B	38 D	39 D	40 A	41 D	42 B	43 D	44 A	45 A
	46 A	47 A	48 B	49 D	50 B	51 B						

Q 52. Transverse fracture of medial malleolus is caused by:
[Essential Orthopedics/Maheshwari/3rd Ed./Pg. 137]
A. Abduction
B. Adduction
C. Rotation of foot
D. Dorsiflexion of foot

Q 53. Most common bone fracture in body is:
[Essential Orthopedics/Maheshwari/3rd Ed./Pg. 73]
A. Radius
B. Clavicle
C. Femur
D. Vertebra
E. Pelvis

Q 54. After a fall from a height calcaneal fracture is associated with fracture of:
[Essential Orthopedics/Maheshwari/3rd Ed./Pg. 144]
A. Tibia
B. Vertebra
C. Pelvis
D. Femur

Q 55. Commonest site of fracture scaphoid:
[Essential Orthopedics/Maheshwari/3rd Ed./Pg. 96]
A. Waist
B. Proximal third
C. Distal third
D. Tuberculosis

Q 56. Which of the following is best related to fat embolism?
[Essential Orthopedics/Maheshwari/3rd Ed./Pg. 122]
A. 20% of polytrauma
B. 40% of Bilateral fracture femur
C. 90% of trauma
D. Only 15%

Q 57. Suspected medial epicondylar fracture of humerus in:
[Essential Orthopedics/Maheshwari/3rd Ed./Pg. 81]
A. X-ray both arms with elbow by comparison
B. X-ray same limb only
C. Examination under general anesthesia
D. POP in full flexed position

Q 58. Treatment at choice or fracture neck of humerus in a 70-year-old male:
[Essential Orthopedics/Maheshwari/3rd Ed./Pg. 76]
A. Analgesic with arm sling
B. U-slab
C. Arthroplasty
D. Open reduction + Internal fixation

Q 59. A young adult presenting with oblique, displaced fracture olecranon treatment of choice:
[Essential Orthopedics/Maheshwari/3rd Ed./Pg. 88]
A. Plaster cast
B. Percutaneous wiring
C. Tension band wiring
D. Removal of displaced piece with triceps repair

Q 60. The treatment of choice for non-union of extracapsular fracture neck femur:
[Essential Orthopedics/Maheshwari/3rd Ed./Pg. 119]
A. Hip spica
B. Intramedullary nailing
C. Internal fixation
D. Compression plating

Q 61. Least correction in remodeling of bone in children is seen in:
[Essential Orthopedics/Maheshwari/3rd Ed./Pg. 48]
A. Fracture shaft of humerus
B. Fracture shaft of femur
C. Subtrochanteric fracture

Q 62. Late complication of acetabular fracture:
[Essential Orthopedics/Maheshwari/3rd Ed./Pg. 118]
A. Avascular necrosis of head of femur
B. Avascular necrosis at iliac crest
C. Fixed deformity of the hip joint
D. Secondary osteoarthritis of hip joint

Q 63. In Colle's fracture what is not seen in:
[J. Ebnazar/1st Ed./Pg. 108]
A. Proximal impaction
B. Lateral rotation
C. Dorsal angulation
D. Medial rotation

Q 64. In the case of 65-year-old person with fracture neck of femur the treatment of choice is:
[Essential Orthopedics/Maheshwari/3rd Ed./Pg. 116]
A. Close reduction
B. Close reduction with internal fixation
C. Open reduction
D. Replacement of head and neck of the femur with prosthesis

Q 65. Least Common complication of Colle's fracture:
[Essential Orthopedics/Maheshwari/3rd Ed./Pg. 96]
A. Malunion
B. Nonunion
C. Stiffness of fingers
D. Sudeck's dystrophy

Q 66. Meyer's operation is done for:
[Essential Orthopedics/Maheshwari/3rd Ed./Pg. 298]
A. Recurrent dislocation of patella
B. Dislocation of shoulder joint
C. Dislocation of hip joint
D. Fracture of scaphoid

Q 67. Fracture blisters commonly appear on how many days?
[Orthopaedics and Applied physiotherapy/Jayant Joshi/Pg. 65]
A. 1 – 3 days
B. 3 – 5 days
C. 5 – 7 days
D. 5 – 9 days

Q 68. Most common site of fracture in osteoporosis:
[Essential Orthopedics/Maheshwari/3rd Ed./Pg. 261]
A. Fracture neck femur
B. Vertebra
C. Hip bone
D. Humerus

Q 69. Which fracture neck of femur has a poor prognosis?
[Essential Orthopedics/Maheshwari/3rd Ed./Pg. 118]
A. Intracapsular
B. Extracapsular
C. Both
D. None

Q 70. Multiple bone fracture in a new born is seen in:
[Essential Orthopedics/Maheshwari/3rd Ed./Pg. 269]
A. Scurvy
B. Syphilis
C. Osteogenesis imperfecta
D. Morquio's syndrome

Q 71. A segmental compound fracture of tibia with 1cm skin wound is classified as:
[Orthopaedics and Applied Physiotherapy/Jayant Joshi/Pg. 56]
A. Type I
B. Type II
C. Type IIIA
D. Type IIIB

Answer	52 A	53 B	54 B	55 A	56 B	57 A	58 A	59 C	60 C	61 A	62 A	63 D
	64 D	65 B	66 C	67 B	68 B	69 A	70 C	71 A				

Q 72. A Bennet's fracture is difficult to maintain in reduced position because of the pull of:
[Clinical Orthopedic Rehabilitation/Brotzman 2nd Ed.]
A. Extensor pollicis longus   B. Extensor pollicis brevis
C. Abductor pollicis longus   D. Abductor pollicis brevis

Q 73. Ideal treatment with fracture neck of humerus in a lady will be:
[Essential Orthopedics/Maheshwari/3rd Ed/Pg. 76]
A. Triangular sling   B. Hemiarthroplasty
C. Chest arm bandage   D. Internal fixation

Q 74. What is the position of immobilization in fracture of both bones of the forearm in an adult male?
[Refer to Text]
A. Prone   B. Mid-prone
C. Full supine   D. 10 degree supine

Q 75. Avascular necrosis is commonest in one of the following fractures:
[Jayant Joshi/Prakash Katwal/Pg. 522]
A. Gorden 1 & 2 fracture of femoral neck
B. Gorden 3 & 4 fracture of femoral neck
C. Subtrochanteric fracture of femoral neck
D. Basotrochanteric fracture

Q 76. Carpal bone which fractures commonly:
[Refer to Text]
A. Scaphoid   B. Lunate
C. Hamate   D. Pisiform

Q 77. Treatment of fracture head of Radius in young patients:
[Orthopaedics and Applied Physiotherapy/Jayant Joshi/Pg. 98]
A. Excision of head of Radius,
B. Immobilization in cast
C. Late excision after trial immobilization,
D. None of the above

Q 78. March fracture affects:
[Essential Orthopedics/Maheshwari/3rd Ed./Pg. 3]
A. Neck of 2nd metatarsal
B. Body of 2nd metatarsal
C. Neck of 1st metatarsal
D. Fracture of lower end of tibia
E. Fracture of lower end of fibula

Q 79. In supracondylar fracture, the segment is often displaced:
[Orthopaedics and Applied Physiotherapy/Jayant Joshi/Pg. 89]
A. Laterally   B. Medially
C. Anteriorly   D. Posteriorly

Q 80. Osteotomy done for malunited supracondylar fracture is:
[Essential Orthopedics/Maheshwari/ 3rd Ed./Pg. 68]
A. French   B. Shan's
C. McMurray's   D. McAllister

Q 81. Treatment of choice in an elderly lady with fracture shaft of humerus is:
[Essential Orthopedics/Maheshwari/Pg. 77]
A. Open reduction and internal fixation
B. External fixation
C. Traction
D. Pop immobilization

Q 82. The last step in the healing a fracture is:
[Essential Orthopedics/Maheshwari/Pg. 9]
A. Hematoma formation   B. Consolidation
C. Remodeling   D. Callus formation
E. Demineralization of bones

Q 83. Transverse fracture of patella in a young adult. What is the treatment of choice?
[Essential Orthopedics/Maheshwari/Pg. 126]
A. Tension band wiring   B. Cylinder cast
C. Patellectomy   D. Conservative

Q 84. An army recruit, smoker and 6 months into training started complaining of pain at posterior medial aspect of both legs. There was acute point tenderness and the pain was aggravated on physical activity. The most likely diagnosis is:
[Essential Orthopedics/Maheshwari/Pg. 261]
A. Buerger's disease   B. Gout
C. Lumbar canal stenosis   D. Stress fracture

Q 85. Shepherd's Crooke's deformity is seen in:
[Medicine/Davidson/20th Ed./Pg. 748]
A. Achondroplasia   B. Gaucher's disease
C. Hypothyroidism   D. Fibrous dysplasia

Q 86. In transverse fracture of the patella, the treatment is:
[Orthopaedics and Applied Physiotherapy/Jayant Joshi/Pg. 167]
A. Excision of a small fragment
B. Wire fixation
C. Plaster cylinder
D. Patellectomy

Bone Disease

Q 87. Which is the most common site of osteoclastoma?
[Essential Orthopedics/Maheshwari/2005/Pg. 216]
A. Lower end of femur   B. Upper end tibia
C. Lower humerus   D. Upper radius

Q 88. Commonest site for Osteogenic sarcomas:
[Essential Orthopedics/Maheshwari/2005/Pg. 218]
A. Upper end of femur   B. Lower end of femur
C. Upper end of tibia   D. Lower end of tibia

Q 89. In multiple myeloma which of the following is seen:
[Essential Orthopedics/Maheshwari/2005/Pg. 223]
A. Raised serum calcium
B. Raised alkaline phosphatase
C. Raised acid phosphatase
D. All

Q 90. Commonest benign bone tumor is:
[Essential Orthopedics/Maheshwari/2005/Pg. 225]
A. Bone cyst   B. Chondroma
C. Chordoma   D. Osteoma

Q 91. Commonest tumor arising from the metaphysis is:
[Essential Orthopedics/Maheshwari/2005/Pg. 222]
A. Osteoclastoma   B. Osteosarcoma
C. Ewing's sarcoma   D. Synovial sarcoma

Answer	72 C	73 A	74 D	75 B	76 A	77 B	78 A	79 D	80 A	81 D	82 C	83 A
	84 D	85 C	86 B	87 A	88 B	89 A	90 B	91 B				

Q 92. Which is true regarding acute osteomyelitis:
[Essential Orthopedics/Maheshwari/2005/Pg. 157-160]
A. Staphylococcus is the usual organism
B. Rest and elevation relieves pain
C. Parenteral antibiotics are given
D. Surgery is the only treatment

Q 93. Increased density of skull vault is seen in:
[Samuell L. turek/4th Ed./Pg. 742]
A. Hyperparathyroidism   B. Multiple myeloma
C. Fluorosis   D. Renal osteodystrophy

Q 94. Treatment of solitary bone cyst is:
[Apley and Soloman/7th Ed./Pg. 174]
A. Curettage
B. Excision
C. Curettage and bone grafting
D. Irradiation

Q 95. The 1st sign of TB is:
[Essential Orthopedics/Maheshwari/2005/Pg. 175]
A. Narrowing of intervertebral space
B. Rarefaction of vertebral bodies
C. Destruction of laminae
D. Fusion of spinous processes

Q 96. The following are radiological signs of Paget's disease of bone except:
[Turek's SL, Lippincot Raven/Pg. 737-738]
A. "Cotton Wool" appearance
B. "Picture Window Frame" appearance
C. "Hair-on-end" appearance
D. "Blade of grass" appearance

Q 97. Following are features of Paget's disease except:
[Turek'SSL Lippincot Raven/4th Ed./Pg. 737-738]
A. Deformity of bones
B. Secondary osteosarcoma
C. Lowered serum alkaline phosphatase
D. Increased urinary excretion of hydroxyl-proline

Q 98. Commonest organism causing osteomyelitis in children under 3 years is:
[Essential Orthopedics/Maheshwari/2005/Pg. 157]
A. Hemophilus   B. Staphylococcal
C. Streptococcal   D. Salmonella

Q 99. Commonest site for acute osteomyelitis in infants is:
[Turk's Lippincott and Raven/4th Ed./Pg. 258]
A. Hip joint   B. Tibia
C. Femur   D. Radial

Q 100. Sun ray appearance is seen in:
[Turek'sl, Lippincott Ravan/4th Ed./Pg. 737-738]
A. Osteogenic sarcoma   B. Ewing's sarcoma
C. Multiple myeloma   D. Osteoclastoma

Q 101. Tumor arising from Diaphysis:
[Turek'sl, Lippincot Raven/Ed. 4th/Pg. 644]
A. Osteogenic sarcoma   B. Ewing's sarcoma
C. Osteoclastoma   D. Osteochondroma

Q 102. Tumor most sensitive to radiotherapy is:
[Turek'sl, Lippincott Raven/4th Ed./Pg. 645]
A. Osteogenic sarcoma   B. Ewing's sarcoma
C. Chondrosarcoma   D. Osteoclastoma

Q 103. Most radiosensitive bone tumor is:
[Essential Orthopedics/Maheshwari/3rd Ed./Pg. 221]
A. Chondrosarcoma   B. Osteoclastoma
C. Ewing sarcoma   D. Osteosarcoma

Q 104. Bony ankylosis result from:
[Essential Orthopedics/Maheshwari/3rd Ed./Pg. 164]
A. Pyogenic arthritis   B. TB arthritis
C. Osteoarthritis   D. Rheumatic arthritis

Q 105. Osteogenic sarcoma can develop in:
[J. Ebnezar/1st Ed./Pg. 425]
A. Osteoblastoma   B. Paget's disease
C. Osteoid osteoma   D. All of the above

Q 106. Sunray appearance in X-rays suggest:
[J. Ebnezar/1st Ed./Pg. 425]
A. Paget's disease   B. Chondrosarcoma
C. Osteogenic sarcoma   D. Osteoclastoma

Q 107. Onion peel appearance in X-ray suggests:
[Essential Orthopedics/Maheshwari/3rd Ed./Pg. 221]
A. Osteogenic sarcoma   B. Ewing's sarcoma
C. Osteoclastoma   D. Chondrosarcoma

Q 108. Soap bubble appearance in X-ray suggests:
[Essential Orthopedics/Maheshwari/3rd Ed./Pg. 210]
A. Osteogenic sarcoma   B. Ewing's sarcoma
C. Osteoclastoma   D. Chondrosarcoma

Q 109. Infarction of the distal epiphysis of the second metatarsal bone is:
[Essential Orthopedics/Maheshwari/3rd Ed./Pg. 269]
A. Kienbock's disease   B. Kohler's disease
C. Freiburg's disease   D. Perthe's disease

Q 110. Senile osteoporosis is radiologically manifest only when ....% of skeleton has been lost:
[Essential Orthopedics/Maheshwari/3rd Ed./Pg. 261]
A. 20%   B. 30%
C. 40%   D. 80%

Q 111. Involvement of regional lymph nodes is seen in:
[Essential Orthopedics/Maheshwari/3rd Ed./Pg. 224]
A. Osteogenic sarcoma   B. Synovial sarcoma
C. Osteoclastoma   D. Fibrosarcoma

Q 112. The gold standard for the diagnosis of osteoporosis is:
[Essential Orthopedics/Maheshwari/3rd Ed./Pg. 262]
A. Dual energy X-ray absorptiometry
B. Single energy X-ray absorptiometry
C. Ultrasonography
D. Quantitative computed tomography

Q 113. Increased bone density occurs in:
[Essential Orthopedics/Maheshwari/3rd Ed./Pg. 266]

Answer	92 D	93 C	94 C	95 B	96 C	97 C	98 B	99 B	100 A	101 B	102 B	103 C
	104 A	105 B	106 C	107 B	108 C	109 C	110 B	111 B	112 A			

A. Cushing syndrome   B. Hypoparathyroidism
C. Fluorosis   D. Hypoparathyroidism

Q 114. Commonest site of a bone cyst:
[Essential Orthopedics/Maheshwari/3rd Ed./Pg. 226]
A. Upper end of humerus   B. Lower end of tibia
C. Lower end of femur   D. Upper end of femur

Q 115. Drug of choice for senile osteoporosis is:
[Essential Orthopedics/Maheshwari/3rd Ed./Pg. 358]
A. Estrogens   B. Androgens
C. Calcitonin   D. Alendronate

Q 116. The lytic lesion in the epiphysis in children is seen in:
[Essential Orthopedics/Maheshwari/3rd Ed./Pg. 215]
A. Osteogenic sarcoma   B. Osteoclastoma
C. Aneurismal bone cyst   D. Chondroblastoma

Q 117. Sclerotic lesion in the bone is seen in all except:
[Neurology and Neurosurgery/Lindsay/4th Ed./Pg. 545]
A. Osteitis fibrosa   B. Osteopetrosis
C. Myelomeostosis   D. Caffey's disease

Q 118. A 70-year-old lady presented with mild low back pain tenderness in L3 vertebra. On examination Hb 8 gm, ESR 110 mm/hr, A/G ratio of 2:4, likely diagnosis is:
[Essential Orthopedics/Maheshwari/3rd Ed./Pg. 223]
A. Walder storms   B. Multiple myeloma
C. Bone secondaries   D. None

Q 119. All are seen in chronic osteomyelitis except:
[J. Ebnezar/1st Ed./Pg. 365]
A. Sequestrum   B. Amyloidosis
C. Myositis ossificans   D. Metastatic abscess

Q 120. Osteochondritis dissecans occurs at:
[Essential Orthopedics/Maheshwari/3rd Ed./Pg. 97]
A. Lateral surface lateral condyle
B. Medial surface of lateral condyle
C. Medial surface medial condyle
D. Lateral surface medial condyle

Q 121. Rare site of metastasis in bone:
[J. Ebnezar/1st Ed./Pg. 430]
A. Skull   B. Spine
C. Upper end of humerus   D. Below elbow and knee

Q 122. The quality in bone formation in transplanted bone is best improved in:
[Essential Orthopedics/Maheshwari/3rd Ed./Pg. 70]
A. Autogenic cortical bone graft
B. Allogenic cancellous bone graft
C. Allogenic composite bone graft
D. Autogenic cancellous bone graft

Q 123. Which one of the following Odontomes is a locally invasive malignant tumor?
[J. Ebnezar/1st Ed./Pg. 420]
A. Odontogenic myxoma   B. Fibromatous opulis
C. Dentigerous cyst   D. Ameloblastoma

Q 124. Bone graft with maximum osteogenic potential is:
[Essential Orthopedics/Maheshwari/3rd Ed./Pg. 70]
A. Fresh autograft   B. Fresh cortical autograft
C. Osteoperiosteal graft   D. Vascular bone graft

Q 125. Deafness in cases of Paget's disease is due to:
[J. Ebnezar/1st Ed./Pg. 352]
A. Thickened cranium
B. Narrowing of foramina of skull
C. Brain compression
D. Otosclerosis

Q 126. Sclerosis of bone is seen in all except:
[J. Ebnezar/1st Ed./Pg. 256]
A. Flourosis   B. Osteopetrosis
C. Secondaries from prostate   D. Hyperparathyroidism

Q 127. Most reliable method for defecting bony metastasis is:
[J. Ebnezar/1st Ed./Pg. 419]
A. MRI   B. CT scan
C. Radiography   D. SPECT

Q 128. Phocomelia is best described as:
[Refer to Text]
A. Defect in development of long bones
B. Defect in development of flat bones
C. Defect of intramembranous ossification
D. Defect of cartilage replacement by bone

Q 129. Most common cause of pathological fracture in a child is:
[Essential Orthopedics/Maheshwari/3rd Ed./Pg. 226]
A. Malignancy   B. Bone cyst
C. Fibrous dysplasia   D. Paget's disease

Q 130. True statement of regarding osteogenic sarcoma is:
[Essential Orthopedics/Maheshwari/3rd Ed./Pg. 218]
A. Affects middle aged people
B. X-ray shows honey combing
C. Can be a complication of Paget's disease of bone
D. All of the above

Q 131. Commonest benign tumor under 21 years of age:
[Essential Orthopedics/Maheshwari/3rd Ed./Pg. 225]
A. Aneurysmal bone cyst   B. Osteochondroma
C. Giant cell tumor   D. Osteoid osteoma

Q 132. A boy presenting with swelling of lower end femur with calcified, nodular shadow in lung has:
[J. Ebnazar/1st Ed./Pg. 425]
A. Osteosarcoma
B. Osteochondroma
C. Tuberculosiss femur lower end
D. Osteomyelitis

Q 133. Densely calcified metastatic shadows are found in:
[Essential Orthopedics/Maheshwari/3rd Ed./Pg. 218]
A. Synovial cell carcinoma   B. Osteosarcoma
C. Chondrosarcoma   D. Chondroblastoma

Q 134. Sever's disease refers to:
[Essential Orthopedics/Maheshwari/3rd Ed./Pg. 269]

Answer	113 C	114 A	115 D	116 D	117 C	118 B	119 C	120 D	121 D	122 C	123 D	124 D
	125 D	126 D	127 B	128 A	129 B	130 C	131 B	132 A	133 B			

A. Calcaneum
B. Radius
C. Talus
D. Capitulum

Q 135. Dysplasia epiphysis Medicine is:
[Medicine/Davidson/20th Ed./Pg. 1191]
A. Trevor's disease
B. Blount's disease
C. Streeter's dysplasia
D. Leri's disease

Q 136. Commonest cause of Medicine osteomyelitis:
[Essential Orthopedics/Maheshwari/3rd Ed./Pg. 157]
A. Streptococcus
B. Staphylococcus aureus
C. Salmonella
D. Haemophilus influenzae

Q 137. Marker for bone formation:
[Medicine/Davidson/20th Ed./Pg. 1068]
A. Osteocalcin
B. TRAP
C. 5 nucleotidase
D. Parathormone

Q 138. Most common joint where arthroscopy is performed is:
[Essential Orthopedics/Maheshwari/3rd Ed./Pg. 130]
A. Hip
B. Knee
C. Ankle
D. Shoulder
E. Elbow

Q 139. Earliest feature of TB vertebra:
[Essential Orthopedics/Maheshwari/3rd Ed./Pg. 175]
A. Decreased joint space
B. Soft tissue swelling
C. Decreased movements
D. Pain

Q 140. Marble bone disease is also known as:
[Essential Orthopedics/Maheshwari/3rd Ed./Pg. 269]
A. Osteogenesis imperfecta
B. Osteopetrosis
C. Perthe's disease
D. Ochronosis

Q 141. Engelman's disease is:
[Essential Orthopedics/Maheshwari/3rd Ed./Pg. 271]
A. Multiple epiphyseal dysplasia
B. Infantile cortical hyperostosis
C. Cleidocranial dysplasia
D. Progressive diaphyseal dysplasia

Q 142. Acute osteomyelitis can best be distinguished from soft tissue infection by:
[Essential Orthopedics/Maheshwari/3rd Ed./Pg. 158]
A. Clinical examination
B. X-ray
C. CT scan
D. MRI

Q 143. A man was diagnosed to have myositis ossificans progressiva at the age of 20 yes. He died 5 years later. What is the most probable cause of death?
[Refer to Text]
A. Starvation and chest infection
B. Myocarditis
C. Hypercalcemia
D. Hyperphosphatemia

Q 144. A 50 year old patient presents with a lesion in the midline involving the sacrum which is sclerotic, what is the likely diagnosis?
[Essential Orthopedics/Maheshwari/3rd Ed./Pg. 216]
A. Osteosarcoma
B. Chordoma
C. Metastasis
D. Osteoclastoma

Q 145. Commonest site of chondroblastoma:
[Essential Orthopedics/Maheshwari/3rd Ed./Pg. 215]
A. Epiphysis
B. Diaphysis
C. Metaphysis
D. Soft tissues
E. Periosteum

Q 146. Subperiosteal new bone formation is seen in all except:
[Essential Orthopedics/Maheshwari/3rd Ed./Pg. 158]
A. Scurvy
B. Osteosarcoma
C. Osteomyelitis
D. Eosinophilic granuloma

Q 147. Hand Schuller Christian disease, which is correct?
[Essential Orthopedics/Maheshwari/3rd Ed./Pg. 269]
A. Proliferation at reticuloendothelial cells
B. Foam cells seen
C. Punched out lesions in X-ray
D. Diabetes insipidus and Exophthalmos present
E. All are correct

Q 148. A 8-year-old child has a swelling in diaphysis of femur. Histology reveals small clear round symmetrical cells, minimum cytoplasm, necrotic areas, minimum osteoid and chondroid material cells. Most likely, it contains
[Medicine/Davidson/20th Ed./Pg. 442]
A. Mucin
B. Lipid
C. Iron
D. Glycogen

Q 149. Drug therapy of Paget's disease (osteitis deformans) include all except:
[Essential Orthopedics/Maheshwari/3rd Ed./Pg. 269]
A. Alendronate
B. Etidronate
C. Calcitonin
D. Plicamycin

Q 150. Histology of myositis ossificans mimics:
[Essential Orthopedics/Maheshwari/3rd Ed./Pg. 42]
A. Osteosarcoma
B. Osteochondroma
C. GCT
D. Ewing's tumor

Q 151. Avascular neurosis does not occur in one of the following bones:
[Essential Orthopedics/Maheshwari/3rd Ed./Pg. 270]
A. Talus
B. Femoral head
C. Scaphoid
D. Calcaneum

Q 152. Therapeutic program for gout could include administration of:
[Essential Orthopedics/Maheshwari/Pg. 151]
A. Heavy dose of vit C
B. Phenyl butazone
C. Furadatin
D. Gold therapy

Q 153. Arthroplasty means:
[Essential Orthopedics/Maheshwari/Pg. 68]
A. The joint is made of plastic material
B. The articular parts of bone forming the joint are excised and made to fuse together
C. Joint are excised and made to fuse together as to avoid fusion
D. Any of the above

Q 154. A recessive form of osteogenesis imperfecta may closely resemble:
[Essential Orthopedics/Maheshwari/Pg. 268]
A. Alkaptonuria
B. Cretinism
C. Hypophosphatasia
D. Homocysteine

Answer	134 A	135 A	136 B	137 A	138 B	139 A	140 B	141 D	142 A	143 A	144 D	145 A
	146 C	147 E	148 D	149 C	150 A	151 D	152 B	153 B	154 B			

Dislocation

Q 155. The following is true in the treatment of posterior dislocation:
[Essential Orthopedics/Maheshwari/2005/Pg. 75]
A. Closed reduction under anesthesia
B. Open reduction
C. Skeletal traction
D. Soft tissue release and then internal reduction in 2nd stage

Q 156. Commonest type of dislocation of the hip is:
[J. Ebnezar 2004/Pg. 126]
A. Anterior
B. Posterior
C. Central
D. Dislocation with fracture of the shaft

Q 157. Re-implantation is not possible in:
[J. Ebnezar/1st Ed./Pg. 70-76]
A. Gridstone amputation   B. Thumb amputation
C. Crush injury with avulsion   D. Single digit amputation

Q 158. Gaenslen's operation is done for:
[Essential Orthopedics/Maheshwari/3rd Ed./Pg. 297]
A. Cervical spondylosis
B. Recurrent shoulder dislocation
C. Tubercular arthritis of knee Joint
D. Sacroiliac subluxation

Q 159. Flexion, adduction and internal rotation is characteristic posture in:
[J. Ebnezar/1st Ed./Pg. 128]
A. Anterior dislocation of hip joint
B. Posterior dislocation of hip joint
C. Fracture of femoral head
D. Fracture shaft of femur

Q 160. Dislocation of which one of the following carpal bones can present as median nerve palsy?
[Karim Khan, Mcg Raw.hill/3rd Ed./Pg. 318]
A. Scaphoid   B. Hamate
C. Lunate   D. Trapezium

Q 161. Commonest cause for recurrent shoulder dislocation is:
[Essential Orthopedics/Maheshwari/3rd Ed./Pg. 75]
A. Shallow glenoid labrum
B. Bankart's lesion
C. Weakness of subscapularis muscle
D. Injury to humeral head

Q 162. Treatment of anterior dislocation of shoulder is by:
[Essential Orthopedics/Maheshwari/3rd Ed./Pg. 75]
A. Kocher's maneuver   B. Dennis Browne splint
C. Barlow's maneuver   D. Surgery

Q 163. Dislocation of hip joint palpable on per rectal examination:
[Essential Orthopedics/Maheshwari/3rd Ed./Pg. 111]
A. Congenital dislocation of hip
B. Posterior dislocation of hip
C. Fracture neck of femur
D. Anterior dislocation of hip

Q 164. Recurrent dislocation of patella in an adolescent could be treated by:
[Essential Orthopedics/Maheshwari/Pg. 127]
A. Patellectomy   B. Excision arthopalsty
C. Putti plat operation   D. Lateral release

Q 165. Pulled elbow is:
[Essential Orthopedics/Maheshwari/Pg. 88]
A. Disarticulation of elbow
B. Subluxation of distal radioulnar joint
C. Subluxation of proximal radioulnar joint
D. None of the above

Q 166. Recurrent dislocation of patella is most often associated with:
[Essential Orthopedics/Maheshwari/Pg. 131]
A. Abnormally high patella   B. Abnormally low patella
C. Bow leg   D. Quadriceps contracture

Q 167. Commonest type of shoulder dislocation:
[Essential Orthopedics/Maheshwari/Pg. 74]
A. Subcoracoid   B. Subglenoid
C. Posterior   D. Suboclavicular

Congenital/Infection Disease

Q 168. Phacomelia is caused by ingestion of ......during Pregnancy:
[Turek/4th Ed./Pg. 286]
A. Steroids   B. Tetracycline
C. Thalidomide   D. Barbiturates

Q 169. Which of the following is seen in bilateral congenital dislocation of hip?
[Essential Orthopedics/Maheshwari 2005/ Pg. 200-203]
A. Waddling Gait
B. Shenton's line is broken
C. Trendelenberg test positive
D. Allis test positive

Q 170. Bilateral symmetrical idiopathic fractures are most commonly seen in:
[J. Ebnezar/1st Ed./Pg. 348]
A. Osteogenesis Imperfecta   B. Stress fracture
C. Polytrauma   D. Osteoporosis

Q 171. Metaphyseal fracture is commonly seen in:
[J. Ebnezar/1st Ed./Pg. 354]
A. Osteogenesis imperfecta   B. Scurvy
C. Rickets   D. None of these

Q 172. Viral osteomyelitis seen usually to be due vaccination of:
[J. Ebnezar/1st Ed./Pg. 362]
A. Small pox virus infection   B. Influenza virus infection
C. Coxsackie infection   D. Dengue fever

Q 173. Tuberculous arthritis in advanced cases leads to:
[J. Ebnezar 1st Ed./Pg. 403]
A. Bony ankylosis   B. Fibrous ankylosis
C. Loose joints   D. Charcot's joints

Answer	155 A	156 B	157 C	158 D	159 B	160 C	161 B	162 A	163 B	164 D	165 D	166 A
	167 B	168 C	169 C	170 A	171 C	172 B	173 B					

Q 174. Tuberculosis of the spine starts in:
[J. Ebnezar/1st Ed./Pg. 368]
A. Vertebral body
B. Nucleus pulposus
C. Annulus fibrosis
D. Paravertebral fascia

Q 175. Organism causing osteomyelitis in sickle cell anemia:
[J. Ebnezar/1st Ed./Pg. 361]
A. Salmonella
B. Staphylococcus
C. Pneumonia
D. Streptococcus

Q 176. A 25-year-old lady sustained a lacerated wound on the back of right thigh by the horn of a butt. The wound was sutured. Two months later she developed foot drop and an ulcer on the dorsum of the foot. The most likely diagnosis is:
[Essential Orthopedics/Maheshwari/3rd Ed./Pg. 56]
A. Chronic ischemic to limbs due to popliteal artery injury
B. Partial injury to sciatic nerve
C. Complete division of sciatic nerve
D. Injury to hamstring muscles

Q 177. Limb salvage primarily depends on:
[Essential Orthopedics/Maheshwari/3rd Ed./Pg. 278]
A. Vascular injury
B. Skin cover
C. Bone injury
D. Nerve injury

Q 178. Pathological changes in Caisson's disease is due to:
[Pathology/Harsh Mohan/5th Ed./Pg. 126]
A. N_2
B. O_2
C. CO_2
D. CO

Q 179. Caffey's disease occurs in:
[Essential Orthopedics/Maheshwari/3rd Ed./Pg. 271]
A. Infants below 6 months
B. Above 5 years
C. Above 10 – 20 years
D. 21 – 40 years

Q 180. Most common lesion of hand is:
[Essential Orthopedics/Maheshwari/3rd Ed./Pg. 228]
A. Enchondroma
B. Synovioma
C. Exostosis
D. Osteoclastoma

Q 181. Treatment of Hypercalcemia is all except:
[Medicine/Davidson/20th Ed./Pg. 772]
A. Riwazul
B. Plicamycin
C. Ritodisnate
D. Gallium nitrate

Q 182. Not associated with osteogenesis imperfecta is:
[Essential Orthopedics/Maheshwari/3rd Ed./Pg. 268]
A. Blue sclera
B. Cataract
C. Deafness
D. Fractures

Q 183. Osteoblastic secondaries can arise from:
[Medicine/Davidson/20th Ed./Pg. 511]
A. Carcinoma prostate
B. Thyroid carcinoma
C. Renal carcinoma
D. Breast carcinoma

Q 184. Epiphyseal dysgenesis:
[Essential Orthopedics/Maheshwari/Pg. 46]
A. Hypothyroidism
B. Hypothyroidism
C. Addison's disease
D. Rickets

Q 185. Weaver's bottom is:
[Essential Orthopedics/Maheshwari/Pg. 256]
A. Eczematous lesion over buttocks of weaver's due to then sedentary position
B. Ischiogluteal bursitis
C. Coccydynia
D. None of the above

Q 186. Anterior ligament calcification of spine and mottling of teeth is seen with:
[Essential Orthopedics/Maheshwari/Pg. 226]
A. Ankylosing spondylitis
B. Rheumatoid arthritis
C. Ochronosis
D. Fluorosis

Q 187. Avascular necrosis is common with:
[Essential Orthopedics/Maheshwari/Pg. 118]
A. Fracture trochanter
B. Fracture shaft of femur
C. Fracture head of humerus
D. Fracture neck of femur

Joint Diseases

Q 188. Commonest cause of loose bodies in joints:
[Apley and Soloman/7th Ed./Pg. 104]
A. Tuberculous tenosynovitis
B. Rheumatoid arthritis
C. Osteoarthritis
D. Osteochondritis dissecans

Q 189. Trouser leg appearance on an ascending myelogram is suggestive of .... tumor.
[Neurology and Neurosurgery/Lindsay/4th Ed./Pg. 393-396]
A. Extradural
B. Extramedullary
C. Intramedullary
D. None of the above

Q 190. Commonest site of skeletal tuberculosis is:
[Essential Orthopedics/Maheshwari/3rd Ed./Pg. 169]
A. Tibia
B. Radius
C. Humerus
D. Vertebrae

Q 191. Osteomyelitis of the spine is mostly caused by:
A. *Salmonella*
B. *Pneumococcus*
C. *Tubercle bacilli*
D. *Staphylococcus*

Q 192. Osteomyelitis in a case of sickle cell anemia is caused by:
[Neurology and Neurosurgery/Lindsay/4th Ed./Pg. 475]
A. *Salmonella*
B. *Pneumococcus*
C. *Streptococcus*
D. *Haemophilus*

Q 193. The joint commonly involved in syphilitic arthritis is:
[Essential Orthopedics/Maheshwari/3rd Ed./Pg. 166]
A. Hip
B. Shoulder
C. Wrist
D. Knee

Q 194. Enchondroma commonly arises from
[Essential Orthopedics/Maheshwari/3rd Ed./Pg. 226]
A. Ribs
B. Vertebra
C. Tibia
D. Phalanges

Q 195. Which joint is not fused in Triple arthrodesis:
[Essential Orthopedics/Maheshwari/3rd Ed./Pg. 198]
A. Tibiotalar
B. Calcaneonavicular
C. Talonavicular
D. Talocalcaneal

Answer	174 A	175 A	176 B	177 A	178 A	179 A	180 A	181 A	182 B	183 A	184 A	185 B
	186 D	187 D	188 D	189 C	190 D	191 C	192 A	193 D	194 D	195 A		

Q 196. Drawer's sign is diagnostic for injuries of:
[Essential Orthopedics/Maheshwari/3rd Ed./Pg. 97]
A. Neck femur
B. Shaft femur
C. Collateral ligaments of knee
D. Cruciate ligaments of knee

Q 197. Viscosity of synovial fluid depends on:
[Refer to Text]
A. Chondroitin sulfate
B. Keratosulfate
C. Hyaluronic acid
D. Heparin sulfate

Q 198. Normal bone remodelling in response to stress was described by:
[Essential Orthopedics/Maheshwari/3rd Ed./Pg. 8]
A. Kuntscher
B. Wolff
C. Pauwels
D. Hugh Owen Thomas

Q 199. Earliest changes in Perthe's disease is seen by:
[Essential Orthopedics/Maheshwari/3rd Ed./Pg. 270]
A. X-ray
B. CT
C. MRI
D. US
E. Nuclear scan

Q 200. Diabetic Charcot's joint affect most commonly:
[J. Ebnezars/1st Ed./Pg. 379]
A. Knee
B. Ankle
C. Hip
D. Foot joint

Q 201. Most common cause of hemarthrosis knee joint is:
[Medicine/Davidson/19th Ed./Pg. 949]
A. Hemophilia
B. Anterior cruciate ligament tear
C. Posterior cruciate ligament tear
D. Medial meniscus tear
E. Lateral meniscus tear

Q 202. In osteoporosis all are seen except:
[Essential Orthopedics/Maheshwari/3rd Ed./Pg. 261]
A. Bending bones
B. Pseudofractures
C. Increase serum Ca 2+
D. Loss of lamina dura

Q 203. Cleidocranial dysostosis may show:
[Essential Orthopedics/Maheshwari/Pg. 271]
A. Wide foramen magnum
B. Absence of clavicles
C. Coxa vara
D. All of the above

Spine

Q 204. The following is true of spondylolisthesis:
[Essential Orthopedics/Maheshwari/2005/Pg. 236]
A. Slipping of S1 over L5
B. Posterior arch defect
C. Congenital defect
D. more in pregnancy

Q 205. Beheaded Scottish Terrier sign is seen in:
[J. Ebnezar/1st Ed./Pg. 247]
A. Disc prolapse
B. Sacarlization of L5
C. Spondylosis
D. Spondylolisthesis

Q 206. Traction injury to epiphyses of the vertebra is known as
[Essential Orthopedics/Maheshwari/3rd Ed./Pg. 269]

A. Osgood Schlatter's disease
B. Sindino Larsen disease
C. Scheurmanns's disease
D. None

Q 207. Fish head appearance of the vertebral bodies is seen in:
[Essential Orthopedics/Maheshwari/3rd Ed./Pg. 262]
A. Paget's disease
B. Rickets
C. Osteomalacia
D. Osteoporosis

Q 208. Tuberculosis of the spine is known as:
[J. Ebnezar/1st Ed./Pg. 368]
A. Pott's disease
B. Scheurmann's disease
C. Perthe's disease
D. Frieberg's disease

Q 209. Commonest site of fracture in senile osteoporosis:
[J. Ebnezar/1st Ed./Pg. 357]
A. Neck of femur
B. Shaft of femur
C. Radius
D. Vertebra

Q 210. Earliest sign in X-ray in TB spine is:
[J. Ebnezar/1st Ed./Pg. 369]
A. Paravertebral shadow
B. Narrowing of disk space
C. Gibbus
D. straightening of the spinal curves

Q 211. Recovery in T B Spine is delayed in Children because of:
[Essential Orthopedics/Maheshwari/3rd Ed./Pg. 180]
A. Inadequate rest
B. Fragile bone
C. More cartilage
D. Increased vascularity

Q 212. Jefferson's fracture occurs at:
[J. Ebnezar/1st Ed./Pg. 181]
A. C1
B. C2
C. C1, C2
D. C2, C3

Q 213. Fall on heel with fracture is associated with commonly:
[J. Ebnezar/1st Ed./Pg. 176]
A. Fracture clavicle
B. Fracture vertebra
C. Fracture femur
D. Any of the above

Q 214. Vertical striations on vertebral bodies are seen in:
[Essential Orthopedics/Maheshwari/3rd Ed./Pg. 215]
A. Hemangioma
B. Paget's disease
C. Vertebral metastasis
D. Osteoporosis

Q 215. Bamboo spine is seen in:
[Essential Orthopedics/Maheshwari/3rd Ed./Pg. 218]
A. Ankylosing spondylosis
B. Rheumatoid arthritis
C. Scheurmann's disease
D. Pott's spine

Q 216. Commonest site of TB spine:
[J. Ebnezar/1st Ed./Pg. 368]
A. Dorsolumbar
B. Lumbar
C. Sacral
D. Cervical

Q 217. The ideal surgical treatment for Pott's paraplegia is:
[Essential Orthopedics/Maheshwari/3rd Ed./Pg. 180]
A. Laminectomy and decompression
B. Anterior decompression
C. Anterolateral decompression
D. Costotransversectomy

Answer	196 D	197 C	198 B	199 E	200 D	201 A	202 B	203 B	204 B	205 D	206 C	207D
	208 A	209 D	210 B	211 B	212 A	213 B	214 A	215 A	216 A	217 C		

Q 218. Schmoni's node is:
[Orthopaedic Medicine/vol-1 Cyriax/5th Ed./Pg. 245]
A. Radiological finding protruded nucleus pulposus into the vertebral body
B. Soft tissue tumor in relation to the vertebral
C. A tumor in the vertebral disk
D. None of the above

Q 219. Steinman pin is used for all except:
[Essential Orthopedics/Maheshwari/3rd Ed./Pg. 22]
A. Fracture of upper end of tibia
B. Fracture through lower end of tibia
C. Fracture through lower end of femur
D. Skull traction

Q 220. What is the diagnostic radiological finding in skeletal fluorosis:
[Essential Orthopedics/Maheshwari/3rd Ed./Pg. 266]
A. Sclerosis sacroiliac joint
B. Interroseous membrane ossification
C. Osteoscelerosis of vertebral body
D. Ossification of ligaments of knee joint

Q 221. Commonest site of TB spine is:
[Essential Orthopedics/Maheshwari/3rd Ed./Pg. 172]
A. C8-T2
B. T2-T6
C. T10-L1
D. L1-L4

Q 222. Most unstable spinal injury is:
[Essential Orthopedics/Maheshwari/Pg. 144]
A. Flexion injury
B. Flexion rotation injury
C. Extension injury
D. Flexion distraction injury

Others

Q 223. Commonest site for acute osteomyelitis in infants is:
[Tureks/4th Ed./Pg. 258]
A. Hip joint
B. Tibia
C. Femur
D. Radial

Q 224. Osteitis fibrosa cystica is seen in:
[J. Ebnezar/2004/Pg. 356)]
A. Hyperparathyroidism
B. Hypoparathyroidism
C. Hypothyroidism
D. Hyperthyroidism

Q 225. In Burton's disease there is:
[J. Ebnezar/1st Ed./Pg. 359]
A. Scurvy and Rickets
B. Scurvy and Syphilis
C. Syphilis and Rickets
D. Scurvy and Pellagra

Q 226. Most common cause of pressure sore in the foot in India is
[Essential Orthopedics/Maheshwari/3rd Ed./Pg. 196]
A. Diabetes
B. Syringomyelia
C. Leprosy
D. Thorn prick

Q 227. The treatment of enchondroma is:
[Essential Orthopedics/Maheshwari/ 3rd Ed./Pg. 226]
A. Amputaion
B. Irradiation
C. Local excision
D. Curettage and bone chip filling

Q 228. In Volkman's ischemia, surgery should be done:
[Essential Orthopedics/Maheshwari/3rd Ed./Pg. 84]
A. Immediately
B. After 6 hours
C. 24 hours
D. 72 hours

Q 229. Pain in Paget's disease is relieved best by:
[J. Ebnezar/1st Ed./Pg. 35]
A. Simple anesthetics
B. Narcotic analgesics
C. Radiation
D. Calcitonin

Q 230. Complications of Paget's disease is:
[Essential Orthopedics/Maheshwari/3rd Ed./Pg. 269]
A. Osteogenic sarcoma
B. Deafness
C. Heart failure
D. All of these

Q 231. Pain in osteoid osteoma is specifically relieved by:
[Essential Orthopedics/Maheshwari/3rd Ed./Pg. 215]
A. Salicylates
B. Narcotic analgesics
C. Radiation
D. Splinting

Q 232. Osteogenic sarcoma metastasizes to commonly:
[Essential Orthopedics/Maheshwari/3rd Ed./Pg. 218]
A. Liver
B. Lung
C. Brain
D. Regional lymph nodes

Q 233. Pectus carinatus a seen in:
[Medicine/Daivdson/19th Ed./Pg. 574]
A. Cretinism
B. Senile osteoporosis
C. Osteogenesis imperfecta
D. Chronic asthma

Q 234. Multiple myeloma is most frequently encountered in the .... decade:
[Essential Orthopedics/Maheshwari/3rd Ed./Pg. 223]
A. Third
B. Fourth
C. Fifth
D. Seventh

Q 235. Intervertebral disc prolapse is treated chemically by:
[Essential Orthopedics/Maheshwari/3rd Ed./Pg. 232]
A. Hylase
B. Chymotrypsin
C. Chymopapain
D. Elastase

Q 236. Chemical synovectomy is done by:
[Essential Orthopedics/Maheshwari/3rd Ed./Pg. 232]
A. Osmic acid
B. Chymopapain
C. Chymotrypsin
D. Trypsin

Q 237. Fat embolism is associated with:
[Essential Orthopedics/Maheshwari/3rd Ed./Pg. 34]
A. Petechial hemorrhages
B. Hemarthrosis
C. Hematuria,
D. Bruise below the line of lesion

Q 238. Age group of osteogenic sarcoma is:
[Essential Orthopedics/Maheshwari/3rd Ed./Pg. 218]
A. 1 – 10
B. 10 – 20
C. 20 – 30
D. 20 – 40

Q 239. The following is false of Achondroplasia:
[J. Ebnezar/1st Ed./Pg. 347]
A. Autosomal dominant
B. Mental Retardation
C. due to gene mutation
D. Shortening of limbs present

Answer	218 A	219 D	220 C	221 C	222 B	223 B	224 A	225 A	226 C	227 D	228 A	229 D
	230 C	231 A	232 B	233 D	234 C	235 C	236 B	237 A	238 B	239 B		

Q 240. Avascular necrosis of the head of femur is not seen in:
[Essential Orthopedics/Maheshwari/3rd Ed./Pg. 42]
A. Subcapital Fracture
B. Intertrochanteric fracture
C. Transcervical fracture
D. Central dislocation of hip

Q 241. Osteomyelitis of jaw is seen in:
[Essential Orthopedics/Maheshwari/3rd Ed./Pg. 271]
A. Osteomalacia
B. Osteopoikilosis
C. Osteoporosis
D. Caffey's disease

Q 242. Bone growth is influenced maximally by:
[Essential Orthopedics/Maheshwari/3rd Ed./Pg. 265]
A. Estrogen
B. Thyroxine
C. Growth hormone
D. Testosterone

Q 243. Injury to the popliteal artery in fracture lower end of femur is due to:
[J. Ebnezar/1st Ed./Pg. 133]
A. Distal fragment pressing the artery
B. Proximal fragment pressing the artery
C. Tight plaster
D. Hematoma

Q 244. Which tumor does not arise from cartilage?
[J. Ebnezar/1st Ed./Pg. 420]
A. Osteoblastoma
B. Osteochondroma
C. Chondrosarcoma
D. Enchondroma

Q 245. Resorption of the terminal phalanx is not seen in:
[J. Ebnezar/1st Ed./Pg. 181]
A. Hyperparathyroidism
B. Reiter's syndrome
C. Scleroderma
D. Psoriasis

Q 246. Trident hand is seen in:
[J. Ebnezar/1st Ed./Pg. 347]
A. Achondroplasia
B. Scurvy
C. Mucopolysaccharidosis
D. None

Q 247. Treatment of choice for Carffey's disease:
[Essential Orthopedics/Maheshwari/3rd Ed./Pg. 271]
A. Multiple drilling
B. Tetracycline
C. Penicillin
D. Curettage

Q 248. Bone remodeling responds to stress is by:
[J. Ebnezar/1st Ed./Pg. 420]
A. H Q Thomas
B. Griffith
C. Galen
D. None

Q 249. Most common Site of Ivory Osteoma:
[J. Ebnezar/1st Ed./Pg. 420]
A. Orbit
B. Maxilla
C. Frontal sinus
D. Mandible

Q 250. Avascular necrosis of bone is most common in:
[Essential Orthopedics/Maheshwari/3rd Ed./Pg. 97]
A. Scapula
B. Scaphoid
C. Calcaneus
D. Cervical Spine

Q 251. During the surgical procedure:
[J. Ebnezar/1st Ed./Pg. 36]
A. Tendons should be repaired before nerves
B. Nerves should be repaired before tendons
C. Tendons should be repaired at the same time
D. None is true

Q 252. Adult bone trabeculae are differentiated from foetal bone trabaeculae histologically by the presence of:
[J. Ebnezar/1st Ed./Pg. 21]
A. Haversian system
B. Lamellar structure
C. Certain special straning characteristics
D. Different type of bone cells in each

Q 253. Tetanus is noticed usually in:
[Essential Orthopedics/Maheshwari/3rd Ed./Pg. 117]
A. Burn cases
B. Wounds contaminated with fecal matter
C. Open fracture
D. Gunshot wounds
E. All the above

Q 254. Which of the following causes acute compartment syndrome most frequently?
[J. Ebnezar/1st Ed./Pg. 39]
A. Fractures
B. Postischemic swelling
C. Exercise initiated syndrome
D. Soft tissue injury

Q 255. Large vacuolated cells on histopathology are characteristics of:
[J. Ebnezar/1st Ed./Pg. 420]
A. Osteosarcoma
B. Osteoclastoma
C. Liposarcoma
D. Chondrosarcoma
E. Chondroma

Q 256. McMurray's osteotomy operation is based on the following principle:
[J. Ebnezar/1st Ed./Pg. 121]
A. Mechanical
B. Biological
C. Biomechanical
D. None of these

Q 257. Complications of an amputation stump may be:
[Essential Orthopedics/Maheshwari/3rd Ed./Pg. 280]
A. Phantom limb
B. Stump neuroma
C. Ring sequestrum
D. All the above

Q 258. Bone tumor metastasizing to bone is:
[J. Ebnezar/1st Ed./Pg. 420]
A. Giant cell tumor
B. Ewing's sarcoma
C. Chondrosarcoma
D. Osteosarcoma

Q 259. Osteoclastoma is common in age group of:
[Essential Orthopedics/Maheshwari/3rd Ed./Pg. 117]
A. Below 10 years
B. 10 to 20 years
C. All age groups
D. 20 to 40 years

Q 260. When osteomyelitis disseminates by hematogenous way the most affected part of bone is:
[Essential Orthopedics/Maheshwari/3rd Ed./Pg. 157]
A. Metaphysis
B. Epiphysis
C. Diaphysis
D. Any of the above

Answer	240 B	241 D	242 C	243 A	244 A	245 B	246 A	247 C	248 A	249 C	250 B	251 B
	252 B	253 E	254 B	255 C	256 C	257 D	258 D	259 D	260 A			

Q 261. When a person reports with vertebral fracture, hemiplegia and urinary retention the acute measure to be taken is:
[Orthopaedics and Applied Physiotherapy/Jayant Joshi/Pg. 139]
A. Suprapubic cystostomy   B. Catheterization
C. Hot fermentation   D. Condom drainage

Q 262. Not a complication of menopause:
[Essential Orthopedics/Maheshwari/3rd/Pg. 82]
A. Fracture spine
B. Colle's fracture
C. Fracture neck of femur
D. Supracondylar fracture humerus

Q 263. Soft tissue calcification occurs in all except:
[J. Ebnezar/1st Ed./Pg. 356]
A. Hyperparathyroidism   B. Scleroderma
C. Hyperthyroidism   D. Hypervitaminosis

Q 264. Osteosarcoma has a very poor prognosis because:
[Essential Orthopedics/Maheshwari/3rd Ed./Pg. 218]
A. Highly malignant
B. Resistant to radiotherapy
C. Inoperable
D. Spreads to lung very fast

Q 265. Which of the following arises from epiphysis?
[Essential Orthopedics/Maheshwari/3rd Ed./Pg. 216]
A. Osteosarcoma   B. Ewing's Sarcoma
C. Osteoclastoma   D. Multiple myeloma

Q 266. All of following conditions may be responsible for osteoporosis except:
[Essential Orthopedics/Maheshwari/3rd Ed./Pg. 261]
A. Steroid therapy
B. Prolonged weightlessness in space ship
C. Hyperparathyroidism
D. Hypoparathyroidism

Q 267. The type of displacement of fractured fragment in which bone is not remodeled:
[Essential Orthopedics/Maheshwari/3rd Ed./Pg. 10]
A. Anterior angulation   B. Posterior angulation
C. Lateral angulation   D. Rotation

Q 268. Pseudoarthrosis of tibia is best treated by:
[J. Ebnezar/1st Ed./Pg. 137]
A. Internal fixation
B. Internal fixation & bone grafting
C. Above knee POP cast
D. Above knee POP cast

Q 269. All the following requires open reduction and internal fixation almost always except:
[Essential Orthopedics/Maheshwari/3rd Ed./Pg. 86]
A. Lateral condyle of humerus   B. Olecranon
C. Patella   D. Volar Barton's fracture

Q 270. Multiple exostosis usually presents at:
[J. Ebnezar/1st Ed./Pg. 349]
A. Birth   B. Puberty
C. After 21 years   D. At 5 years of age

Q 271. Accessory navicular is called:
[Neumann/Mosby/1st Ed./Pg. 481]
A. Os trigonum   B. Os tibiale internum
C. Os tibiale externum   D. Os navicular

Q 272. Ideal site for bone graft harvesting:
[Essential Orthopedics/Maheshwari/3rd Ed./Pg. 70]
A. Iliac crest   B. Skull bones
C. Femur cortex   D. Tibial cortex

Q 273. Treatment based on Gate theory is:
[Clayton's Electrotherapy/9th Ed./Pg. 102]
A. Short wave diathermy
B. Ultrasound
C. Electrical nerve stimulation
D. Infrared therapy

Q 274. Ewing's tumor arises from:
[Essential Orthopedics/Maheshwari/3rd Ed./Pg. 221]
A. Mesothelial cells   B. Endothelial cells
C. Epithelial cells   D. None of these

Q 275. Osteosclerotic rim is seen in:
[Davidson/20th Ed./Pg. 1132]
A. Growing epiphysis   B. Giant cell tumor
C. Enchondroma   D. Old people

Q 276. In a 8-year-old child the least common cause of lytic bone lesion in:
[J. Ebnazar/1st Ed./Pg. 429]
A. Plasmacytoma   B. Histiocytoma
C. Metastasis   D. Brown tumor

277. The cause of short fourth metacarpal bone is:
[Medicine/Davidson/19th Ed./Pg. 717]
A. Down's syndrome   B. Edward's syndrome
C. Turner's syndrome   D. Pseudohypoparathyroidism

Q 278. Most reliable method for detecting bony metastases is:
[Essential Orthopedics/Maheshwari/3rd Ed./Pg. 225]
A. MRI   B. CT scan
C. Radiography   D. SPECT

Q 279. Ivory osteoma commonly arises in the:
[Essential Orthopedics/Maheshwari/3rd Ed./Pg. 215]
A. Skull   B. Ribs
C. Pelvis   D. Vertebra

Q 280. Commonest site of multiple myeloma:
[Essential Orthopedics/Maheshwari/3rd Ed./Pg. 223]
A. Skull   B. Ribs
C. Vertebra   D. Long bones
E. Pelvis

Q 281. Commonest benign tumor of the bone is:
[Essential Orthopedics/Maheshwari/3rd Ed./Pg. 225]
A. Osteoma   B. Osteochondroma
C. Osteoid osteoma   D. Chondroma

Q 282. A painter after a day's strenuous work complaints of pain in the shoulder, most likely diagnosis is:
[Essential Orthopedics/Maheshwari/Pg. 38]

Answer	261 B	262 D	263 C	264 D	265 C	266 D	267 D	268 B	269 D	270 B	271 C	272 A
	273 C	274 B	275 A	276 A	277 D	278 B	279 A	280 C	281 B			

A. Subacromial bursitis
B. Frozen shoulder
C. Biceps tendinosis
D. Myositis

Q 283. Gallow's traction is given for fracture of:
[Essential Orthopedics/Maheshwari/Pg. 122]
A. Femur
B. Tibia
C. Humerus
D. Spine

Q 284. Who is acclaimed worldwide for total joint replacement?
[Essential Orthopedics/Maheshwari/Pg. 287]
A. Paul Brand
B. John Charnley
C. Paul Harrington
D. Huckstep

Q 285. Ossification in fetus starts in:
[Human Anatomy B.D.Chaurasia/Vol. 1/4th Ed./Pg. 9]
A. 1 week of intrauterine life
B. 3rd week of intrauterine life
C. 5th week of intrauterine life
D. 5th month of Intrauterine life

Q 286. In Psoriatic arthroplasty the characteristic joint involved is:
[Essential Orthopedics/Maheshwari/Pg. 251]
A. Proximal interphalangeal joint
B. Distal interphalangeal joint
C. Metacarpophalangeal joint
D. Wrist joint

Q 287. Aseptic loosening in cemented total hip replacement, occurs as a result of hypersensitivity response to:
[J. Joshi/Pg. 204]
A. Titanium debris
B. High density polythene debris
C. N N - Dimethyltryptamine (DMT)
D. Free radicals

Q 288. Young man with a tibia of left side 2 months ago is having popliteal cast. Now needs mobilization with single crutch. Which will be the preferred site?
[Principles of Exercise Therapy/Dina Gardiner/ 4th Ed./Pg. 260,605]
A. Left sided crutch
B. Right sided
C. Any side
D. Both sides

Q 289. Slipped femoral epiphysis is commonly seen in the:
[Essential Orthopedics/Maheshwari/Pg. 274]
A. 1st decade
B. 2nd decade
C. 3rd decade
D. 4th decade

290. A therapist reviews the surgical report of a patient that sustained extensive burns in a fire. The report indicates that at the time of primary excision cadaver skin was utilized to close the wound. This type of graft is termed as/an:
[Physical Agent in Rehabilitation Sullivan/5th Ed./Pg. 1103]
A. Allograft
B. Autograft
C. Heterograft
D. Xenograft

Deformities

Q 291. Rocker bottom foot results from:
[Essential Orthopedics/Maheshwari/3rd Ed./Pg. 196]
A. Congenital vertical talus
B. Poliomyelitis

C. Club foot over correction
D. both A and C

Q 292. Coxa vara is found in:
[Essential Orthopedics/Maheshwari/3rd Ed./Pg. 263]
A. Perthe's disease
B. Tuberculosis
C. Rickets
D. Rheumatoid arthritis

Q 293. A patient presented with claw hand, after supracondylar fracture was reduced and plaster applied. The diagnosis is:
[Essential Orthopedics/Maheshwari/3rd Ed./Pg. 85]
A. Median Nerve injury
B. Volkmann's ischemic contracture
C. Ulnar nerve injury
D. Dupuytren's contracture
E. Both B and C

Q 294. Hill Sach's lesion is:
[J. Ebnezar/1st Ed./Pg. 87]
A. Avulsion of glenoid labrum
B. Rupture of capsule near scapula
C. Bony defect in humeral head
D. Rupture of capsule near humerus

Q 295. Airplane splint is used for:
[Essential Orthopedics/Maheshwari/3rd Ed./Pg. 20]
A. Brachial plexus palsy
B. Myositis ossificans
C. Volkman's ischemic contracture
D. Fracture talus

Q 296. Arthrodesis of which is not done to correct flat foot:
[Essential Orthopedics/Maheshwari/3rd Ed./Pg. 198]
A. Talus
B. Cuboid
C. Navicular
D. Calcaneum

Q 297. Open reduction for supracondylar fracture in a child is not preferred because of the fear of:
[J. Ebnezar/1st Ed./Pg. 92]
A. Injury to nerves and vessels in that region
B. Myosistis ossificans traumatica
C. Permanent stiffness of the elbow
D. Infection

Q 298. Macewen's osteotomy is performed in cases of:
[J. Ebnezar/1st Ed/Pg. 258]
A. Coxa vara
B. Tibia vara
C. Genu valgum
D. Tom smith disease

Q 299. CTEV is should be treated at the age of:
[Essential Orthopedics/Maheshwari/3rd Ed./Pg. 196]
A. 10 – 12 years
B. From the date of birth
C. 2 – 3 years
D. After epiphyseal fusion

Q 300. Syme's amputation is contraindicated in:
[J. Ebnezar/1st Ed./Pg. 436]
A. Malignancy of big toe
B. Diabetic foot
C. Madhura mycosis foot
D. Crush injury

Q 301. Earliest sign of Volkmann's ischemic contracture is:
[J. Ebnezar/1st Ed./Pg. 140]
A. Pain during passive extension
B. Pulselessness

Answer												
	282 C	283 A	284 B	285 C	286 B	287 C	288 A	289 B	290 A	291 D	292 A	293 E
	294 C	295 A	296 B	297 C	298 C	299 B	300 B	301 A				

C. Necrosis of muscles
D. Loss of adduction

Q 302. Treatment for chronic cases of club foot is:
[Essential Orthopedics/Maheshwari/3rd Ed./Pg. 198]
A. Triple arthrodesis   B. Dorsomedial release
C. Amputation   D. None

Q 303. Treatment for CTEV should start at the age of:
[Essential Orthopedics/Maheshwari/3rd Ed./Pg. 196]
A. 2 weeks   B. 1 month
C. Soon after birth   D. 9 months

Q 304. The "Card Test" tests the function of:
[J. Ebnezar/1st Ed./Pg. 195]
A. Median nerve   B. Ulnar nerve
C. Axillary nerve   D. Radial nerve

Q 305. Triple deformity of knee is seen in:
[Essential Orthopedics/Maheshwari/3rd Ed./Pg. 207]
A. Polio   B. Tuberculosis
C. Villonodular synovitis   D. Rheumatoid arthritis

Q 306. Causes of painful limb are all except:
[J. Ebnezar/1st Ed./Pg. 253]
A. Perthe's disease   B. Congenital coxa vara
C. Slipped femoral epiphysis   D. TB hip

Q 307. The complication not common in Colle's fracture is:
[J. Ebnezar/1st Ed./Pg. 108]
A. Malunion   B. Nonunion
C. Sudeck's atrophy   D. Stiffness of wrist

Q 308. Treatment of triple deformity is:
[Essential Orthopedics/Maheshwari/3rd Ed./Pg. 207]
A. ATT
B. ATT + immobilization
C. ATT + immobilization + Debridement
D. None

Q 309. Tendon transfer in polio is done after age of:
[Essential Orthopedics/Maheshwari/3rd Ed./Pg. 208]
A. Less than 6 months   B. 6 months to 1 year
C. 2 years   D. 5 years

Q 310. In Hallux valgus surgery, the patients who are likely to be most satisfied are:
[Kinesiology of Musculoskeletal System/Mostby/4th Ed./Pg. 505]
A. Those with pain
B. Those with hammer toe
C. Those with metatarsus primus varus
D. Young age

Q 311. Triple deformity is a complication of:
[Essential Orthopedics/Maheshwari/3rd Ed./Pg. 245]
A. Rheumatoid arthritis   B. Tuberculosis
C. Osteoarthritis   D. Septic arthritis

Q 312. Fracture which most often requires open reduction and internal fixation:
[Essential Orthopedics/Maheshwari/3rd Ed./Pg. 86]

A. Lateral condyle of humerus
B. Femoral condyle
C. Distal tibial epiphyseal separation
D. Fracture both bones forearm

Q 313. Child aged 3 and 1/4 years is treated for CTEV by:
[Essential Orthopedics/Maheshwari/3rd Ed./Pg. 97]
A. Triple arthrodesis
B. Posteromedial soft tissue release
C. Lateral wedge resection
D. Tendo-Achilles lengthening and posterior capsulotomy

Q 314. One of the following fractures requires plaster of Paris cast with equinus position:
[Essential Orthopedics/Maheshwari/3rd Ed./Pg. 142]
A. Distal fracture both bones leg
B. Distal fracture fibula
C. Bimalleolar
D. Fracture Talus

Q 315. The cause of the gun stork deformity is:
[J. Ebnazar/3rd Ed./Pg. 92]
A. Supracondylar fracture
B. Fracture both bones forearm
C. Fracture surgical head of humerus
D. Fracture fibula

Q 316. Which among the following benefits from cervical sympathectomy:
[Orthopaedics and Applied Physiotherapy/Jayant Joshi/Pg. 112]
A. Sudeck's dystrophy
B. Compound palmar ganglion
C. Osteoarthritis of first MCP joint
D. De Quervain's tenosynovitis

Q 317. Nondynamic splint is:
[Orthopaedics and Applied Physiotherapy/Jayant Joshi/Pg. 493]
A. Banjo   B. Opponens
C. Cock-up   D. Brand

Q 318. Mallet finger is:
[Broteman/2nd Ed/Pg. 20]
A. Avulsion fracture of extensor tendon of distal phalanx
B. Fracture of distal phalanx
C. Fracture of middle phalanx
D. Fracture of proximal phalanx

Q 319. Triradiate pelvis is seen in:
[Essential Orthopedics/Maheshwari/3rd Ed./Pg. 265]
A. Paget's disease   B. Rickets
C. Osteoporosis   D. Chondroma

Q 320. Pes Cavus is caused by:
[Orthopaedics and Applied Physiotherapy/Jayant Joshi/Pg. 346]
A. Weakness of intrinsic muscles of the foot
B. Excessive tone of intrinsic muscles
C. Collapse of the arch
D. Fracture of calcaneum

Answer	302 A	303 C	304 B	305 A	306 B	307 B	308 B	309 D	310 D	311 E	312 A	313 B
	314 D	315 A	316 A	317 C	318 A	319 B	320 B					

5

CHAPTER

Medical

Objective Questions with Answers

Physiology

Q 1. The Bohr's effect causes:
[Textbook of Physiology/A. K. Jain/3rd Ed./Pg. 458]
A. Increase of the hemoglobin level
B. Loading of CO_2 and unloading of O_2 in blood
C. Loading of O_2 and unloading of CO_2 in blood
D. Loading of CO_2 and unloading of O_2 in blood

Q 2. Physiological neonatal jaundice is caused due to:
[Textbook of Physiology/A. K. Jain/3rd Ed./Pg. 81]
A. Hypoxia   B. Splenomegaly
C. Hepatic immaturity   D. Anemia

Q 3. Which of the following blood groups is called universal donor:
[Textbook of Physiology/A. K. Jain/3rd Ed./Pg. 115]
A. Blood group A   B. Blood group B
C. Blood group O   D. Blood group AB

Q 4. Raised serum acid phosphates suggest:
[Textbook of Physiology/A. K. Jain/3rd Ed./Pg. 574]
A. Carcinoma prostate   B. Liver disease
C. Paget's disease   D. All of these

5. In normal healthy Indian adult male, daily urinary calcium excretion is:
[Textbook of Physiology/A. K. Jain/3rd Ed./Pg. 702-723]
A. 50 mg   B. 100 mg
C. 150 mg   D. 200 mg

Q 6. Hyperbaric oxygen is indicated in:
[Textbook of Physiology/A. K. Jain/3rd Ed./Pg. 491]
A. Aerobic infections   B. Anaerobic infections
C. Viral infections   D. Fungal infections

Q 7. The life span of a red blood cell is:
[Textbook of Physiology/A. K. Jain/3rd Ed./Pg. 47]
A. 12 weeks   B. 12 days
C. 60 days   D. 120 days

Q 8. Cryptorchidism is a condition in which:
[Medicine/Davidson/20th Ed./Pg. 765]
A. Thyroid gland is enlarged
B. Parathyroid hormone function is increased
C. Incomplete descend of testes in newborn
D. Benign tumor of prostate gland

Q 9. The level of concentration of following hormone reaches peak levels at 10 weeks of pregnancy and used for the confirmation of pregnancy:
[Medicine/Davidson/20th Ed./Pg. 766]
A. HCG   B. BCG
C. TSH   D. LMP

Q 10. The volume of urine excreted by a healthy adult is:
[Textbook of Physiology/A. K. Jain/3rd Ed./Pg. 560]
A. 1500 – 2000 mL/day
B. 500 – 550 mL/day
C. 1.5 – 2 gallons/day
D. 4000 – 4500 mL/day

Q 11. The commonest variety of renal stone is:
[Medicine/Davidson/20th Ed./Pg. 473]
A. Uric acid stone   B. Oxalate stone
C. Phosphate stone   D. Mixed stone

Q 12. A therapist monitors a patient's blood pressure using the brachial artery. What effect would you expect to see on the measured blood pressure value if the therapist selects blood pressure cuff that is too narrow in relation to the circumference of the patient's arm?
[Physical Rehabilitation/Sullivan/5th Ed./Pg. 115]
A. Systolic values will be higher and diastolic values will be lower
B. Systolic values will be lower and diastolic values will be higher
C. Systolic and diastolic values will be higher
D. Systolic and diastolic values will be lower

Answer   1 C   2 C   3 C   4 D   5 D   6 B   7 D   8 C   9 A   10 D   11 B   12 C

Q 13. A patient with suspected cardiac dysfunction is placed on a continuous ambulatory ECG monitor. Which of the following is the name commonly used for this type of monitoring?

[Medicine/Davidson/20th Ed./Pg. 529]

A. Hemodynamic   B. Holter
C. Phonocardiography D. Pulmonic

Q 14. Dysrhythmias can result in varying degrees of abnormal hemodynamics. Which of the following dysrhythmias would have the most significant effect on hemodynamics?

[Medicine/Davidson/20th Ed./Pg. 560]

A. Sinus rhythm with first degree A-V block
B. Sinus rhythm with premature atrial contractions
C. Sinus rhythm with short episodes of paroxysmal supraventricular tachycardia
D. Ventricular tachycardia

Q 15. After administration, many drugs are stored at specific locations in the body. What is the primary site for drug storage in the body?

[Medicine/Davidson/20th Ed./Pg. 24]

A. Adipose tissue   B. Bone
C. Muscle   D. Organs

Q 16. A therapist examines an electrocardiogram of a patient during exercise. What change in the electrocardiogram would be indicative of myocardial ischemia?

[Medicine/Davidson/20th Ed./Pg. 528]

A. P wave changes   B. PR interval changes
C. QRS changes   D. ST segment changes

Q 17. A therapist employed in a large medical center reviews the chart of a 63-year-old male referred to physical therapy for pulmonary rehabilitation. The chart indicates the patient has smoked 1–2 packs of cigarettes a day since the age of 25. the admitting physician documented that the patient's thorax was enlarged with flaring of the costal margins and widening of the costochondral angle. Which pulmonary disease does the chart most accurately describe?

[Medicine/Davidson/20th Ed./Pg. 653]

A. Asthma   B. Bronchiectasis
C. Chronic bronchitis D. Emphysema

Q 18. A patient is instructed by the nursing staff to increase dietary consumption of food sources that are rich in vitamin A. Which of the following food groups would be the most appropriate to meet this goal?

[Medicine/Davidson/20th Ed./Pg. 121]

A. Green leaves, nuts, seafood
B. Fish liver oils, butter, yellow vegetables
C. Milk, cheese, liver
D. Vegetable oil, wheat germ, dried yeast

Q 19. An acute myocardial infarction can often be diagnosed by analyzing the characteristic pattern and duration of selected enzymes in the blood. Which of the following enzymes is not commonly elevated following a acute myocardial infarction?

[Medicine/Davidson/20th Ed./Pg. 592]

A. Aspartate aminotransferase
B. Creatine phosphokinase
C. Lactate dehydrogenase
D. Alkaline phosphatase

Q 20. A patient is placed on a 12 lead ECG following a suspected myocardial infarction. What ECG finding is the best indicator of an acute myocardial infarction?

[Medicine/Davidson/20th Ed./Pg. 528]

A. ST segment elevation
B. QRS complex elevation
C. P wave elevation
D. T wave elevation

Q 21. Patients often progress through a predictable series of stages after being diagnosed with a terminal illness. According to Elizabeth Kubler Ross' Stages of Dying, what is the stage patients will first experience?

[Physical Rehabilitation/Sullivan/5th Ed./Pg. 31,36]

A. Acceptance   B. Anger
C. Denial and isolation D. Depression

Q 22. A therapist monitors the blood pressure of a 28-year-old male during increasing levels of physical exertion. Assuming a normal physiologic response, which of the following best describes the patients' blood pressure response to exercise?

[Textbook of Physiology/A. K. Jain/Pg. 365, 505]

A. Systolic pressure decreases, diastolic pressure increases
B. Systolic pressure remains the same, diastolic pressure decreases
C. Systolic pressure and diastolic pressure remains the same
D. None

Q 23. A patient with chronic arterial insufficiency may demonstrate which of the following signs?

[Medicine/Davidson/20th Ed./Pg. 1278]

A. Edema   B. Brown skin pigment
C. Gangrene   D. Warm skin temperature

Q 24. While discussing a patient's progress with a referring physician the physician asks if the patient has demonstrated any signs of thoracodynia. Thoracodynia can best be described as:

[Medicine/Davidson/20th Ed./Pg. 534-539]

A. Hypoventilation
B. Inadequate chest expansion
C. Diaphragmatic spasm
D. Chest pain

Q 25. A therapist reviews the medical chart of a patient with a history of recurrent dysrhythmias. The therapist is concerned about the past medical history and would like to monitor the patient during all activities. Which of the following monitoring devices would be the most beneficial?

[Physical Rehabilitation/Sullivan/5th Ed./Pg. 603]

A. Pulmonary artery catheter
B. Electrocardiogram
C. Intracranial pressure monitor
D. Pulse oximeter

Answer   13 B   14 D   15 A   16 D   17 D   18 B   19 D   20 A   21 C   22 D   23 C   24 D   25 B

Q 26. A therapist monitors a patient's blood pressure using the brachial artery. What effect would you expect to see on the measured blood pressure value if the therapist selects blood pressure cuff that is too narrow in relation to the circumference of the patient's arm?

[Physical Rehabilitation/Sullivan/5th Ed./Pg. 115]

A. Systolic valves will be higher and diastolic valves will be lower
B. Systolic valves will be lower and diastolic valves will be higher
C. Systolic and diastolic valves will be higher
D. Systolic and diastolic valves will be lower

Q 27. Therapists must be aware of a variety of factors that can influence a patient's pulse rate. Which of the following factors would not have a tendency to increase a patient's pulse rate?

[Physical Rehabilitation/Sullivan/5th Ed./Pg. 96]

A. Infection
B. Low temperatures
A. Hypotension
B. Stress or anxiety

Rehabilitation

Q 28. A patient is admitted to a phase I cardiac rehabilitation program after sustaining a myocardial infarction. Assuming an uncomplicated medical course, how long would a patient typically stay in a phase I program?

[Physical Rehabilitation/Sullivan/20th Ed./Pg. 617]

A. 3 – 5 days
B. 7 – 12 days
C. 16 – 20 days
D. 24 – 30 days

Others

Q 29. Diclofenac sodium is used as an:

[Medicine/Davidson/20th Ed./Pg. 973]

A. Antibiotic
B. Antiepileptic
C. Anti-inflammatory
D. Antimalarial

Q 30. Salbutamol is a pharmaceutical agent used as:

[Medicine/Davidson/20th Ed./Pg. 677]

A. Bronchodilator
B. Anticonvulsant
C. Antihypertensive
D. Antiemetic

Q 31. Which of the following inhibit bone calcification maximally?

[Medicine/Davidson/20th Ed./Pg. 153]

A. Tetracycline
B. Oxytetracyclin
C. Chloromycetin
D. Ampicillin

Q 32. The correct dose of ethambutol in Indian adult weighing 80 kg is:

[Medicine/Davidson/20th Ed./Pg. 903]

A. ½ gram per day
B. 1 gram per day
C. 2 gram per day
D. 3 gram per day

Q 33. The correct dose of rifampicin in Indian adult weighing 80 kg is:

[Medicine/Davidson/20th Ed./Pg. 701]

A. 200 mg per day
B. 600 mg per day
C. 1000 mg per day
D. 2 g per day

Q 34. A patient rehabilitating from a myocardial infarction prepares for a graded exercise test. Which of the following pharmacological agents would lower heart rate and blood pressure during an exercise test?

[Medicine/Davidson/20th Ed./Pg. 585]

A. Antidepressants
B. Diuretics
C. Beta blockers
D. Bronchodilators

Q 35. A frequently administered treatment for cancer in which high doses of energy are administered to the body to stop cell replication is termed:

[Medicine/Davidson/20th Ed./Pg. 264]

A. Immunotherapy
B. Radiation therapy
C. Chemotherapy
D. Surgical intervention

Q 36. Certain types of drugs such as nitroglycerin can be metabolized and destroyed by the liver. What route of administration would best allow nitroglycerin to each the systemic circulation?

[Medicine/Davidson/20th Ed./Pg. 597]

A. Oral
B. Rectal
C. Nasal
D. Sublingual

Q 37. Acetaminophen is a commonly encountered drug seen frequently in patients requiring physical therapy. What is the primary benefit of acetaminophen compared to aspirin and other nonsteroidal anti-inflammatory medications?

[Medicine/Davidson/20th Ed./Pg. 27]

A. Increased analgesic effects
B. Increased antipyretic effects
C. Decreased upper gastrointestinal tract irritation
D. Decreased irritation of the oral mucosa

Q 38. A therapist reviews a patient's medical chart to determine when they were last medicated. The chart indicates the patient received medication at 2300 hours. Assuming it is now 8:00 AM, how long ago did the patient receive the medication?

[Medicine/Davidson/20th Ed./Pg. 25]

A. 5 hours
B. 9 hours
C. 15 hours
D. 18 hours

Q 39. A physical therapy department attempts to develop a clinical education program. Which of the following criteria would be considered the most essential?

[Medicine/Davidson/20th Ed./Pg. 21]

A. The clinical family's philosophy and objectives for patient care should be identical with those of the affiliating physical therapy education program.
B. The clinical staff should have a strong desire to participate in the education of future therapists.
C. The clinical staff should develop a specific plan to meet the objectives of individual students.
D. The clinical facility should have a variety of learning experiences available during the clinical practicum.

Answer

| 26 C | 27 B | 28 A | 29 C | 30 A | 31 A | 32 C | 33 B | 34 C | 35 B | 36 D | 37 C |
| 38 B | 39 B | | | | | | | | | | |

Q 40. A therapist often works with a variety of patients with known or suspected communicable diseases or infections. Depending on the type of disease or infection, these patients may be placed in isolation. What type of isolation would require a therapist to wear a gown?

[Medicine/Davidson/20th Ed./Pg. 286]

A. Enteric precautions
B. Contact
C. Respiratory
D. Strict

Q 41. A patient indicates that she is currently taking medication to control high blood pressure. Which of the following classifications of drug would be helpful in the treatment of hypertension?

[Medicine/Davidson/20th Ed./Pg. 613]

A. Diuretics
B. Narcotics
C. Nonsteroidal anti-inflammatories
D. Stimulants

Q 42. A physician completes a physical examination on 16-year-old male who injured his knee while playing in a soccer contest yesterday. The physician's preliminary diagnosis is a grade II anterior cruciate ligament injury with probable meniscal involvement. Which of the following diagnostic tools would be the most appropriate in the immediate medical management of the patient?

[Essential of Orthopedics/Maheshwari/3rd Ed./Pg. 135]

A. Bone scan
B. Computerized tomography
C. Magnetic resonance imaging
D. X-rays

Q 43. A physician suspects a stress fracture in a 16- year-old distance runner after completing a physical examination. Assuming the physician's preliminary diagnosis is correct, which of the following diagnostic tests would be the most appropriate to identify the stress fracture?

[Medicine/Davidson/20th Ed./Pg. 1010]

A. Bone scan
B. Magnetic resonance imaging
C. Telethermography
D. Ultrasound scan

Pathology and Pharmacology

Q 44. For prophylactic immunization of poliomyelitis OPV used is:

[Medicine/Davidson/20th Ed./Pg. 138-139]

A. Salk + sabin vaccine given by injection
B. Salk vaccine given by mouth
C. Sabin vaccine given by injection
D. Sabin vaccine given by mouth

Q 45. Essential basic treatment of domestic dog bites are all of the following except:

[Medicine/Davidson/20th Ed./Pg. 318]

A. Anti tetanus and antirabies injection
B. Irrigation and debridement
C. Prophylactic antibiotics
D. Hydrocortisone therapy

Q 46. A patient with a lengthy history of substance abuse is referred to physical therapy after sustaining multiple injuries in a motor vehicle accident. Which of the following controlled substances does not foster physical dependence?

A. Depressants
B. Hallucinogen
C. Narcotics
D. Stimulants

Q 47. Most commonly the isolated organism from domestic animal bite is:

[Medicine/Davidson/Churchill/20th Ed./Pg. 312]

A. Staphylococcus aureus
B. Pasteurella multocida
C. Streptococcus pyogenes
D. E coli

Q 48. Normal running speed of ECG is:

A. 30 mm/sec
B. 20 mm/sec
C. 25 mm/sec
D. 40 mm/sec

Q 49. Three types of polio virus isolated are:

[Medicine/Davidson/20th Ed./Pg. 1230]

A. Brunhilde, Mcmurray, and Newton
B. Leon, Mcburney and Voldik
C. Brunhilde, Lansing and Leon
D. Mchilde, Salk and Newton

Q 50. A patient with a lengthy history of substance abuse is referred to physical therapy after sustaining multiple injuries in a motor vehicle accident. Which of the following controlled substances does foster physical dependence?

A. Depressants
B. Hallucinogen
C. Narcotics
D. All of above

Answer   40 D   41 A   42 D   43 A   44 D   45 D   46 D   47 C   48 C   49 B   50 D

6

Research and Analysis

Objective Questions with Answers

Ethics

Q1. A therapist supervising a physical therapy student observes the student performing an initial examination. During the examination the patient appears to be uncomfortable with the student and reports to the supervision therapist. The most appropriate therapist action is to:

[Physical Rehabilitation/Sullivan/Pg. 68]

A. Attempt to convince the patient to accept the student.
B. List the student's academic accomplishments.
C. Inform the patient that the student is qualified to complete the examinations
D. Complete the examination for the student.

Q 2. A therapist treats a 61-year-old male at home following thoracic surgery. As part of treatment, the therapist designs a general exercise program for the patient. The patient is extremely eager to begin a formal exercise program however his spouse expresses serious doubt about protocols importance. The most appropriate therapists action is to:

[Tidy's Physiotherapy/12th Ed./Pg. 215]

A. Explain to the patient and spouse why the exercise program is an essential part of rehabilitation.
B. Redesign the exercise program to address the spouse's concerns
C. Ask the spouse to leave the room during treatment sessions
D. Discharge the patient from physical therapy

Q 3. A patient seen at home requires assistance with tub transfers using a tub bench. The physical therapist is scheduled to treat the patient three times a week, but there is a six-day waiting period for occupational therapy service. The therapist would best assist the patient by:

[Physical Rehabilitation/Sullivan, 5th Ed./Pg. 1151]

A. Practicing tub transfers during physical therapy treatment sessions
B. Waiting until an occupational therapist can examine the patient

C. Giving the patient written information on tub transfers
D. Calling another agency and requesting the services of an occupational therapist

Q 4. As part of a community outreach program, a therapist conducts an in service for expectant mothers. During the presentation the therapist identifies several potential effects of maternal substance abuse. Which of the following would not be considered a neonatal complication of cigarette smoking?

[Tidy's Physiotherapy/12th Ed./Pg. 390]

A. Low birth weight
B. Increased risk of sudden infant death syndrome
C. Increased neonatal mortality
D. Placenta previa

Q 5. A 45-year-old female involved in a phase II cardiac rehabilitation program refuses to take part in a group exercise session. The most appropriate therapist action is to:

[Refer to Text]

A. Ask the patient why she is unwilling to participate
B. Inform the patient that she is only hurting herself
C. Notify the patient's insurance provider
D. Discharge the patient from therapy

Q 6. A physician refers a patient rehabilitating from an intertrochanteric fracture to physical therapy. On the referral form the physician specifies the use of continuous ultrasound at 2.4 W/cm² over the fracture site. The most appropriate therapist action is to:

[Physical agents in Rehabilitation/ Cameroon/ Pg. 280]

A. Treat the patient as indicated on the referral form
B. Request that the patient obtain a new referral from the physician
C. Use another more acceptable modality
D. Contact the referring physician

Answer   1 D   2 A   3 A   4 D   5 A   6 D

Q 7. A patient being treated in an outpatient physical therapy clinic explains that he has felt nauseating since having his methotrexate medication level altered. The most appropriate therapist action is to:

[Physical Rehabilitation/Sullivan 5th Ed./Pg. 74]

A. Explain to the patient that nausea is very common when altering medication levels
B. Ask the patient to stop taking the prescribed medication
C. Request that the patient make an immediate appointment with the physician
D. Request that the patient contact the physician's office to discuss the situation

Q 8. A group of health care professionals participate in a family conference for a patient with a cord injury. During the conference one of the participants summarizes the patient's program bathing and dressing activities. This type of information is typically conveyed by a/an

[Physical Rehabilitation/Sullivan 5th Ed./Pg. 1151]

A. Nurse   B. Physical therapist
C. Occupational therapist   D. Case manager

Q 9. There are a variety of different isolation categories which require the use of specific techniques designed to reduce or prevent the transmission of disease. Which of the following is required regardless of the specific isolation category?

[Physical Rehabilitation/Sullivan/5th Ed./Pg. 68/]

A. Mask   B. Gown
C. Gloves   D. Handwashing

Q 10. A former patient calls to ask for advice immediately after injuring his lower back in a work related accident. The patient explains that he cannot bend down and touch his toes without severe pain and has muscle spasm throughout the entire lower back. You work in a state without direct access, but would like to help your former patient. The most appropriate response would be:

[Physical Rehabilitation/Sullivan/5th Ed./Pg. 74/]

A. Explain to the patient that you would be happy to treat him, however since you have not completed a formal examination it would be unfair to prescribe treatment over the phone
B. Arrange a time for the patient to come into your clinic for immediate treatment
C. Prescribe flexion exercises and ice every three hours
D. Refer the patient to a qualified physician.

Q 11. A patient rehabilitating from congestive heart failure is examined in physical therapy department. During the examination the patient begins to complain of pain. The most immediate therapist action is to:

[Tidy's Physiotherapy/12th Ed./Pg. 229]

A. Notify the nursing staff to administer pain medication
B. Contact the referring physician
C. Discontinue the treatment session
D. Ask the patient to describe the location and severity of the pain

Q 12. A therapist treating a patient in a special care unit notices a marked increase in fluid on the dorsum of a patient's hand around an IV site. The therapist recognizing the possibility that the IV has become dislodged should immediately:

[Physical Rehabilitation/Sullivan/5th Ed./Pg. 903]

A. Continue with the present treatment
B. Contact the primary physician
C. Turn of the iv
D. Reposition the peripheral iv line.

Q 13. Policies and procedures are necessary tools to carry out effective and efficient management. Which of the following statements describing policies is not accurate?

[Physical Rehabilitation/Sullivan/5th Ed./Pg. 18]

A. Polices should be assembled into a manual for quick and easy reference
B. Existing policies should be reviewed at regular intervals and revised as indicated
C. Policies should be established on an oral basis
D. Final approval of policies is the responsibility of the chief administrator

Q 14. A therapist treating a patient overhears two of his colleagues discussing another patient's case in the charting area. The therapist is concerned that this patient may overhear the same conversation. The most appropriate action is to:

[Physical Rehabilitation/Sullivan/5th Ed. Pg. 68]

A. Discuss the situation with the director of rehabilitation
B. Confront the therapists and ask them if their behavior is professional
C. Move the patient away from the charting area
D. Inform the therapists that their conversation may be audible to patients

Q 15. A therapist completes a family training session with a patient rehabilitating from a spinal cord injury. During the training the family asks a question regarding the functional ability of the patient following rehabilitation. The most appropriate therapist response is to:

[Physical Rehabilitation/Sullivan/5th Ed./Pg. 942]

A. Explain to the family that it is difficult to predict since all patients progress differently
B. Provide information on the expected prognosis based on the nature and severity of the injury
C. Refer the family to the director of rehabilitation
D. Refer the family to the patient's referring physician

Q 16. A physical therapist and a physical therapist assistant are employed in a skilled nursing facility. Which of the following activities would be appropriate for the physical therapist assistant?

[Physical Rehabilitation/Sullivan/ 5th Ed.Pg. 12]

A. Fitting of an assistive device
B. Development of a plan of care
C. Re-examination of a patient
D. Establishment of a discharge plan

Answer   7 D   8 C   9 D   10 D   11 D   12 C   13 C   14 D   15 B   16 A

Q 17. A physical therapist assistant provides patient coverage for a physical therapist on vacation. The physical therapist assistant should be allowed to perform all of the following except:

[Physical Rehabilitation/Sullivan/ 5th Ed./Pg. 11]

A. Supervision of exercise activities
B. Modification of the plan of care
C. Gait training activities
D. Daily progress notes

Q 18. An effective manager will rely on well established policies and procedures when disciplining an employee. Which of the following action would be considered inappropriate?

[Refer to Text]

A. Begin with a clear description of the unacceptable behavior
B. Indicate what action should be taken by the employee
C. Set a follow up date to discuss the situation
D. Focus the discussion on the individual and not on a performance discrepancy

Q 19. A patient receiving physical therapy treatment complains that he is experiencing a great deal of pain around the I V site. The therapist's most appropriate would be to:

[Refer to Text]

A. Reposition the I V
B. Remove the I V
C. Turn off the I V
D. Contact nursing

Q 20. A work site examination is scheduled for a patient rehabilitating from a closed head injury eight weeks ago. The patient presents with mild dysarthria, right-sided hemiparesis with moderate upper extremity involvement, and utilizes a straight cane for mobility. The patient's job is secretarial including: answering phones, filing, and organizing the office. The most appropriate clinician to participate in the work site examination is a/am:

[Physical Rehabilitation/Sullivan/ 5th Ed./Pg. 1151]

A. Physical therapist
B. Occupational therapist
C. Speech therapist
D. Social worker

Q 21. An 18-year-old male status of post fractured right femur with open reduction and internal fixation is referred to physical therapy. After the initial therapy session the patient states that therapy is a waste of time and he will not return for any additional treatment. The most immediate response would be to:

[Physical Rehabilitation/Sullivan/5th Ed./Pg. 71]

A. Inform the referring physician of the patient's decision
B. Instruct the patient to return for one additional treatment session
C. Discuss the importance of physical therapy with the patient
D. Discharge the patient from physical therapy

Q 22. A therapist suspects a patient may be under the influence of alcohol during a treatment session. The therapist has been treating the patient for over five weeks and during that time has failed to recognize any signs or symptoms of substance abuse. The therapist's most immediate action would be to:

[Physical Rehabilitation/Sullivan/5th Ed./Pg. 71]

A. Contact the referring physician and discuss the patient's problem
B. Ask the patient if he/she has been drinking
C. Discharge the patient from physical therapy
D. Refer the patient to a local Alcoholics Anonymous group

Q 23. The parents of a patient with a C4 spinal cord injury request projected outcome information on their 18-year- old son. The most appropriate health care professional to answer the parents' question is the:

[Physical Rehabilitation/Sullivan/5th Ed./Pg. 962]

A. Primary nurse
B. Psychiatrist
C. Case manager
D. Social worker

Q 24. Therapists are often faced with ethical issues. In their daily clinical practice. Which of the following would be the most appropriate initial step when faced with an ethical dilemma:

[Physical Rehabilitation/Sullivan/5th Ed./Pg. 72]

A. Determine an action plan
B. Seek external support
C. Gather relevant information
D. Complete the action plan

Q 25. A risk management committee identifies several examples of physical therapy malpractice. Which of the following would not be considered a potentially negligent act?

[Physical Rehabilitation/Sullivan/5th Ed./Pg. 65]

A. Failure to follow a physician's order
B. Application of faulty equipment
C. Sexual misconduct
D. Failure to achieve an established long term goal

Q 26. A physical therapist and physical therapist assistant work as a team in an acute care medical facility. Which of the following responsibilities would be appropriate for the physical therapist to delegate to the therapist assistant?

[Tidy's Physiotherapy/12th Ed./Pg. 373]

A. Develop a patient treatment plan based on an initial examination
B. Revise an established patient plan
C. Implement a therapeutic exercise program
D. Write a discharge summary

Q 27. A therapist describes an exercise program to a patient using terms such as flexion, extension, and abduction. The patient informs the therapist that she does not understand the instruction. The most appropriate action is to:

[Physical Rehabilitation/Sullivan/5th Ed./Pg. 14]

A. Verbally define each term
B. Provide a written definition of each term
C. Define each term without using medical terminology
D. Select a different exercise

Q 28. A patient rehabilitating from a laminectomy informs a therapist that his work schedule has prohibited him from completing the prescribed home exercise program. The therapist is frustrated with the patient's admission, particularly since the home exercise program takes only 10 minutes to complete. The most appropriate therapist action is to:

[Tidy's Physiotherapy/12th Ed./Pg. 157]

Answer   17 B   18 D   19 D   20 B   21 C   22 B   23 B   24 C   25 D   26 C   27 C

A. Emphasize the importance of the home exercise program is part of the patient's rehabilitation program
B. Ask the patient to make a specific effort to complete the home exercise program
C. Inform the referring physician that the patient has been noncompliant
D. Discharge the patient from physical therapy

Q 29. A physical therapist assistant completes daily documentation in the medical record. Which of the following documentation activities would be inappropriate for a physical therapist assistant?
[Physical Rehabilitation/Sullivan/5th Ed./Pg. 12]
A. A reaction to treatment
B. Patient compliance
C. Discharge summary
D. Treatment of services provided

Q 30. A physical therapist is a member of a interdisciplinary team in a rehabilitation center. One of the patients in the pediatric unit is a 5-year-old boy who sustained a head injury and multiple fractures in a motor vehicle accident. The patient is scheduled to be treated by the team, but there is no information in the medical chart which specifies the patient's current weight bearing status. Which member of the interdisciplinary team would be responsible for determining the patient's weight bearing status?
[Physical Rehabilitation/Sullivan/5th Ed./Pg. 2]
A. Physical therapist   B. Occupational therapist
C. Speech therapist   D. Physician

Q 31. A therapist attempts to take a history from a patient who is acutely ill. In an attempt to conserve the patient's energy the therapist should ask questions that are:
[Physical Rehabilitation/Sullivan/5th Ed./Pg. 4]
A. Thought provoking and reflective
B. Easily answered with brief statements
C. Stimulating and invigorating
D. Sympathetic and endearing

Q 32. A patient is informed that her condition is terminal shortly before her scheduled therapy session. During the treatment session, the patient asks the therapist if she believes the physician's assessment is accurate. The most appropriate therapist response is:
[Physical Rehabilitation/Sullivan/5th Ed./Pg. 29]
A. Physicians are not infallible
B. Your present condition is very serious
C. Channel your energy towards getting better
D. Focus on your therapy goals

Q 33. A physical therapist notices a student physical therapist using improper guarding techniques on a patient that appears to be unstable. The most immediate therapist action should be:
[Physical Rehabilitation/Sullivan/5th Ed./Pg. 68]
A. discuss the situation with the student's clinical instructor
B. Leave the student an anonymous note describing proper guarding technique

C. Offer suggestions to improve the student's guarding technique
D. Ignore the situation since you are not the clinical instruction

Q 34. A patient three weeks status post right total knee replacement complains of pain in the right calf. The patient's pain increases with ambulation and with quick passive range of motion into dorsiflexion. The patient's lower extremity is warm to touch. The most appropriate response would be to:
[Tidy's Physiotherapy/5th Ed./Pg. 273]
A. Disregard the findings as postoperative pain
B. Continue with ambulation to tolerance
C. Perform active calf stretching
D. Request a physician to rule out deep venous thrombosis

Q 35. An increasing number of states offer consumers the ability to enter the health care system by going directly to a physical therapist. Which statement describing the effects of direct access is accurate?
[Physical Rehabilitation/Sullivan/5th Ed./Pg. 28]
A. Physical therapists' malpractice rates have sharply risen as a result of direct access.
B. Insurance carriers may deny claims without a physician's signature in states with direct access
C. Physical therapy has been over utilized in states with direct access.
D. Physicians are being alienated by physical therapists in states with direct access.

Q 36. A male therapist prepares to treat a female patient using a soft tissue massage technique. The therapist would like to reassure that the patient does not misinterpret the purpose of the treatment technique. The most appropriate action is to:
[Tidy's Physiotherapy/12th Ed./Pg. 443]
A. Transfer the patient to another therapist's schedule
B. Request a female staff member to be present during treatment
C. Select another less invasive technique
D. Discharge the patient from physical therapy

Q 37. A therapist develops a list of behavioral objectives for a new employee working in hydrotherapy. Which of the following is not considered to be a behavioral objective?
[Physical Rehabilitation/Sullivan/5th Ed./Pg. 47]
A. The therapist will perform wound debridement to remove necrotic material
B. The therapist will identify two commonly used antibacterial agents
C. The therapist will apply sterile dressing to an open would
D. The therapist will understand the stages of tissue inflammation and repair

Q 38. A therapist examines a patient bedside, when suddenly the patient's I V becomes disconnected. The therapist's most appropriate response would be to:
[Refer to Text]
A. Reconnect the I.V.
B. Contact the primary physician
C. Contact nursing
D. Continue with your present treatment

Answer   28 A   29 C   30 D   31 B   32 B   33 C   34 D   35 B   36 B   37 D   38 C

Biostatics

Q 39. A group of senior physical therapy students attempt to determine if there is a relationship between intelligence and academic achievement. Which of the following correlation coefficients would indicate the strongest positive correlation?
[Research Methods for Clinical Therapist/Hicks/4th Ed./Pg. 77]
A. +.65
B. +.81
C. −.26
d. −.91.

Q 40. The reliability of goniometric measurements taken by different therapists is measured by interrater reliability. Which join motion would you expect to have the poorest interrater reliability?
[Physical Rehabilitation/Sullivan/5th Ed./Pg. 173]
A. Ankle eversion
B. Elbow flexion
C. Knee flexion
D. Shoulder lateral rotation

Q 41. A physical therapy program designs study that uses performance on the scholastic aptitude test as a prediction of grade point average in a physical therapy academic program. The results of the study identify that the overall correlation between the variables is r=.87. Which statement is most accurate based on the results. of the study?
[Research Methodology for Clinical Therapists/Hicks/4th Ed./Pg. 101]
A. Grade point average in a physical therapy program is a function of performance on the scholastic aptitude test
B. A student that performs well on the scholastic aptitude test is likely to have a high grade point average in a physical therapy academic program
C. There is no relationship between grade point average in a physical therapy program and performance on the scholastic aptitude test
D. There is an inverse relationship between grade point average in a physical therapy program and performance on the scholastic aptitude test

Q 42. A therapist attempts to determine that a selected set of data can be statistically analyzed using a parametric test. Which of the following conditions is essential when using a parametric test?
[Research Methods for Clinical Therapists/Hicks/4th Ed./Pg. 112]
A. The data should be interval or ration level
B. The data should be normally distributed
C. The variance in the results from each condition should be similar
D. The subjects should be normally distributed

Q 43. A group of therapists utilize a statistical test to determine whether two means differ significantly from each other. Which parametric test of statistical significance is the most appropriate?
[Research Methods for Clinical Therapists/Hicks/4th Ed./Pg. 112]
A. Test
B. Analysis of variance
C. Chi-square test
D. Manu-Whitney test

Research Methodology

Q 44. As part of a total quality management program, a physical therapy department decides to collect patient satisfaction data. The most appropriate initial action is to:
[Research Methods for Clinical Therapist/Hicks/4th Ed./Pg. 23]
A. Identify appropriate statistical techniques to analyze the data
B. Design a questionnaire for therapists
C. Design a patient satisfaction survey
D. Modify patient care standards based on the collected date

Q 45. A therapist designs a research study which examines the effect of functional knee bracing on speed and agility. In this study speed and agility are the:
[Research Methods for Clinical Therapist/Hicks/4th Ed./Pg. 70]
A. Dependent variables
B. Independent variables
C. Criterion variables
D. Extraneous variables

Q 46. A group of physical therapy students develops a physical activity survey as part of a community health screening. The survey consists of a series of question in which subjects must respond year or no. This type of survey utilizes a/an ___ level of measurement?
[Research Methods for Clinical Therapists/Hicks/4th Ed./Pg. 34]
A. Nominal
B. Ordinal
C. Interval
D. Ration

Q 47. A group of physical therapy students gather data on the public's perception of physical therapy. The students use a questionnaire of closed end questions with is randomly distributed to individuals throughout the country. All of the following are advantages of using closed end questions except:
[Research Methods for Clinical Therapists/Hicks/4th Ed./Pg 22]
A. Quicker and relatively inexpensive to analyze
B. Helps to ensure that answers are given in a frame of reference relevant to the research
C. Forces the respondent to choose an answer even if the choice that corresponds to that of the respondents not listed
D. Makes the meaning of the question clearer.

Q 48. A physical therapy practice attempts to demonstrate appropriate allocation of its resources. The process is bet accomplished by:
[Refer to Text]
A. Utilization review
B. Quality assurance program
C. Program examination
D. Peer assessment.

Q 49. A therapist prepares a research article which will be submitted to a national monthly physical therapy publication. Which of the following components of the research article will be the last to appear?
[Research Methods for Clinical Therapists/Hicks/4th Ed./Pg. 140]
A. Abstract
B. Discussion
C. Methods
D. Results

Answer 39 B 40 A 41 B 42 A 43 A 44 C 45 A 46 A 47 C 48 A 49 B

Q 50. Therapists routinely assess the amount of assistance a patient needs to complete a selected activity. Categories of assistance include maximal, moderate, minimal, standby or independent. This type of measurement scale is best classified as:
[Research Methods for Clinical Therapists/Hicks/4th Ed./Pg. 35]
A. Interval
B. Nominal
C. Ordinal
d. Ratio

Q 51. A therapist measures the vertical leap of members of a basketball team. The therapist then calculates the difference between the highest and lowest values in the distribution. What measure of variability has the therapist determined?
[Research Methods for Clinical Therapists/Hicks/4th Ed./Pg. 54]
A. Mode
B. Range
C. Standard deviation
D. Variance

Q 52. A group of senior physical therapy students utilizes ten patients from a local rehabilitation center with decubitus ulcers for a research project. This type of sampling most accurately describes:
[Research Methods for Clinical Therapists/Hicks/4th Ed./Pg. 27]
A. Cluster sampling
B. Convenience sampling
C. Stratified sampling
D. Systematic sampling

Q 53. A therapist example a patient rehabilitating from a traumatic brain injury. The therapist makes the following entry in the medical record. The patient is able to respond to simple commands fairly consistently, however has difficulty with increasingly complex commands or lack of any external structure. Responses are nonpurposeful, random, and fragmented. According to the Ranchoes Los Amigos Cognitive functioning Scale the patient is most representative of level:
[Physical Rehabilitation/Sullivan/5th Ed./Pg. 901]
A. III—localized response
B. IV—confused agitated
C. V—confused inappropriate
D. VI—confused appropriate

Q 54. A therapist compares the significance of the mean vertical leap difference between samples of 12 athletes and 10 nonathletes. How many degree of freedom are there in study?
[Research Methods for Clinical Therapists/Hicks/4th Ed./Pg. 119]
A. 20
B. 21
C. 22
D. 23

Q 55. Therapists utilize a variety of sampling designs when conducting research. Which design is most likely to result in the greatest degree of sampling error?
[Research Methods for Clinical Therapists/Hicks/4th Ed./Pg. 27]
A. Simple random sample
B. Systematic sample
C. Cluster sample
D. Stratified random sample

Q 56. A group of physical therapy students present a research project entitled "Effects of Ultrasound on Blood Flow and Nerve Conduction Velocity." The dependent variable in the student' study is:
[Research Methods for Clinical Therapists/Hicks/4th Ed./Pg. 32]
A. Ultrasound
B. Ultrasound and blood flow
C. Ultrasound and nerve conduction velocity
D. Blood flow and nerve conduction velocity

Q 57. A therapist participates in a study which examines knee range of motion at selected postoperative intervals. After collecting the necessary data, the therapist prepares to measure the spread or dispersion of the range of motion at each interval. Which statistical measure would be the most appropriate to meet he therapist's objective:
[Research Methods for Clinical Therapists/Hicks/4th Ed./Pg. 55]
A. Median
B. Mode
C. Mean
D. Variance

Q 58. What percentage of physical therapy students taking their state board examination would you expect to score within plus and minus one standard deviation of the mean?
[Research Methods for Clinical Therapists/Hicks/4th Ed./Pg. 49]
A. 48%
B. 58%
C. 68%
D. 88%

Q 59. A therapist is asked to indicate on a five point scale how competent a patient is in a selected transfer technique. The scale ranges from totally incompetent to extremely competent. The type of scale utilizes a/an _______ level of measurement?
[Research Methods for Clinical Therapists/Hicks/4th Ed./Pg. 35]
A. Nominal
B. Ordinal
C. Interval
D. Ration

Q 60. The middle score of a distribution which divides a group of scores into equal parts with half of the scores falling above and half of the scores falling below describes the:
[Research Methods for Clinical Therapists/Hicks/4th Ed./Pg. 50]
A. Mean
B. Median
C. Mode
D. Quota

Q 61. A group of therapists conduct a research study which examines the effect of functional keen bracing on speed and agility. As part of the study the therapists determine measures of central tendency for each measured test. Which of the following would not be considered a measure of central tendency?
[Research Methods for Clinical Therapists/Hicks/5th Ed./Pg. 55]
A. Median
B. Mode
C. Mean
D. Range

Q 62. A physical therapy department plans a study to examine rehabilitation outcomes in patients who have undergone anterior cruciate ligament reconstruction. The study will include a sample of patients from 25 orthopedic surgeons in the local region. If the therapists compile a list of all eligible patients and select every third patient to participate in the study, what type of sampling was used?
[Research Methods for Clinical Therapists/Hicks/4th Ed./Pg. 27]
A. Simple random sampling
B. Stratified sampling
C. Systematic sampling
D. Cluster sampling

Q 63. A therapist conducts a study which measures knee flexion range of motion two weeks following arthroscopic surgery. Assuring a normal distribution what percentage of patients participating in the study would you expect to achieve a goniometric measurement value greater than one standard deviation below the mean:
[Research Methods for Clinical Therapists/Hicks/4th Ed./Pg. 49]

Answer 50 C   51 B   52 B   53 C   54 A   55 C   56 B   57 D   58 C   59 B   60 B   61 D
62 C

A. 49%   B. 64%
C. 68%   D. 84%

Q 64. A therapist presents the results of a research project entitled "Effect of an Aerobic Exercise Program on Heart Rate and Blood Pressure." The independent variable in the therapist's study is:

[Research Methods for Clinical Therapists/Hicks/Pg. 32]

A. Exercise program
B. Exercise program and heart rate
C. Exercise program and blood pressure
D. Heart rate and blood pressure

Assessment and Examination

Q 65. A therapist works with a 70-year-old patient diagnosed with generalized deconditioning. The patient is pleasant and cooperative however has short term memory deficits. The therapist the following home exercise program would be the most beneficial for the patient?

[Physical Rehabilitation/Sullivan/
5th Ed./Pg. 1167]

A. A program that allows for individual exercise selection
B. A program that requires significant attention to detail
C. A program that alternates exercises on consecutive days
D. A program that varies based on results from a subjective pain scale

Q 66. A therapist treats a five-year-old with cerebral palsy. Initially, the therapist was frustrated by the child's poor participation in therapy and as a result developed a reward system that enables the child to earn a sticker for good behavior. Since the therapist initiated the reward system the child has earned a sticker in each of the last five treatment sessions. This type of associated learning is termed:

[Refer to Text]

A. Classical conditioning
B. Operant conditioning
C. Procedural learning
D. Declarative learning

Q 67. A therapist working in an oncology unit reviews the medical chart of a patient prior to initiating an exercise program. The patient's cell counts are as follows: hematocrit 24 mL/dL, white blood cells 400/mm², platelet 4,0000/mm³, hemoglobin levels 7 g/dL. Based on the patient's blood counts, which of the following would be the most accurate statement regarding the patient's allowable exercise level?

[Refer to Text]

A. No exercise is allowed
B. Light exercise is allowed
C. Active exercise is allowed
D. Resistive exercise is allowed

Q 68. A therapist examines a patient diagnosed with rotator cuff tendonitis in physical therapy. The physician referral indicates the patient should be seen three times a week, however after examining the patient the therapist feels once a week is adequate. The most appropriate therapist action is to:

[Physical Rehabilitation Sullivan/5th Ed./Pg. 74]

A. Schedule the patient once a week and notify the referring physician of your rationale
B. Schedule the patient as indicated on the physician referral
C. Ask the patient how often he/she would like to be seen in physical therapy
D. Attempt to determine if the patient's insurance will cover physical therapy visits three times a week.

Q 69. A therapist working in an acute care hospital attempts to determine the effectiveness of treating psoriatic lesions with ultraviolet. The most appropriate initial action is to:

[Research Methods for Clinical Therapists/Hicks/4th Ed./Pg. 124]

A. Design a research study which examines the effectiveness of treating psoriatic lesions with ultraviolet
B. Determine if the current patient population would allow for an adequate sample size for a research study
C. Submit a research proposal to the hospital's institutional review board
D. Conduct a literary search for research related to treating psoriatic lesions with ultraviolet

Q 70. A five-year-old patient is examined in physical therapy. Department The patient seems very uncomfortable during the examination and offers little useful information concerning her injury. The most appropriate therapist action is to:

[Physical Rehabilitation/Sullivan/5th Ed./Pg. 68]

A. Speak loudly and direction to the patient
B. Request that the patient parents come into the treatment room
C. Explain to the patient the importance of physical therapy
D. Inform the patient that effective communication involves more than one individual

Q 71. A patient rehabilitating from a grade I medial collateral ligament injury questions a therapist; his expected functional activity level is the:

[Tidy's Physiotherapy/Pg. 46/12th Ed.]

A. Patient's age and past medical history
B. Patient's previous functional activity level
C. Duration of physical therapy services
D. Patient's compliance with the established home exercise program

Q 72. A patient with vertigo is referred to physical therapy for a balance assessment. When testing kinesthesia, the most reliable method is to:

[Physical Rehabilitation/Sullivan/5th Ed./Pg. 1007]

A. Have the patient describe the position of his/her extremity once it is placed in a static position
B. Have the patient describe the direction and position of his/her extremity during movement
C. Have the patient describe the if the stimuli are sharp or dull
D. Have the patient name the object in his/her hand without visual input

Q 73. During a balance assessment of a patient with left hemiplegia, it is noted that in sitting the patient requires minimal assistance to maintain the position and cannot accept any additional challenge. The therapist would appropriately document the patient's sitting balance as:

[Physical Rehabilitation/Sullivan/5th Ed./Pg. 181]

Answer   63 D   64 A   65 A   66 B   67 D   68 A   69 D   70 B   71 B   72 B

A. Normal   B. Good
C. Fair   D. Poor

Q 74. A complete medical history should be conducted on all patients prior to initiating treatment. Questions asked during the patient. Which of the following questions would not be considered leading?

[Orthopaedic, Physical Assessment/Magee/5th Ed./Pg. 5]

A. Does this increase your pain?
B. Does this alter your pain in anyway?
C. Does your pain increase at night?
D. Does your pain decrease with activity?

Q 75. When two therapists give drastically different manual muscle testing results on the same patient, it is an example of poor:

[Research Methods for Clinical Therapists/Hicks/4th Ed./Pg. 771]

A. Intrarater reliability   B. Interrater reliability
C. Internal validity   D. External validity

Q 76. A therapist measures a patient's respiration rate at rest. In order to obtain the most accurate value the therapist should measure the inspirations or expirations for _________ seconds?

[Human Physiology and Biochemistry for PT and OT/ A.K. Jain/1st Ed./Pg. 133]

A. 10   B. 15
C. 30   D. 60

Q 77. During an initial examination a physical therapist examines a patient's general willingness to use an affected body part. What objective information would provide the most useful information:

[Joint Structure and Function/Norkin/3rd Ed./Pg. 95]

A. Bony palpation   B. Active movement
C. Passive movement   D. Sensory testing

Q 78. A male physical therapist examines a female diagnosed with subacromial bursitis. After taking a though history, the therapist ask the patient to change into a gown. The patient seems very uneasy about this suggestion, but finally agrees to use the gown. The most appropriate course of action would be to:

[Physical Rehabilitation/Sullivan/5th Ed./Pg. 68/]

A. Continue treatment as planned
B. Attempt to treat the patient without using the gown
C. Bring a female staff member into the treatment room and continue with treatment
D. Offer to transfer the patient to a female therapist.

Q 79. There are many guidelines that are useful for clinicians attempting to avoid unnecessary litigation. Which of the following, would be considered the most essential?

[Refer to Text]

A. Conduct a thorough initial examination
B. Instruct patients carefully in all exercise activities
C. Keep the referring physician informed
D. Maintain accurate and timely documentation.

Q 80. Which technique would be the most appropriate when assessing the pulse of a patient after exercise?

[Human Physiology and Biochemistry for PT and OT/A.K. Jain/ Arya Pub./1st Ed./Pg. 447]

A. Placing the palm of the hand firmly over the pulse site
B. Counting the pulse for five seconds and multiplying by twelve to determine the beats per minute
C. Selecting a pulse site that will not cause discomfort and subsequently alter the pulse rate
D. Selecting three to five separate pulse sites to assure an accurate measurement.

Q 81. A therapist prepares to treat a patient in isolation. In what order should the protective clothing be applied?

[Physical Rehabilitation/Sullivan/ 5th Ed./Pg. 19]

A. Gloves, gown, mask   B. Gown, gloves, mask
C. Mask, gown, gloves   D. Gloves, mask, gown

Q 82. A therapist supervising a physical therapy student observes the student performing an initial examination. During the examination the patient appears to be uncomfortable with the student and asks by the supervision therapist. The most appropriate therapist action is to:

[Physical Rehabilitation/Sullivan/5th Ed./Pg. 68]

A. Attempt to convince the patient to accept the student.
B. List the student's academic accomplishments.
C. Inform the patient that the student is qualified to complete the examinations
D. Complete the examination for the Student.

Q 83. A therapist covering for a colleague on vacation examines a patient with a traumatic brain injury. The therapist had read the patient's medical chart, but remains anxious about the examination. The most important area for the therapist to assess immediately is:

[Physical Rehabilitation/Sullivan/5th Ed./Pg. 900]

A. Extent of orthopedic involvement
B. Level of communication
C. Muscle tone
D. Sensation

Q 84. A therapist identifies several inconsistencies between a patient's subjective complaints and the objective findings of an initial examination. A detailed discussion of the identified inconsistencies belongs in the _________ section of a SOAP note?

[Physical Rehabilitation/Sullivan/5th Ed./Pg. 19]

A. Subjective   B. Objective
C. Assessment   D. Plan

Q 85. After examining the respiratory status of a patient with a C6 spinal cord injury, which of the following clinical findings would you expect to be accurate?

[Physical Rehabilitation/Sullivan/5th Ed./Pg. 962]

A. Partial innervation of the diaphragm
B. Full epigastric rise in supine
C. A ventilator is required for assisted breathing
D. Normal ventilatory reserve

Answer   73 D   74 B   75 B   76 D   77 B   78 C   79 D   80 C   81 C   82 B   83 B   84 C
              85 B

Q 86. A therapist develops a problem list after completing an examination of a patient status postarthroscopic medial meniscectomy. The therapist identifies increased edema in the right knee as the first entry in the problem list. Which of the following short term goals would be the most appropriate entry in the medical record?
[Tidy's Physiotherapy/12th Ed./Pg. 52]
A. Decrease edema in the knee by one centimeter
B. Decrease edema in the knee by one centimeter within two weeks
C. Decrease right knee circumferential measurements by one centimeter at a level three centimeters and five centimeters above the knee
D. Decrease right knee circumferential measurements by one centimeter at a level three centimeters and five centimeters above the superior pole of the patella within two weeks.

Q 87. A therapist examines a 24-year-old male recently admitted to the hospital with C3 tetraplegia. During the examination the therapist identifies several areas of reddened and mottled skin over selected bony prominences.
[Physical Rehabilitation/Sullivan/5th Ed./Pg. 950]
A. Discuss the situation directly with the nursing staff
B. Ask the patient to perform pressure relief activities
C. Contact the patient's family
D. Contact the patient's referring physician

Q 88. A therapist attempts to document a patient's inability to achieve weekly goals with the following entry: "Patient may have performed poorly during the last week secondary to recent illness." Entry would belong in the __________ section of a SOAP note?
[Physical Rehabilitation/Sullivan/5th Ed./Pg. 19]
A. Subjective   B. Objective
C. Assessment   D. Plan

Q 89. A patient rehabilitating from a motor vehicle accident complains of pain along the chest wall during inspiration. While palpating the chest wall, the therapist detects grating with associated point tenderness. Which type of injury would best explain the patient's symptoms?
[Physical Rehabilitation/Sullivan/5th Ed./Pg. 168]
A. Rib fracture
B. Subluxation of costal cartilage
C. Intercostals fibrositis
D. Pulmonary embolus

Q 90. A patient, eight weeks, status post right total hip replacement loses his balance and falls to the ground. The patient is visibly shaken by the fall, but insists that he is uninjured. The therapist examines the right hip and although active motion elicits pin, all other findings are inconclusive. The therapist should.
[Physical Rehabilitation/Sullivan/5th Ed./Pg. 18]
A. Continue with the current treatment so the patient does not focus on the incident
B. Notify the supervising therapist about incident
C. Document the incident and contact a physician to examine the patient before resuming treatment

D. Document the incident and gradually resume prior treatment

Q 91. The results of a manual muscle test should be recorded in the __________ section of a SOAP note?
[Physical Rehabilitation/Sullivan/5th Ed./Pg. 19]
A. Subjective   B. Objective
C. Assessment   D. Plan

Q 92. A therapist assesses a patient blood pressure using the brachial artery. Which of the following statements is not accurate when performing this technique?
[Physical Rehabilitation/Sullivan/5th Ed./Pg. 96]
A. Explain the procedure to the patient in terms appropriate to his or her level of understanding
B. Expose the arm and place it at heart level with the elbow extended
C. Wrap and blood pressure cuff around the arm approximately four to six inches above the antecubital fossa
D. Place the diaphragm of the stethoscope over the brachial artery in the antecubital fossa

Q 93. A physical therapist examines a patient with T1 paraplegia. As the therapist and patient perform balance activities in sitting, the patient begins to complain of a pounding headache. The patient also demonstrates profuse sweating above the T1 lesion, and blotching of the skin. The therapist should immediately identify this as:
[Physical Rehabilitation/Sullivan/5th Ed./Pg. 943]
A. Orthostatic hypotension   B. Autonomic dysreflexia
C. Lowe's syndrome   D. Homonymous hemianopsia

Q 94. A therapist examines the developmental status of an infant. Which of the following would not be recommended when treating a child?
[Physical Rehabilitation/Sullivan/5th Ed./Pg. 68]
A. Various therapists should be involved at each visit so that the child feels secure with a variety of social contacts.
B. Treatment should be given in a small area since large spaces are often frightening to children
C. The infant should be encouraged and praised for each success
D. A fall off in performance, an increase in irritability, or a refusal or perform often signals the conclusion of productive treatment

Q 95. A physical therapist examines a 22-year-old soccer player who suffered an inversion ankle sprain 24 hours ago. The therapist notices the athlete's right ankle is moderately edematous. What valuable information has the therapist already acquired:
[Tidy's Physiotherapy/12th Ed./Pg. 41]
A. The athlete will probably be out of competitive soccer for at least two weeks because of the severity of the sprain
B. The athlete should be nonweight bearing at all times due to the amount of effusion in the ankle
C. The sprain is a third degree ligament sprain although no timetable for recovery is available based on the information given
D. The therapist still does not have an accurate indication as to the severity of the injury

---

Answer   86 D   87 A   88 C   89 A   90 C   91 B   92 C   93 B   94 A   95 D

Q 96. A therapist records grip strength measurements on a patient diagnosed with bilateral carpal syndrome. Which description does not accurately describe typical results when using a hand dynamometer?

[Tidy's Physiotherapy/12th Ed./Pg. 357]

A. A bell curve is seen when charting multiple recordings from adjustable hand spacing in consecutive order
B. Twenty to twenty five percent differences in grip strength may be seen between the done and non-dominant hand
C. Discrepancies of more than twenty- five percent in a test-retest situation may indicate the patient is not exerting maximal force
D. An individual who does not exert maximal force for each test will not show that typically curve

Q 97. A therapist examines a patient there days following lumbar laminectomy. The most accurate predictor of the patient's functional status following rehabilitation is based on the patient's.

[Tidy's Physiotherapy/12th Ed./Pg. 157]

A. Age
B. Previous functional status
C. Level of family community support
D. Postsurgical history

Q 98. A short term goal for a patient status post CVA is to perform a stand pivot transfer from a bed to a wheelchair. The goal should be recorded in the _______ section of a SOAP note?

[Physical Rehabilitation/Sullivan/5th Ed./Pg. 19]

A. Subjective   B. Objective
C. Assessment   D. Plan

Q 99. When writing daily progress notes using the SOAP format, a therapist records her professional judgment in the _______ section?

[Physical Rehabilitation/Sullivan/5th Ed./Pg. 15]

A. Subjective   B. objective
C. Assessment   D. Plan

Q 100. A therapist completes a series of special tests designed to examine the ligamentous integrity of a patient's knee. After completing the tests, the therapist is unsure if the laxity is normal for the patient or if it is indicative of a ligamentous injury. The most appropriate step to gather more information is to:

[Physical Rehabilitation/Sullivan/5th Ed./Pg. 14]

A. Attempt to quantify the millimeters of laxity and compare the values with established norms
B. Contact the physician and suggest a referral for magnetic resonance imaging
C. Directly compare the laxity in the involved knee to the laxity in the uninvolved knee
D. Attempt to identify other special test which can offer more information on the ligamentous integrity of the knee

Q 101. A physical therapy problem list is often developed following an initial examination. The problem list can be a useful tool for therapists to develop an effective and organized treatment plan. The physical therapy problem list should be recorded in the _______ section of a SOAP note?

[Physical Rehabilitation/Sullivan/5th Ed./Pg. 20]

A. Subjective   B. Objective
C. Assessment   D. Plan

Personality Development

Q 102. A patient diagnosed with spinal stenosis is referred to physical therapy three times a week for six weeks. During the initial examination the patient informs the therapist that the commute to therapy is over 90 miles. The most appropriate action is to:

[Physical Rehabilitation/Sullivan/5th Ed./Pg. 68]

A. Schedule the patient once a week
B. Schedule the patient three times a week
C. Attempt to locate a physical therapy clinic closer to the patient's home
D. Discharge the patient with a home exercise program

Q 103. A therapist is treating a head injured patient who begins to perseverate. In order to refocus the patient and achieve the desired therapeutic outcome, the therapist should:

[Physical Rehabilitation/Sullivan/5th Ed./Pg. 909]

A. Focus on the topic of perseveration for a short period of time in order to appease the patient
B. Guide the patient into an interesting new activity and reward successful completion of the task
C. Take the patient back to his room for quiet time and attempt to resume therapy once he has stopped perseverating
D. Continue with repetitive verbal cues to cease perseveration

Q 104. A therapist works on bed mobility exercise with a patient recently diagnosed with terminal cancer. The patient is extremely upset and tells the therapist, "I know I will never get better." The therapist most appropriate response would be:

[Physical Rehabilitation/Sullivan/5th Ed./Pg. 71]

A. Radiation treatments will make you feel better
B. Many people have overcome larger obstacles
C. Having cancer must be very difficult for you to deal with
D. Physical therapy can improve your condition

Q 105. A therapist examines a patient referred to physical therapy diagnosed with a medial collateral ligament sprain. During the examination the patient appears to be relaxed and comfortable, however is extremely withdrawn. Which of the following questions would be the most appropriate to further engage the patient?

[Physical Rehabilitation/Sullivan/5th Ed./Pg. 73]

A. Is this the first time you have injured your knee?
B. Have you ever been to physical therapy before?
C. How long after your injury did you see a physician?
D. What do you hope to achieve in physical therapy?

Q 106. A therapist working on an orthopedic floor notices that a particular patient recently diagnosed with pulmonary disease appears to be depressed. When training the patient the therapist should:

[Physiotherapy/Tidys/12th Ed./Pg. 197]

Answer   96 B   97 B   98 C   99 C   100 C   101 C   102 C   103 B   104 C   105 D

A. Provide additional information on the patient's medical condition
B. Create an environment that promotes internal motivation
C. Avoid activities that require prolonged verbal interaction
D. Explain to the patient that his/her prognosis is very good

Special Test

Q 107. A patient which vertigo is refined to physical therapy for a balance assessment. When testing kinesthesia, the most reliable method is to:
[Physical Rehabilitation/Sullivan/5th Ed./Pg. 1007]
A. Have the patient describe the position of his/her extremity once it is placed in a static position
B. Have the patient describe the direction and position of his/her extremity during movement
C. Have the patient describe the if the stimuli are sharp or dull
D. Have the patient name the object in his/her hand without visual input

Medicolegal Seefi

Q 108. A patient in a rehabilitation hospital confides to her therapist that she has been physically abused by her husband in the past and is concerned about returning home following discharge. The most appropriate therapist action is on:
[Physical Rehabilitation/Sullivan/5th Ed./Pg. 68]
A. Call adult protective services
B. Contact the patient's case manager
C. Ask the patient to leave her husband
D. Contact the patient's spouse

Q 109. An orthopedic surgeon instructs a patient to remain nonweight bearing for three weeks following a medial meniscus repair. During the patient's initial examination it becomes obvious that the patient has not adhered to the prescribed weight bearing stats. The most immediate therapist action to:
[Tidy's Physiotherapy/12th Ed./Pg. 52]
A. Contact the orthopedic surgeon
B. Explain to the patient the potential consequences of ignoring the weight bearing restrictions
C. Draft a letter to the patient's third party payer
D. Complete an incident report.

Q 110. A therapist provides an in-service to the rehabilitation department on the Americans with Disabilities Act. Which of the following individuals would not be covered under the act?
[Physical Rehabilitation/Sullivan/5th Ed./Pg. 25]
A. A 28-year-old with a documented learning disability
B. A 46-year-old with severe mental retardation
C. A 14-year-old that is blind
D. A 36-year-old homosexual

Q 111. A physical therapist treats a patient using high voltage galvanic stimulation. During treatment the therapist observes smoke rising from the machine and smells an unusual odor. The most appropriate immediate response is to:
[Physical Rehabilitation/Sullivan/5th Ed./Pg. 68]
A. Unplug the machine and label it "Defective-Do Not Use"
B. File an incident report
C. Contact the appropriate service group
D. Request an investigation by the biomedical instrumentation department

Q 112. A therapist treats a 26 year old male with complete C6 tetraplegia. During treatment the patient makes a culturally insensitive remark that the therapist feels is offensive. The most appropriate therapist action s to:
[Physical Rehabilitation/Sullivan/5th Ed./Pg. 68/]
A. Document the incident in the medical record
B. Transfer the patient to another therapist's schedule
C. Discharge the patient from physical therapy
D. Inform the patient that the remark was offensive and continue with treatment

Q 113. An employee with a disclosed disability informs her employer that she is unable to perform an essential function of her job unless her workstation is modified. Which of the following would provide the employer with a legitimate reason for not granting the employee's request?
[Refer to Text]
A. The accommodation would cost hundreds of dollars
B. The accommodation would require an expansion of the employee's present workstation
C. The accommodation would fundamentally alter the operation of the business
D. The accommodation would not address the needs of other employees

Q 114. Evaluative forms, diagnostic studies, and written medical information completed by those caring for a patient are all part of the medical record in an acute care setting. Who is the owner of the official medical record?
[Refer to Text]
A. The government
B. Third party payers
C. The patient
D. The health care facility.

Q 115. The practice of physical therapy in a given state is often defined according to the state physical therapy practice act. Which source of law is responsible for formalizing a practice act?
[Refer to Text]
A. Constitutional law
B. Statutory law
C. Common law
D. Administrative law

Q 116. Health maintenance organizations have been more successful than the majority of private health insurance companies in controlling escalating medical costs. The primary method used by health maintenance organizations to contain medical costs is:
[Refer to Text]
A. Increasing premiums to discourage the unnecessary use of health care

---

Answer   106 B   107 B   108 A   109 B   110 D   111 A   112 D   113 C   114 D   115 B

B. Restricting the duration of physical therapy services
C. Limiting services to specific health care providers
D. Having the providers of care share in some aspect of the financial risk

Q 117. A health care provider negotiates with an insurance company to provide health care services. As part of the agreement, the insurance company agrees to pay the health care provider a predetermined amount for each member in the plan on an annual basis. This type of arrangement is best termed:

[Refer to Text]

A. Capitation
B. Fee for service
C. Case pricing
D. Negotiated compensation

Q 118. A child is referred to physical therapy with physician orders to examine and treat the left knee. During the examination the patient describes diffuse pain throughout the area of the patella and proximal tibia/fibula. The mother states that the child has been extremely tired and has had a significant reduction in her appetite during the past two months. The medical record shows no evidence of any special testing and all other evaluative finding are inconclusive. The most appropriate therapist action is to:

[Tidy's Physiotherapy/12th Ed./Pg. 47]

A. Utilize superficial modalities in an attempt to reduce the patient's pain
B. Call the physician to discuss the patient's care
C. Design an exercise program for the patient
D. Inform the physician that the patient is not a candidate for physical therapy

Q 119. Health maintenance organizations differ from typical fee for service insurance providers in a variety of ways. Which of the following does not accurately describe health maintenance organizations?

[Physical Rehabilitation/Sullivan/5th Ed./Pg. 11]

A. Members are limited to receiving services from specific providers
B. Payment to providers is often on a capitated or prospective basis
C. Health maintenance organizations provide services for a monthly fee which varies based on the amount of services utilized by each member.
D. Health maintenance organizations are responsible for the provision and accessibility of care.

Others

Q 120. While performing high level balance activities, a patient falls into a piece of equipment that causes a deep laceration the calf. Immediate first aid includes direct pressure to the area and elevation, however the bleeding does not stop. The therapist should continue to administer first aid by providing:

[Refer to Text]

A. Eat to the laceration site
B. Ice to the laceration site
C. Pressure to the posterior tibial artery pressure point
D. Pressure to the femoral artery pressure point.

Q 121. A 20-year-old women rehabilitating from a head injury is unable to bathe and dress herself independently. This would correctly be identified as a/an:

[Physical Rehabilitation/Sullivan/5th Ed./Pg. 8/]

A. Handicap
B. Indirect impairment
C. Composite impairment
D. Disability

Q 122. A physical therapist examines a five-year-old child's gait. The therapist notes that the child is unsteady and uses a wide base of support. The child appears to lurch at times with minimal truncal bobbing in an anterior and posterior direction. The child cannot maintain a standing position with the feet placed together for more than five seconds. The area of the brain most likely affected is the:

[Neurology and Neurosurgery Illustrated/
Lindsay/4th Ed./Pg. 189/]

A. Corticospinal tracts
B. Basal ganglia
C. Substantia nigra
D. Cerebellar hemisphere

Q 123. While talking to a patient about a previous exercise program, the patient mentions that he used to exclusively perform negative work. Negative work or a negative muscular contraction is best defined as:

[Jt. Structure and Function/Norkin/3rd Ed./Pg 99/]

A. The muscle develops tension and increases in length
B. The muscle develops tension and decrease in length
C. Muscle length remains constant as tension is develop
D. Purposeful voluntary motion.

Q 124. A 45-year-old obese woman in a long leg cast attempts to transfer to a mat table using a sliding board. Which of the following instructions would be incorrect?

[Refer to Text]

A. Lean away from the mat and place the sliding board under your buttocks
B. Perform a series of small pushups gradually moving closer to the mat
C. Grasp the edge of the sliding board with your fingers to secure additional support
D. Maintain a slight forward trunk position while transferring

Q 125. A patient is given a prescription for a nonsteroidal anti-inflammatory which is to be taken three times a day with meals. What is the most common side effect of nonsteroidal anti-inflammatory medications?

[Neurology and Neurosurgery Illustrated/
Medicine/Davidson/5th Ed./Pg. 1090]

A. Convulsions
B. Fever
C. Nausea and vomiting
D. Stomach discomfort

Q 126. A patient is unable to take in an adequate supply of nutrients by mouth due to the side effects of radiation therapy. As a result the patient's physician orders the implementation of tube feeding. What type of tube is most commonly used for short term feeding?

[Neurology and Neurosurgery Illustrated/
Medicine/Davidson/20th Ed./Pg. 119]

A. Endobronchial
B. Nasogastric
C. Otopharyngeal
D. Tracheostomy

Answer   116 D   117 A   118 B   119 C   120 D   121 D   122 D   123 A   124 C   125 D   126 B

Q 127. A physical therapy manager is responsible for enforcing employee compliance with departmental policies and procedures. Which of the following would be the most appropriate action for an employee who has violated the departmental dress code policy for the first time?

[Refer to Text]

A. Private oral warning   B. Written warming
C. Probation   D. Suspension

Q 128. Interim progress notes are typically required following each patient treatment session. These notes often add to the information presented in the initial note and provide detailed information on the patient's physical therapy treatment session. Which of the following would not be included in an interim note?

[Physical Rehabilitation/Sullivan/5th Ed./Pg. 4]

A. Compliance with a home exercise program
B. Recent medical problems which could explain a patient's failure to progress
C. Response to selected treatment techniques
D. Past medical history

Q 129. While working with a patient with a T6 spinal cord injury a physical therapist identifies a small reddened area over the patient's right ischial tuberosity. The therapist should immediately:

[Physical Rehabilitation/Sullivan/5th Ed./Pg. 950]

A. Notify nursing and remind the patient of his/her role in proper skin care
B. Order a water mattress for the patient
C. Alert the patient to the potential dangers of skin breakdown
D. Notify the primary physician

Q 130. A patient falls to the ground during gait activities and appears to be in cardiac arrest. After performing a primary survey, the therapist calls for help and begins cardiopulmonary resuscitation. CPR should be continued until all of the following except:

[Neurology and Neurosurgery Illustrated/ Medicine/Davidson/20th Ed./Pg. 556]

A. The patient regains full consciousness
B. The patient reviews
C. A second rescuer in CPR takes over
D. The therapist is too exhausted to continue

Q 131. After completing an initial examination, it is determined that a patient exhibits disability behaviors that are out of proportion to the physical therapist's clinical findings. The therapist's next course of action should be to:

[Physical Rehabilitation/Sullivan/5th Ed./Pg. 11]

A. Confront the patient with the finding before initiating the treatment plan
B. Immediately contact the patient's physician and explain the findings
C. Initiate the treatment plan, however consider the possibility that the disease state is being maintained by external consequences
D. Continue with the current treatment plan and dismiss the findings

Q 132. A patient with cardiac pathology is scheduled for a cardiac catheterization. This diagnostic technique identifies specific lesions, areas of low perfusion, and ventricular aneurysms through:

[Physical Rehabilitation/Sullivan/5th Ed./Pg. 604]

A. The heart's resistance to the presence of the catheter
B. The catheter releasing dye into the coronary arteries
C. The catheter monitoring the pressure within the arteries
D. The catheter obtaining samples of cell which line the arteries

Q 133. While treating a patient, a therapist notices a mixture of blood and urine in the patient's collection bag. The most immediate therapist response would be to:

[Refer to Text]

A. Temporarily disconnect the collection bag
B. Continue with the patient's treatment program
C. Contact a member of the nursing staff
D. Document the observation in the physical therapy record

Q 134. A therapist employed in an acute care hospital attempts to identify a standardized instrument that measures level of consciousness. The most appropriate standardized instrument is the:

[Physical Rehabilitation/Sullivan/5th Ed./Pg. 900]

A. Glasgow coma Scale   B. Rankin Scale
C. Barthel Index   D. Sickness Impact Profile

Q 135. According to guidelines for effective handwashing it would be inappropriate to _______ in a patient's home?

[Refer to Text]

A. Use an existing bar of soap in the bathroom
B. Use paper towels for drying
C. Use liquid soap from a dispenser
D. Turn off the faucets with a paper towel

Q 136. A postoperative rigid dressing provides a patient status post amputation with all of the following advantages except:

[Refer to Text]

A. Allows for daily inspection and dressing changes
B. Allows for earlier ambulation with a pylon attachment
C. Limits postoperative edema
D. Reduces the length of time necessary for shrinking of the limb

Q 137. Communication and perceptual problems are extremely common in patients with hemiplegia. Which clinical problem would be characterizes of a right CVA?

[Physical Rehabilitation/Sullivan/5th Ed./Pg. 725

A. Inability to recognize symbols and perform basic math problems
B. Inability to plan and perform serial steps in activities
C. Distorted awareness of self image
D. Diminished functional speech

Q 138. A physician places a patient with moderate hypertension on diuretics. What is the most serious side effect of diuretics?

[Neurology and Neurosurgery Illustrated/ Medicine/Davidson/20th Ed./Pg. 427]

Answer   127 A   128 D   129 A   130 A   131 C   132 B   133 C   134 A   135 A   136 A   137 C

A. Fluid depletion and electrolyte imbalance
B. Gastrointestinal disturbances
C. Orthostatic hypotension
D. Weakness and fatigue

Q 139. A nurse takes the temperature of a patient before a scheduled physical therapy session. Which of the following temperatures would be classified as normal?

[Physical Rehabilitation/Sullivan/5th Ed./Pg. 92]

A. 35 degrees Celsius
B. 36 degrees Celsius
C. 37 degrees Celsius
D. 38 degrees Celsius

Q 140. A therapist is growing increasingly concerned about a patient that is demonstrating symptoms they are consistent with neoplastic activity. What is the most significant symptom of a rapidly growth neoplasm?

*[Neurology and Neurosurgery Illustrated/
Medicine/Davidson/5th Ed./Pg. 257]*

A. Fatigue
B. Swelling
C. Tenderness to palpation
D. Pain

Q 141. A person who is able to verbalize, but cannot comprehend verbal commands is best described as having:

[Physical Rehabilitation/Sullivan/5th Ed./Pg. 721]

A. Expressive aphasia
B. Receptive aphasia
C. Global aphasia
D. Agraphia

Q 142. A physical therapy department sponsors a program called "Health Heart" for individuals who have been identified as high-risk candidates for developing coronary artery disease. One of the requirements of the course is that upon completion program participants must be able to list three modifiable risk factors associated with coronary artery disease. Which domain of learning is emphasized with this particular requirement:

[Physical Rehabilitation/Sullivan/5th Ed./Pg. 1150]

A. Affective
B. Basilic
C. Cognitive
D. Psychomotor

Q 143. A patient with neurological involvement is able to understand instructions and conversation, but cannot verbalize. The best term to describe this condition is:

[Physical Rehabilitation/Sullivan/5th Ed./Pg. 721]

A. Global aphasia
B. Receptive aphasia
C. Expressive aphasia
D. Agraphia

Q 144. A therapist attempts to have a patient with right hemiplegia brush his teeth while working on standing tolerance. The therapist that the patient attempts to put the toothpaste directly in his mouth and hair. The therapist would document this finding as:

[Physical Rehabilitation/Sullivan/5th Ed./Pg. 721]

A. Ideomotor apraxia
B. Ideational apraxia
C. Constructional apraxia
D. Conduction aphasia

Q 145. A therapist reviews the medical chart of a patient with a history of recurrent dysrhythmias. The therapist is concerned about the past medical history and would like to monitor the patient during all activities. Which of the following monitoring devices would be the most beneficial?

[Physical Rehabilitation/Sullivan 5th Ed./Pg. 603]

A. Pulmonary artery catheter
B. Electrocardiogram
C. Intracranial pressure monitor
D. Pulse oximeter

Q 146. A patient diagnosed with low back pain is referred to physical therapy. During the initial examination the therapist ask if the patient has any formal diagnostic screening. The patient states that she had X-rays and a test where dye was injected into the spinal canal. This description most closely resembles:

[Medicine/Davidson/20th Ed./Pg. 1242]

A. Arthrography
B. Myelography
C. Computed tomography
D. Magnetic resonance imaging

147. Which clinical finding would you expect to see from a patient diagnosed with right-sided heart failure?

[Medicine/Davidson/20th Ed./Pg. 546]

A. Dyspnea
B. Cough
C. Dependent edema
D. Orthopnea

Q 148. Which statement best describes a patient with a traumatic brain injury who is at level VII, "Automatic-Appropriate", of the Ranchos Los Amigos levels of cognitive functioning?

[Physical Rehabilitation/Sullivan/5th Ed./Pg. 906]

A. The patient is in a heightened state of activity with a severe impairment in the ability to process information.
B. The patient has gross attention to the environment, is highly distractible, and lacks ability focus on a task without redirection
C. The patient is able to go through his/her daily routing is a robot like fashion with little to confusion and has an increased awareness of the environment
D. The patient shows goal directed behavior, but relies on external input for direction

Q 149. A therapist passively moves a patient's upper extremity through a selected range of motion with the patient's eyes closed. The patient is the asked to describe verbally the direction and rang of movement of the upper extremity. This technique can be used to examine:

[Physical Rehabilitation/Sullivan/5th Ed./Pg. 145]

A. Barognosis
B. Graphesthesia
C. Kinesthesia
D. Stereognosis

Q 150. Bandaging a residual limb is one methods of postoperative dressing. The purpose of bandaging includes all of the following except:

[Physical Rehabilitation/Sullivan/5th Ed./Pg. 1101]

A. Provides complete protection against accidental bruising and bumping
B. Reduces edema
C. Supports the surgical wound
D. Aids in preventing contractures

Answer   138 A   139 C   140 D   141 B   142 C   143 C   144 B   145 B   146 B   147 C   148 C   149 C
150 A

Q 151. A patient status post total hip replacement indicates to her therapist that she was instructed to avoid hip flexion greater than 90 degrees, adduction, and medial rotation. The most likely sum approach utilized by the surgeon is:
[Tidy's Physiotherapy/12th Ed./Pg. 123]
A. Anterolateral
B. Anteromedial
C. Posterolateral
D. Posteromedial

Q 152. A therapist uses patient care gloves to prevent the transmission of infection. When is it appropriate to reuse patient care gloves?
[Physical Rehabilitation/Sullivan/5th Ed./Pg. 12]
A. When the gloves are used to treat same patient
B. When the gloves are used by the same therapist
C. When the gloves do not come in contact with any potentially infections material
D. Gloves should not be reused

Q 153. A therapist employed in a community health practice presents an in-service to group of expectant mothers. As part of the in-service the therapist facilitates a discussion on cesarean sections. Which of the following would not be an indication for a cesarean section?
[Tidy's Physiotherapy/12th Ed./Pg. 406]
A. Cephalo-pelvic disproportion
B. Prolonged labor
C. Transverse lie of the baby
D. Full effacement and dilation of the cervix

Q 154. A laboratory report indicates that a patient's hematocrit and hemoglobin levels are decreased when compared to expected values. Which condition would not typically be associated with decreased hematocrit and hemoglobin levels?
[Neurology and Neurosurgery Illustrated/
Medicine/Davidson/20th Ed./Pg. 823]
A. Anemia
B. Hypoglycemia
C. Trauma
D. Iron deficiency

Q 155. A therapist examines a 62-years-old female status poststroke with left hemiparesis. Which of the following perceptual deficits in not commonly associated with left hemiparesis?
[Physical Rehabilitation/Sullivan/5th Ed./Pg. 720]
A. Denial of disability
B. Rigidity of thought
C. Short attention span
D. Sequencing deficits

Q 156. A nurse on a cardiac unit describes a patient's pulse is thready. This description most accurately describes a pulse that is:
[Physical Rehabilitation/Sullivan/5th Ed./Pg. 95]
A. Slow and rhythmical
B. Slow and forceful
C. Weak and irregular
D. Intermittent and pronounced

Q 157. A therapist examines a patient recently admitted to the hospital with uncontrolled diabetes mellitus. The physical therapy referral is for daily whirlpool treatments for a decubitus ulcer. Which of the following signs and symptoms might the therapist expect based on the supplied information?
[Tidy's Physiotherapy/12th Ed./Pg. 276]

A. Fever and convulsions
B. Tremors and rigidity
C. Polydipsia and polyuria
D. Nausea and vomiting

Q 158. A therapist reviews the results of a research study that examined intratester reliability of selected goniometric measurements. Which of the following goniometric measurements would you expect to have the poorest intratester reliability?
[Physical Rehabilitation/Sullivan/5th Ed./Pg. 175]
A. Shoulder flexion
B. Shoulder abduction
C. Knee flexion
D. Ankle inversion

Q 159. When reviewing a medical record, a therapist identifies an entry which classifies the patient's pulse rate as bradycardia. This should be interpreted as:
[Physical Rehabilitation/Sullivan/5th Ed./Pg. 96]
A. An increased pulse rate
B. A decreased pulse rate
C. An increase in the size of the heart
D. An underdeveloped atria

Q 160. A therapist records the vital signs of a 45-year-old male prior to beginning treatment. The therapist palpates the patient's radial pulse for 15 seconds, but has difficulty computing the actual pulse rate since the rhythm is irregular. The most appropriate method to identify the actual pulse rate is to:
[Physical Rehabilitation/Sullivan/5th Ed./Pg. 95]
A. Recheck hand positioning and palpate the radial pulse for an additional 15 seconds
B. Select another pulse site and palpate for 15 seconds
C. Palpate the radial pulse for one minute
D. record the original pulse rate and document the rhythm

Q 161. A patient is notable to whistle on command, but you have heard him whistling while listening to music. The same patient is unable to walk in the gym after demonstration, but is observed walking across the room to get his dinner tray. This condition is termed:
[Physical Rehabilitation/Sullivan/5th Ed./Pg. 721]
A. Ideational apraxia
B. Ideomotor apraxia
C. Constructional apraxia
D. Dressing apraxia

Q 162. The SAID principle stands for:
[Physical Rehabilitation/Sullivan/5th Ed./Pg. 403]
A. Specific adaptations to imposed demands
B. Severe and incurable disability
C. Shock after infusion of drugs
D. Specific amputation for impairment and disability

Q 163. as per the WHO's ICIDH classification impairment means:
[Physical Rehabilitation/Sullivan/5th Ed./Pg. 1337]
A. Pathological processes due to microbes attacking a human body
B. Inability to perform activities of daily living with physiological dysfunction
C. Disabled, ambulatory on wheelchair with psychological impairment
D. Any loss or abnormality of psychological, physiological or anatomical structure or function

---

Answer 151 C 152 D 153 D 154 B 155 D 156 C 157 C 158 D 159 B 160 C 161 B 162 A
163 B

Q 164. A therapist examines a patient placed in respiratory isolation. Which of the following diseases would require respiratory isolation?

[Tidy's Physiotherapy/12th Ed./Pg. 210]

A. Diphtheria
B. Pharyngitis
C. Pertussis
D. Hepatitis

Q 165. Typically drugs are administered through central administration. Which of the following is an example of central administration?

[Physical Rehabilitation/Sullivan/5th Ed./Pg. 903]

A. Inhalation
B. Injection
C. Topical
D. Oral

Q 166. A patient completing an exercise program starts to demonstrate signs of an insulin reaction including dizziness, vision difficulties, and a change in the level of consciousness. The most appropriate response for a conscious victim would include:

[Physical Rehabilitation/Sullivan/5th Ed./Pg. 694]

A. Give the patient sugar, candy, or juice
B. Monitor airway, breathing, and circulation
C. Treat the patient for shock
D. Continue to supervise the patient, however do not intervene

Q 167. A therapist designs an exercise program to increase muscle strength and endurance in a patient rehabilitating from knee surgery. Which type of pharmacological agent would have an antagonistic effect on the desired objective?

[Physical Rehabilitation/Sullivan/5th Ed./Pg. 830]

A. Nonnarcotic analgesics
B. Nonsteroidal anti-inflammatory medications
C. Peripheral vasodilators
D. Skeletal muscle relaxants

Q 168. A physical therapist participates in a community based screening program designed to identify individuals with osteoporosis. Which group would have the highest risk for developing osteoporosis?

[Physical Rehabilitation/Sullivan/5th Ed./Pg. 858]

A. White females over the age of 60
B. Black females over the age of 60
C. White females over the age of 40
D. Black females over the age of 40

Q 169. A therapist positions a patient in the Trendelenburg position in preparation for postural drainage. Which of the following is not a relative precaution for the use of the Trendelenburg position?

[Physical Rehabilitation/Sullivan/5th Ed./Pg. 580]

A. Nausea
B. Obesity
C. Pulmonary edema
D. Secretion retention

Q 170. Pharmacological agents can be an important component of a treatment program designed to treat rheumatoid arthritis. Which of the following is not commonly used to treat rheumatoid arthritis?

[Physical Rehabilitation/Sullivan/5th Ed./Pg. 1069]

A. Calcium channel blockers
B. Compounds containing elemental gold
C. Glucocorticoids
D. Nonsteroidal anti-inflammatory medications

Q 171. Which category specific isolation precaution would be to most appropriate for a patient, diagnosed with acquired immunodeficiency syndrome?

[Physical Rehabilitation/Sullivan/5th Ed./Pg. 593]

A. Blood/body fluid isolation
B. contact isolation
C. Respiratory isolation
D. Strict isolation

Q 172. A physician orders the nursing staff to administer digitalis to patient diagnosed with congestive heart failure. The physician's primary goal using this medication is to:

[Physical Rehabilitation/Sullivan/5th Ed./Pg. 540]

A. Increase cardiac pumping ability
B. Increase cellular metabolism
C. Regulate fluid and electrolyte levels
D. Regulate glucose metabolism

Q 173. A therapist identifies a bluish discoloration of the skin and nail beds of a 55-year-old male referred to physical therapy for pulmonary rehabilitation. What does this objective finding indicate?

[Physical Rehabilitation/Sullivan/5th Ed./Pg. 564]

A. Hyperoxemia
B. Hyperoxia
C. Hypokalemia
D. Hypoxemia

Q 174. A therapist is scheduled to treat a patient with meaning it is in respiratory isolation. What precautions are necessary when treating the patient?

[Physical Rehabilitation/Sullivan/5th Ed./Pg. 571]

A. Mask
B. Mask, gown
C. Gloves, gown
D. Mask, gloves, gown

Ex Program Design

Q 175. A therapist prepares to instruct a patient rehabilitating from a CVA in bed mobility activities. The most important initial step when designing an instructional program is to:

*[Physical Rehabilitation/Sullivan/
5th Ed./Pg. 746]*

A. Assess the patient's cognitive status
B. Utilize a variety of teaching methods
C. Avoid using medical jargon
D. Speak loudly and directly to the patient

Q 176. A postoperative patient can reduce the risk of acquiring a deep vein thrombosis by performing all of the following except:

[Tidy's Physiotherapy/12th Ed./Pg. 274]

A. Repeated deep breathing exercises
B. Frequently turning from side to side in bed
C. Sitting with the legs in a dependent position
D. Active flexion and extension of the toes, ankles, knees, and hips

---

Answer 164 C   165 D   166 A   167 D   168 A   169 D   170 A   171 A   172 A   173 D   174 A   175 D
176 C

Q 177. A short term goal for a patient with a neurological deficit is follows: The patient will transfer from tall kneeling to half kneeling with supervision. This activity is a example of:

[Physical Rehabilitation/Sullivan/5th Ed./Pg. 749/]

A. Mobility
B. Stability
C. Controlled mobility
D. Skill

Q 178. A home visit is conducted for a patient status post total hip replacement who will be discharged to a two story home using a walker. All of the following therapist recommendations are appropriate except:

[Jayant Joshi/1st Ed./Pg. 208]

A. Use area rugs smaller than 5 feet by 7 feet
B. Use nonskid rubber cups under bed posts
C. Use a tub bench and hand held shower
D. Place frequently used items on the kitchen counter top

Q 179. A therapist is treating a patient status post left knee replacement with goals of general conditioning and independence for household mobility. Which component of the patient's treatment program would be the most appropriate to delegate to physical therapy aide?

[Jayant Joshi/1st Ed./Pg. 213]

A. Stair training
B. Progressive gait training with a straight cane
C. Patient education regarding the surgical procedure
D. Ambulation with a walker for endurance

Q 180. A patient is referred to a cardiac rehabilitation program following a cardiac event, which of the following is not a realistic goal of a phase I cardiac rehabilitation program?

[Tidy's Physiotherapy/12th Ed./Pg. 231]

A. Adhere to a prescribed diet
B. Learn self-monitoring techniques
C. Recognized signs and symptoms of stress
D. Conduct a job site analysis.

Q 181. A therapist observes that a number of aids appear to be unfamiliar with appropriate guarding techniques. The most appropriate remedial strategy to improve their performance is to:

[Physical Rehabilitation/Sullivan/Pg. 54]

A. Offer assistance to the aids when the inappropriate behavior is observed
B. Refer the aids to textbooks that explain proper guarding technique
C. Develop a mandatory in-service on guarding techniques for the aids
D. Inform the director of rehabilitation that the aids are incompetent

Q 182. A 32-year-old male of Portuguese descent is referred to physical therapy for instruction in a home exercise program. The physician referral indicates the patient is approved for one visit. What is the likelihood the patient will comprehend the home exercise program in the allotted time?

[Physical Rehabilitation/Sullivan/5th Ed./Pg. 13]

A. The patient will require external assistance such as the use of an interpreter to comprehend the home exercise program
B. the patient will comprehend the home exercise program
C. The patient will not be able to comprehend the home exercise program
D. The therapist cannot make a prediction based on the supplied information

Q 183. A therapist develops a list of goals for a developing phase I cardiac rehabilitation program. Which of the following goals would not be appropriate for a phase I program?

[Physical Rehabilitation/Sullivan/5th Ed./Pg. 612]

A. Initiate low levels of activity
B. Educate patients and then families
C. Measure the effectiveness of medication in controlling the patient's cardiovascular status
D. Return the patient to safe vocational and recreational activities

Q 184. A therapist discusses risk factors associated with coronary artery disease with a patient in a phase I cardiac rehabilitation program. Which of the following risk factors in not modifiable?

[Physical Rehabilitation/Sullivan/5th Ed./Pg. 612]

A. Family history of coronary artery disease
B. Elevated serum cholesterol
C. Hypertension
D. Sedentary lifestyle

Q 185. A therapist presentation on preseason conditioning for a group of high school athletes. To maximize the effectiveness of the presentation the therapist should:

[Physical Rehabilitation/Sullivan/5th Ed./Pg. 21]

A. Develop specific learning objectives
B. Utilize a variety of audiovisual equipment
C. Assess the needs of the target audience
D. Provide a typewritten outline

Q 186. A therapist responsible for developing a cardiac rehabilitation program lists goals for a phase I program. Which of the following goals would not be appropriate for this program?

[Physical Rehabilitation/Sullivan/5th Ed./Pg. 617]

A. Ensure the continuity of the exercise program with a transition to the home environment
B. Establish a patient and family education program
C. Collect clinical data that contributes to the patient's prognosis and thus medical management
D. Assess hemodynamic responses to self care and progressive ambulation activities

Q 187. Treatment for a child diagnosed with cerebral palsy must be individualized to each child's need. In planning a treatment program that will remain effective overtime, all of the following guidelines should be incorporated except:

[Tidy's Physiotherapy/12th Ed./Pg. 365]

A. Treatment goals should be designed to address specific problems
B. Play should not be integrated into therapy since it distracts from direct movement respect
C. Therapy should encourage active responses from the child
D. Repetition is an important component of motor learning

Answer 177 C   178 A   179 D   180 D   181 C   182 D   183 D   184 A   185 C   186 A   187 B

Q 188. A therapist designs an exercise program for a patient rehabilitating from a myocardial infarction. During the exercise session the patient's blood pressure and pulse remarkably exceed typical levels. The most appropriate course of action is to:
[Tidy's Physiotherapy/12th Ed./Pg. 28]
A. Consult with the referring physician
B. Ask the director of rehabilitation to examine the patient
C. Continue the exercise program when the patient indicates he/she is ready
D. re-examine the patient prior to the beginning of the next treatment session

Documentation and Management

Q 189. A variety of health care providers make entries in the daily medical record. Which of the following health care provider would require his/her entry to be cosigned?
A. Physical therapist assistant
B. Physical therapist assistant and graduate physical therapist
C. Physical therapist assistant and student physical therapist
D. Student physical therapist and graduate physical therapist

Q 190. A therapist monitors a patient's blood pressure by auscultation. When recording the patient's blood pressure in the medical record, which of the following is usually not required?
[Physical Rehabilitation/Sullivan/5th Ed./Pg. 114]
A. Systolic blood pressure value
B. Extremity used
C. Patient position
D. Type of stethoscope used

Q 191. Gloves can be an effective means of protective asepsis. What type of isolation requires the use of gloves by all individuals entering the room?
[Physical Rehabilitation/Sullivan/5th Ed./Pg. 571]
A. Enteric precautions   B. Contact
C. Respiratory   D. Strict

Q 192. Health care facilities utilize a variety of employees including physical therapists, physical therapist assistants, and physical therapy aids. Which activity would be inappropriate for a physical therapy aid?
[Refer to Text]
A. Assist patients in preparation for treatment
B. Make daily entries in the patient's medical record
C. Assist patients with exercise activities
D. Perform treatment procedures as determined by the physical therapist

Q 193. A physical therapist is growing more and more disenchanted with her job due to exceptionally high productivity expectations. The most appropriate therapist action is to:
[Refer to Text]
A. Speak to the director rehabilitation
B. Increase utilization of support staff
C. Communicate directly with the supervisor
D. Refrain from addressing the topic for fear of being labeled a troublemaker

Q 194. A physical therapist works as a team with a male physical therapist assistant in a fast paced orthopedic private practice. The therapist is unsure of the physical therapist assistant's orthopedic knowledge and therefore regularly delegates cleaning and filing responsibilities. What step would be the most appropriate to improve the quality of the team's performance?
[Refer to Text]
A. Ask the physical therapist assistant how he feels about his present role in the clinic
B. Schedule a meeting with the physical therapist assistant to learn more about his education career goals, and prior clinical experience
C. Encourage the physical therapist assistant to attend physical therapy school if he wants to become more involved in patient care
D. Continue to delegate various undesirable takes to the physical therapist assistant

Q 195. In what section of a SOAP note would the following entry belong? Patient is not functional in activities of daily living due to lower extremity muscle weakness. Wife is unable to care for spouse at present level of functioning.
[Physical Rehabilitation/Sullivan/5th Ed./Pg. 20]
A. Subjective   B. Objective
C. Assessment   D. Plan

Q 196. A patient ambulating with crutches trips over an object on the floor and falls to the ground. The patient appears to be uninjured, however complains of diffuse pain in the involved knee. The most formal mechanism to document the patient's fall is to:
[Physical Rehabilitation/Sullivan/5th Ed./Pg. 18]
A. Send a memo to the director of rehabilitation
B. Write a litter to the patient's insurance company
C. Complete an incident report
D. Dictate a letter to the referring physician

Q 197. A therapist employed by a home health agency treats a patient in a home that is dirty and unsanitary. When treating the patient in the home, the most appropriate location for the therapist's treatment and supply bag is:
[Tidy's Physiotherapy/12th Ed./Pg. 415]
A. In the car
B. On countertop in the patient's house
C. On a piece of newspaper supplied by the therapist
D. On a chair in the treatment area

Q 198. A patient diagnosed with an acromioclavicular separation explains how the injury occurred. During the explanation the therapist identifies several inconsistencies and begins to question its authenticity. The most appropriate action is to:
[Physical Rehabilitation/Sullivan/5th Ed./Pg. 160]
A. Document the patient's explanation
B. Document the patient's explanation and identify each stated inconsistency
C. Dismiss the patient's explanation
D. Inform the patient that the explanation is difficult to believe

---

Answer   188 A   189 D   190 D   191 D   192 B   193 C   194 B   195 C   196 C   197 C   198 B

Q 199. A patient with superficial partial-thickness burns on the dorsal surface of the right foot refuses physical therapy services after being transported to the hydrotherapy area. The most immediate therapist action is to:
[Physical Rehabilitation/Sullivan/5th Ed./Pg. 1102]
A. Continue with the treatment session
B. Discontinue the treatment session
C. Explain to the patient the expected consequences of refusing treatment
D. Notify the referring physicians

Q 200. A physical therapist is responsible for supervising a physical therapist assistant at an offsite location. Which guideline is most appropriate when determining the frequency of supervisory visits?
[Physical Rehabilitation/Sullivan/5th Ed./Pg. 11]
A. Supervisory visits should take place when convenient for the physical therapist and the physical therapist assistant
B. Supervisory visits should take place in accordance with patient need
C. Supervisory visits should take place on a weekly basis
D. Supervisory visits should take place at least once every third visit

Q 201. A physical therapy department attempts to establish a quality assurance program. The first step I developing the program should be to:
[Physical Rehabilitation/Sullivan/5th Ed./Pg. 11]
A. Identify important aspects of patient care provided by the department
B. Collect and analyze data for each established indication
C. Identify quality indicators that will allow the department to monitor selected aspects of patient care
D. Determine a percentage of occurrence that will dictate a specified action

Q 202. Policies are used to carry out effective and efficient management. Which statement descript policies are not accurate?
[Physical Rehabilitation/Sullivan/5th Ed./Pg. 18]
A. Policies should be written on topics such as dress code, promotions, and discipline
B. Policies should be established on an oral basis and subjected to individual interpretation
C. Policies should be reviewed on a regular basis and revised if indicated
D. Policies should be assembled into a manual for quick and easy reference

Q 203. A therapist completes a discharge summary on a patient following a six week hospital admission. A discharge summary is best described as:
[Physical Rehabilitation/Sullivan/5th Ed./Pg. 21]
A. An explanation of the patient's condition at the time of discharge
B. An overview of the patient's progress during therapy and his/her condition at discharge
C. A document which indicates the reason for discharge and explains the patient's home grogram
D. A record which indicates the frequency and number of appointments from the initial examination until discharge

Q 204. An audit attempts to determine the quality of patient care through a review of patient records. All of the following are recommended to ensure that the results of the audit are accurate except:
[Physical Rehabilitation/Sullivan/5th Ed./Pg. 12]
A. A comparison of the actual practice's level of care to the expected level of care
B. Specific objectives of the audit are defined prior to the collection of data
C. An audit should not exceed a sample size of 15 to 20 charts
D. The study should include records over a six month period to ensure a diverse sample

Q 205. A manager is responsible for motivating staff members to take on the organization's goals as their own. Useful guidelines for a successful manager include all of the following except:
[Refer to Text]
A. Managing by results with emphasis on upward communication
B. Maintaining morale with emphasis on productivity and revenue generated
C. Negotiating ad maintaining a mutual commitment to goals
D. Using performance appraisals for setting future goals

Q 206. A physical therapist debrides a decubitus ulcer after a whirlpool treatment. The therapist should take off sterile patient care gloves after:
[Tidy's Physiotherapy/12th Ed./Pg. 277]
A. Completing debridement and transporting the patient to the patient waiting area
B. Completing debridement
C. Contact with the patient's decubitus ulcer
D. Cleaning the whirlpool at the conclusion of patient treatment

Q 207. A home visit is performed for a patient who resides alone and is three weeks status post total hip replacement. The patient is presently partial weight bearing on the affected side. The most appropriate recommendation to increase safety in the bathroom is:
[Tidy's Physiotherapy/12th Ed./Pg. 123]
A. Carsed toilet seat with rails, tub bench, hand held shower
B. Grab bars on the shower and next to the toilet
C. Handrails for the toilet, tub bench hand held shower
D. The patient should not shower until her weight bearing status increases

Q 208. A therapist working in a special care unit notices a tiny air bubble in a peripheral IV line. The therapist's most immediate response would be to:
[Tidy's Physiotherapy/12th Ed./Pg. 215]
A. Turn off the IV
B. Remove the IV
C. Reposition the peripheral IV line
D. Continue with the present treatment

Answer   199 C   200 B   201 A   202 B   203 B   204 C   205 B   206 B   207 A   208 D

Q 209. A patient with a lengthy cardiac history ambulates on a treadmill as part of a phase II cardiac rehabilitation program. Suddenly, the patient begins to experience signs and symptoms of an angina attack. The therapist's most immediate response should be to:
[Physical Rehabilitation/Sullivan/5th Ed./Pg. 621]
A. Contact emergency medical services
B. Stop the exercise session
C. Contact the patient's physician
D. Document the incident in the medical record

Q 210. A therapist prepares a sterile field for wound debridement. Which of the following methods would be unacceptable when removing an object from the sterile field?
[Physical Rehabilitation/Sullivan/5th Ed./Pg. 665]
A. Using a sterile towel
B. Using sterile gloves
C. Using a bare hand after a thorough scrubbing
D. Using a sterile gauze pad

Q 211. A patient two days status post- cardiac surgery complains of soreness in her right calf. Which of the following actions would be the most appropriate?
[Tidy's Physiotherapy/12th Ed./Pg. 246]
A. Gently massage the calf
B. Notify the patient's nurse of the symptoms
C. Assess the patient's dorsal pedal pulse
D. Have the patient ambulate and reassess the calf

Q 212. A therapist examines a patient diagnosed with thoracic outlet syndrome. During the examination the patient repeatedly uses offensive language. The most appropriate therapist action is to:
[Physical Rehabilitation/Sullivan/5th Ed./Pg. 31]
A. Document the patient's offensive language in the medical record
B. Discharge the patient from physical therapy
C. Inform the patient you find his/her language to be offensive
D. Contact the referring physician

Q 213. A patient rehabilitating from a myocardial infarction expresses to his therapist a desire to quit smoking. The most appropriate therapist action is to:
[Physical Rehabilitation/Sullivan/5th Ed./Pg. 636]
A. Supply the patient with the phone number of the American Heart Association
B. Refer the patient to a smoking cessation program
C. Provide the patient with general information on the dangers of smoking
D. Ask the patient to consider nicotine gum

Q 214. Which of the following statements would probably not increase a patient's compliance with a home exercise program?
[Physical Rehabilitation/Sullivan/5th Ed./Pg. 28]
A. The patient should receive both written and verbal instruction.
B. The program should be goal oriented
C. The program should be individualized to the need of the patient
D. The program should take in excess of thirty minutes to complete

Q 215. A physician request that a therapist report to the orthopedic surgical center to instruct a patient in a preoperative training program. After completing the training program the therapist returns to the outpatient physical therapy area and finds a number of items that require her attention. Which of the following items should be given the highest priority?
[Tidy's Physiotherapy/12th Ed./Pg. 371]
A. An intern progress note for a patient scheduled to see a physician
B. Unfinished documentation from a patient seen earlier in the day
C. A message from a patient that has been discharged from therapy
D. A scheduled patient that has been waiting for 15 minutes

Q 216. A therapist instructs a patient who seems to be disinterested in a home exercise program. Which therapist action would be the most appropriate?
[Physical Rehabilitation/Sullivan/5th Ed./Pg. 15]
A. Allow the patient to select exercise activities
B. Explain to the patient the importance of the home exercise program
C. Explain to the patient the consequences of refusing treatment
D. Discontinue the treatment session

Q 217. To increase patient compliance with a new exercise program, a therapist should:
[Physical Rehabilitation/Sullivan/5th Ed./Pg. 15]
A. Speak strongly and directly to the patient
B. Individualize the program to the particular needs of each patient
C. Lecture the patient on the importance of compliance
D. Use medical terminology to impress the patient

Q 218. A physical therapist prepares a presentation on proper body mechanics for a group of 100 autoworker. Which of the following media would be most effective to maximize learning during the presentation?
[Physical Rehabilitation/Sullivan/5th Ed./Pg. 21]
A. Lecture, handouts
B. Lecture, charts, statistics
C. Lecture, handouts, demonstration
D. Lecture, statistics

Q 219. According to the Standards of Practice for physical therapy as published by the American physical therapy association, who is responsible for the physical therapist's individual professional development and continued competence?
[Physical Rehabilitation/Sullivan/5th Ed./Pg. 21]
A. The individual physical therapist
B. The physical therapist's employer
C. The state chapter of the American Physical Therapy Association
D. The American Physical Therapy Association

Answer   209 B   210 C   211 B   212 C   213 B   214 D   215 D   216 B   217 B   218 C   219 A

Q 220. A 63-year-old female referred to physical therapy for gait training suddenly loses her balance and falls to the floor. After rushing to the scene, it becomes obvious that the patient is unconscious. Which of the following would be the most appropriate immediate response?

[Physical Rehabilitation/Sullivan/5th Ed./Pg. 903]

A. Secure and maintain an airway
B. File an incident report
C. Observe and record vital signs
D. Attempt to define the specific cause for the loss of consciousness

Q 221. A physical therapist working on a team with a physical therapist assistant would be incorrect in asking an assistant to perform which of the following tasks?

[Physical Rehabilitation/Sullivan/5th Ed./Pg. 13]

A. Modify treatment plan or goals
B. Apply and measure assistive or adaptive devices
C. Identify changes in treatment outcome
D. Administer therapeutic modalities

Q 222. Progress notes allow members of all health services to know what the patient is accomplishing in each given area. Which statement regarding physical therapy progress notes is not accurate?

[Physical Rehabilitation/Sullivan/5th Ed./Pg. 13]

A. Observations and recordings should be the result of tangible tests and measurements.
B. The progress not must contain patient identification, the date, and the signature of the therapist
C. Progress notes can include diagrams, graphs, and flow sheets
D. Progress notes should be written by physical therapists and not by other care providers such as physical therapist assistants

Q 223. A fifteen-year-old male is referred to a local orthopedic surgeon after injuring his knee in a football game. The most appropriate initial step in the surgeon's care of the patient is to:

[Physical Rehabilitation/Sullivan/5th Ed./Pg. 160]

A. Complete a physical examination
B. Immobilize the injured knee
C. Aspirate the knee
D. Order X-rays

Q 224. Health care cost containment efforts have created incentives for impatient care providers and hospitals to control the cost and utilization of inpatient services. Which of the following has not resulted as a product of cost containment efforts?

[Refer to Text]

A. A decrease in the average length of impatient hospitalizations
B. An increase in the utilization of home care and skilled long term care
C. A decreased use of routine diagnostic testing during inpatient hospitalization
D. A decreased use of outpatient diagnostic testing and treatment

Q 225. A therapist visits a former patient diagnosed with pneumonic plague in the hospital. The patient is in strict isolation, but the therapist has been granted permission to visit if there is no body contact. What protective measures are necessary when entering the room of a patient in strict isolation?

[Physical Rehabilitation/Sullivan/5th Ed./Pg. 19]

A. Mask
B. Mask, gown
C. Gloves, gown
D. Mask, gown, gloves

Q 226. The clinical instructor and the center coordinator of clinical education both play an integral role in a clinical education program. Which of the following responsibilities is typically completed by the clinical instruction?

[Physical Rehabilitation/Sullivan/5th Ed./Pg. 13]

A. Perform administrative functions between the academic program and the clinical center
B. Serve as a representative of the clinical center to the academic programs
C. Coordinate the assignments and activities of students at the clinical enter
D. Perform formative and summative evaluations of the student's performance

Q 227. Documentation can be an extremely important factor in malpractice litigation. Which of the following statements does not reflect appropriate documentation procedures?

[Physical Rehabilitation/Sullivan/5th Ed./Pg. 18]

A. The complete signature and title of the document's writer should appear at the end of the document
B. Valid objective measurements and terms should be used
C. The date and in some cases, the time of an observation, treatment, or other action should be included
D. Corrections made in record after the notification of a claim should be made by placing single line through the incurred entry

---

Answer   220 A   221 A   222 D   223 D   224 D   225 D   226 D   227 D

7

CHAPTER

PTM and PTS

Objective Questions with Answers

Q 1. A 24-year-old male known epileptic presented with pain in the right shoulder region. Examination revealed that the right upper limb was adducted and internally rotated and the movements could not be performed. Which of the following is the most likely diagnosis?
[Essential Orthopedics/Maheshwari/3rd Ed./Pg. 74]
A. Posterior dislocation of shoulder
B. Luxatio erecta
C. Intrathoracic dislocation of shoulder
D. Subglenoid dislocation of shoulder

Q 2. In neuropraxia of peripheral nerve:
[Essential Orthopedics/Maheshwari/3rd Ed./Pg. 51]
A. The Wallerian degeneration occurs in 3 days
B. No Wallerian degeneration takes place
C. The degenerative changes are completed in 21 days
D. None of the above

Q 3. Onset of articular changes in rheumatic arthritis is seen in:
[Essential Orthopedics/Maheshwari/Pg. 244]
A. Synovial membrane
B. Articular cartilage
C. Capsule
D. Subchondral bone

Q 4. Osteomalacia is caused by the deficiency of:
[Essential Orthopedics/Maheshwari/Pg. 262]
A. Vitamin B
B. Vitamin D
C. Vitamin A
D. Vitamin E

Q 5. The 4th cranial nerve is named as:
[Neurology and Neurosurgery/Lindsay/4th Ed./Pg. 12]
A. Hypoglossal (motor)
B. Olfactory (sensory)
C. Trochlear (motor)
D. Vagus (mixed)

Q 6. Synovial fluid analysis of rheumatoid joints reveal:
[Essential Orthopedics/Maheshwari/Pg. 244-245]
A. High complement level
B. High protein level
C. Low protein level
D. Low complement level

Q 7. Anterior interosseous nerve is a branch of which nerve?
[Human Anatomy/B.D.Chaurasia/Pg. 111]
A. Radial nerve
B. Ulnar nerve
C. Median nerve
D. Musculocutaneous nerve

Q 8. The characteristic attitude of limbs in posterior dislocation of hip is:
[Essential Orthopedics/Maheshwari/Pg. 111]
A. Flexion, adduction and internal rotation with significant shortening of limb
B. Flexion, abduction and external rotation with lengthening of limb
C. Flexion, abduction and external rotation with shortening of limb
D. None of these

Q 9. The cruciate ligament instability is determined best by:
[Essential Orthopedics/Maheshwari/Pg. 313]
A. Anterior drawer test
B. Lachman test
C. Pivot shift test
D. Extension recurvatum test

Q 10. The advantages of Lachman test over anterior drawer test are all except:
[Essential Orthopedics/Maheshwari/Pg. 313]
A. Eliminates posterior meniscus pain
B. Knee is examined within comfortable range and hamstrings do not block motion
C. Rotatory instability can eliminated
D. Difficult to perform

Q 11. The boutonniere deformity of finger is characterized by:
[Essential Orthopedics/Maheshwari/Pg. 246]
A. Inability to completely extend PIP joint
B. Inability to completely flex PIP joint
C. Both (a) and (b)
D. Inability to completely flex MP joint

Q 12. Myoplasty is done in amputations primarily to:
[Physical Rehabilitation/Sullivan/4th Ed./Pg. 621]
A. Produce best cosmetic appearance
B. Restore resting length of muscles and improves circulation

---

Answer   1 D   2 B   3 A   4 B   5 C   6 B   7 C   8 A   9 B   10 C   11 A

C. Improve prosthetic fitting
D. Allow end bearing on stump

Q 13. Maximal functional efficiency is obtained most consistently in prosthetic leg by:
[Physical Rehabilitation/Sullivan/Pg. 664]
A. Proper materials
B. Alignment and lubrication
C. Weight of prosthesis
D. Physical and mental training

Q 14. All of the following refer to pain to the shoulder except:
[Medicine/David J. Magee/3rd Ed./Pg. 190]
A. Elbow
B. Neck
C. Heart
D. Lung

Q 15. A lesion in pyramidal tract causes:
[Cash's/4th Ed./Pg. 73-76]
A. Spasticity in the muscles involved
B. Rigidity in the muscles involved
C. Athetosis in the muscles involved
D. Flaccidity in the muscles involved

Q 16. Piriformis syndrome is caused by piriformis muscle that compresses:
[Medicine/David J.Magee/3rd Ed./Pg. 484]
A. Gluteal nerve
B. Femoral nerve
C. Sciatic nerve
D. Obturator nerve

Q 17. In cerebral palsy the intelligence quotient is:
[Sophie levitt/4th Ed./Pg. 9]
A. Always very low
B. Always borderline
C. May/may not be normal
D. Always exceptionally high

Q 18. Liver is the largest gland in the body weighting about:
[Grays Anatomy/Pg. 285]
A. 5 gms in adult
B. 500 gms in adult
C. 50 gms in adult
D. 5000 gms in adult

Q 19. Exercise causes heart rate to increase in linearity with increase in the physical effort. Maximum heart rate that can be attained during exercise is:
[Macardle/4th Ed./Pg. 266]
A. 72 + 1/2 the age (in years)
B. 100 – 1/4 the age (in years)
C. 220 – age (in years)
D. 220 + 1/4 of the age (in years)

Q 20. The three main orifices in diaphragm:
[Human Anatomy/B.D.Chaurasia/4th Ed./Pg. 185]
A. Aortic, esophageal and vena caval
B. Ureter, splenic and aortic
C. Esophageal, pulmonary and circulatory
D. Phrenic, aortic and renal

Q 21. A therapist attempts to assess the Babinski reflex as part of an initial examination. The effectively elicit the Babinski reflex, the therapist should:
[Orthopedic Physical Assessment/Magee/3rd Ed./Pg. 35]
A. Stroke the lateral aspect of the foot beneath the lateral malleolus
B. Stroke the anteromedial tibial surface
C. Stroke the lateral aspect of the sole of the foot
D. Firmly squeeze the calf.

Q 22. A therapist employed in a nursing home routinely treats patients in excess of 70 years of age. Which of the following physical changes is not associated with aging?
[Mcardle/4th Ed./Pg. 222]
A. Increased residual volume
B. Decreased vital capacity
C. Decreased cardiac output
D. Decreased total lung capacity

Q 23. A therapist discusses the importance of a proper diet to a patient with congestive heart failure. Which of the following substances would most likely be restricted in the patient's diet?
[Physical Rehabilitation/Sullivan/5th Ed./Pg. 626]
A. High density lipoproteins
B. Low density lipoproteins
C. Sodium
D. Triglycerides

Q 24. A patient diagnosed with spastic hemiplegia wears an ankle-foot orthosis set in slight dorsiflexion. If the orthosis was set in excessive dorsiflexion, which of the following would you expect to observe during the stance phase of gait?
[Joint Structure and Function/Norkin/5th Ed/Pg. 478]
A. Increased knee stability
B. Decreased knee stability
C. No effect on knee stability
D. Genu recurvatum.

Q 25. Injury to the lateral cord of the brachial plexus would most likely involve damage to the _____ nerve?
[Human Anatomy/B.D.Chaurasia/Vol. 1/4th Ed./Pg. 52]
A. Musculocutaneous
B. Axillary
C. Radial
D. Ulnar.

Q 26. A therapist observes a patient with a transfemoral prosthesis during ambulation activities. The therapist notes that the patient tends to circumduct the involved lower extremity during ambulation. Which of the following is an anatomic cause for this type of gait deviation?
[Jayant Joshi/Reprint 2004/Pg. 252]
A. Adduction contracture
B. Hip flexion contracture
C. Short amputation limb
D. Weak hip extensors

Q 27. A patient rehabilitating from a medial meniscus repair has been instructed by an orthopedic surgeon to remain nonweight bearing for three weeks following surgery. The patient has no significant past medical history and is expected to make a full recovery. Which of the following would be the most appropriate assistive device for the patient?
[Tidy's Physiotherapy/12th Ed./Pg 52]
A. Straight cane
B. Axillary crutches
C. Parapodium
D. Walker

Q 28. There are a variety of sizes of wheelchairs which can accommodate individuals of almost any size or build. Assuming a full grown adult of average size and build, which of the following wheelchair dimensions would be the most appropriate?
[Physical Rehabilitation/Sullivan/5th Ed/Pg. 1300]
A. Seat width 14 inches, seat depth 12 inches
B. Seat width 14 inches, seat depth 14 inches
C. Seat width 18 inches, seat depth 16 Inches
D. Seat width 20 inches, seat depth 18 inches

Answer

12 D	13 D	14 B	15 A	16 C	17 C	18 B	19 C	20 A	21 C	22 D	23 C
24 D	25 C	26 A	27 D	28 B							

Q 29. A squat pivot transfer is performed by a patient with a diagnosis of CVA, left hemiplegia. The therapist initiates the transfer to the patient's affected side. The benefits of transferring toward affected side include all of the following except:

[Physical Rehabilitation/Sulivan/5th Ed./Pg 757]

A. Retrains motor control through weight shift and weight bearing on the affected side
B. Decreases extensor synergy by weight bearing and maintaining minimal knee flexion
C. Directs attention and vision to the affected side
D. Allows affected upper extremity to remain unsupported which facilitates motion and decreases flexor synergy influence

Q 30. A seven-year-old patient sustains a deep partial-thickness burn to his heel. When teaching the patient a stretching program the greatest emphasis should be placed in the direction of:

[Physical Rehabilitation/Sullivan/5th Ed/Pg 1106]

A. Plantar flexion
B. Dorsiflexion
C. Inversion with plantar flexion
D. Eversion

Q 31. Physical activity has been hypothesized to decrease the occurrence and severity of coronary artery disease. Which of the following does not occur as a result a regular training program?

[Physical Rehabilitation/Sullivan/5th Ed./Pg 609]

A. An increase in coronary collateral vascularization
B. An increase in serum triglyceride level
C. An increase in red blood cell mass and blood volume
D. An increase in myocardial efficiency

Q 32. A therapist conducts a work site examination for a patient rehabilitating from a spinal cord injury. During the examination the therapist determines that the patient's desk height is inadequate for wheelchair. The most cost efficient and acceptable accommodation would be to:

A. Secure a wheelchair with a smaller frame
B. Place bricks under the desk to increase desk height
C. Purchase a new desk
D. Eliminate job duties which require the use of a desk

Q 33. A therapist observes that a patient has an exaggerated heel strike on the left during ambulation activities. Which term is most consistent with heel strike using Rancho Los Amigos nomenclature?

[Joint Structure and Function/Norkin/3rd Ed./Pg. 443]

A. Pressuring   B. Loading response
C. Initial contact   D. Midstance

Q 34. A patient with cerebellar dysfunction exhibits signs of dysmetria. Which of the following activities would be the most difficult for the patient?

[Physical Rehabilitation/Sullivan/5th Ed./Pg 198]

A. Alternate finger to nose
B. Placing feet on floor markers while walking
C. Walking at varying speeds
D. Marching in place

Q 35. A therapist completes a gait analysis on a patient diagnosed with Parkinson's disease. As part of the examination the therapist measures the distance between right heel strike and the next consecutive left heel strike. The measurement is used to measure:

[F.A Davis/Norkin/3rd Ed/Pg. 445]

A. Left stride length   B. Right stride length
C. Left step length   D. Right step length

Q 36. A therapist examines a patient referred to physical therapy with sacroiliac pain. As part of the examination, the therapist assesses the position of the sacrum by palpating the inferior lateral angles. Which spinal level is most consistent with the inferior lateral angles?

[Orthopedic Physical Assessment/Magee/5th Ed/Pg. 22]

A. S2   B. S3
C. S4   D. S5

Q 37. A therapist orders a wheelchair with a reclining back for a patient in a rehabilitation hospital. Which type of leg rests would be the most appropriate for the wheelchair?

Physical Rehabilitation/Sullivan/5th Ed./Pg. 1305]

A. Swing-away   B. Detachable
C. Elevating   D. Fixed

Q 38. A physical therapist transfers a patient in a wheelchair down a curb with a forward approach. Which of the following is an appropriate action for this task?

[Physical Rehabilitation/Sullivan/5th Ed./Pg. 977]

A. Have the patient lean forward
B. Have the wheelchair brakes locked
C. Tilt the wheelchair backwards
D. Position yourself in front for the patient

Q 39. A therapist positions a patient in supine in order to perform a passive stretch to the rectus femoris on the right. In order to effectively stabilize the pelvis in a supine position, the therapist should:

[Kisner/5th Ed./Pg. 674]

A. Passively flex the right hip to the patient's chest
B. Passively flex the right hip and knee to the patient's chest
C. Passively flex the left hip to the patient's chest
D. Passively flex and left hip and knee to the patient's chest

Q 40. Failure to integrate the _________ reflex could explain a child's inability to flex the neck, while in a supine position?

[Sophie Levitt/4th Ed/Pg. 90]

A. Tonic labyrinthine   B. Moro
C. Asymmetrical tonic neck   D. Symmetrical tonic neck

Q 41. A ramp which begins at ground level and ends 18 inches above ground should be at least _________ feet long?

[Physical Rehabilitation/Sullivan/5th Ed./Pg. 409]

A. 9   B. 18
C. 27   D. 36

Answer 29 D   30 B   31 B   32 B   33 C   34 A   35 B   36 B   37 C   38 C   39 C   40 D
41 A

Q 42. The tuberosity of the fifth metatarsal may be avulsed during violent eversion of the foot by the tension of the _________ muscle?

[Human Anatomy/B.D.Chaurasia/Vol. 2/4th Ed./Pg. 106]

A. Posterior Tibialis
B. Peroneus Longus
C. Peroneus Brevis
D. Peroneus Tertius

Q 43. A 47-year-old with a diagnosis of CVA with left hemiplegia is referred for orthotic examination. Significant results of manual muscle testing include: hip flexion 3+/5, hip extension 3/5, knee flexion 3+/5, ankle dorsiflexion 2/5, and ankle inversion and eversion 1/5. Sensation is intact and no abnormal tone is noted. The most appropriate orthosis for this patient is a:

[Physical Rehabilitation/Sullivan/5th Ed./Pg. 1217]

A. Knee-ankle foot orthosis with a locked knee
B. Plastic articulating ankle-foot orthosis
C. Metal upright ankle-foot orthosis locked in neutral
D. Prefabricated posterior leaf orthosis

Q 44. A physical therapist examines a 15 year old female distance runner for foot pain of unknown etiology. As the therapist palpates along the medial aspect of the foot and ankle, she palpates the head of the first metatarsal bone and the metatarsophalangeal joint. Immediately proximal to this she identifies the first cuneiform. What large bony prominence would you expect the therapist to identify next if she continues to move in a proximal direction?

[Joint Structure and Function/Norkin/3rd Ed/Pg. 368]

A. Talar head
B. Navicular
C. Medial malleolus
D. Cuboid

Q 45. A patient with a traumatic brain injury and right hemiplegia receives an ankle for orthosis to assist with ambulation. The patient's knee occasionally buckles during stance phase. A modification to the ankle-foot orthosis that would enhance knee extension during loading and stance on the right is to:

[Physical Rehabilitation/Sullivan/5th Ed./Pg. 1236]

A. Position the ankle joint in 5 degrees of dorsiflexion
B. Shorten the toe plate
C. Extend the foot plate
D. Add a soft anterior shell

Q 46. A therapist treats a patient diagnosed with Parkinson's disease. When working on controlled mobility, which of the following would best describe the therapist's objective?

[Orthopedic Physical Assessment/Sullivan/5th Ed/Pg. 878]

A. Facilitate postural muscle control
B. Promote weight shifting and rotational trunk control
C. Emphasize reciprocal extremity movement
D. Facilitate tone and rigidity

Q 47. A therapist examines a patient for a standard wheelchair. The therapist measures from the patient's posterior buttock along the lateral thing to the popliteal fold. The therapist then subtracts two inches from the measurement. This method can be used to measure:

[Orthopedic Physical Assessment/Physical Rehabilitation/Sullivan/5th Ed/Pg. 1291]

A. Seat height
B. Seat depth
C. Seat width
D. Armrest length

Q 48. A therapist selects an assistive device for a patient rehabilitating from an ankle injury. Which of the following would serve as the most significant obstacle to independent ambulation with axillary crutches?

[Kisner/5th Ed./Pg. 777]

A. Cognitive impairment
B. Weight bearing restrictions
C. Architectural barriers
D. Unilateral lower extremity weakness

Q 49. A developmental examination is performed on an infant. The infant is able to play on extended arms and attempts to reach for objects. The infant can maintain good alignment of the head and truck when pulled to a sitting position. The infant bears weight when placed in supportive standing. The therapist would expect the infant's age to be:

[Sophie Levitt/4th Ed./Pg. 144]

A. 3 months
B. 5 months
C. 7 months
D. 9 months

Q 50. A therapist attempts to obtain in-formation on the integrity of the C7 dermatome. The most appropriate location to assess the dermatome is the:

[Orthopedic Physical Assessment/Magee/5th Ed/Pg. 183]

A. Little Finger and ulnar border of the hand
B. Lateral forearm and thumb
C. Palmar distal phalanx of the middle finger
D. Medial forearm

Q 51. A therapist examines a healthy 12 month old baby. Which activity does not initially develop between the 9th and 12th month

A. Pincer grasp
B. Walking
C. Transfers objects from one hand to the other
D. Stands with high guard

Q 52. A therapist examines a patient with L1 paraplegia for a wheelchair. A wheelchair designed for this patient should include:

[Physical Rehabilitation/Saullivan/5th Ed./Pg. 964]

A. Reclining frame
B. Elevating leg rests
C. Hand rims with 12 vertical projections
D. Removable armrests

Q 53. What functional position should the metacarpophalangeal joint be placed in when designing a splint?

[Joint Structure and Function/Norkin/3rd Ed./Pg. 277]

A. Complete extension
B. 30 – 40 degrees of flexion
C. 60 – 70 degrees of flexion
D. 80 – 90 degrees of flexion

Q 54. A patient with a transfemoral amputation with an abducted gait pattern on the prosthetic side. All of the following may cause this gait deviation except:

[Jayant Joshi/Reprit 2009/Pg. 250]

A. High medial wall
B. Inadequate suspension
C. Abduction contracture
D. Prosthesis is too short

Answer
42 B   43 C   44 B   45 B   46 C   47 B   48 B   49 A   50 B   51 A   52 C   53 B
54 C

Q 55. A patient with C4 tetraplegia requires a custom wheelchair upon discharge from the hospital. The patient's diaphragm is partially innervated. The most appropriate recommendation for proper seating is:

[Physical Rehabilitation/Saullivan/5th Ed./Pg. 91]

A. Light weight manual wheelchair, upright frame, seat and back cushions
B. Folding reclining wheelchair, power chin control, seat and back cushions
C. Nonfolding reclining
D. Wheelchair, power, tongue control understanding tray for ventilator
E. Upright power wheelchair, joystick hand control, seat cushion

Q 56. The sensory system can be divided into protective and discriminative sensations. Which of the following is not considered to be a protective sensation?

[Physical Rehabilitation/Saullivan/5th Ed./Pg. 145]

A. Light touch
B. Pain
C. Proprioception
D. Temperature

Physiotherapy in Surgical Condition

Q 57. Diastasis rectii is:

[Kisner/5th Ed./Pg. 804]

A. Separation of rectus
B. Abdominalis muscle
C. Paralysis of rectal muscles
D. Weakness of rectus femoris muscle cystocoel

Q 58. Sprain is an injury to:

[Essential Orthopedics/Maheshwari/3rd Ed.]

A. A ligament or joint capsule with or without dislocation
B. A joint capsule with dislocation
C. A ligament or joint capsule without dislocation
D. Muscle, ligament or bone

Q 59. Following THR the following position of the hip joint is avoided:

[Jayant Joshi/Pg. 208]

A. Flexion, adduction and internal rotation
B. Flexion, abduction and external rotation
C. Flexion, abduction and internal rotation
D. Flexion, adduction and external rotation

Q 60. The female urethra is:

[Gray's Anatomy/1st Ed./Pg. 401]

A. 3.4 cm in length
B. 3.4 mm in length
C. 12 cm in length
D. 12.5 cm in length

Q 61. A young adult sustained a closed fracture of both bones of right leg in a scooter accident. He was treated by closed reduction and above knee plaster cast for 3 months. His fracture united but on removal of plaster his knee was stiff. Most probable cause of his stiff knee is:

Essential Orthopedics/Maheshwari/3rd Ed/Pg. 41]

A. Intra-articular fibrous adhesions
B. Intra-articular bone

C. Extra-articular bone
D. Extra-articular fibrous adhesions

Q 62. The artificial limb prosthesis is most satisfactory in which of the following amputations:

[Essential Orthopedics/Maheshwari/3rd/Pg. 279]

A. Below knee
B. Mid thigh
C. Hip disarticulation
D. Mid arm

Q 63. A joint least likely to develop recurrent dislocation:

[Orthopedic Physical Assessment/Magee/3rd Ed./Pg 506].

A. Patella
B. Shoulder
C. Hip
D. Knee

Q 64. Muscle hernia's occur most frequently in:

A. Leg
B. Thigh
C. Lumber region
D. Thoracic region

Q 65. A therapist attempts to palpate the tibialis posterior tendon. To facilitate palpation of this structure the therapist should:

[Human Anatomy/B.D. Chaurasia/vol. 2/4th Ed./Pg. 116]

A. Ask the patient to invert and plantar flex his foot
B. Ask the patient to evert and dorsiflex his foot
C. Ask the patient to invert dorsiflex his foot
D. Passively evert and plantar flex the patient's foot.

Q 66. A long term goal for a CVA patient is as follows: The patient will ambulate will ambulate independently with a small base quad cane for household distances using a right ankle-foot orthosis. All of the following are appropriate short term goals to meet the identified long term goal except:

[Essential Orthopedics/Maheshwari/3rd Ed./Pg. 282]

A. Patient will perform 20 repetitions of lower extremity exercise in supine with supervision
B. Patient will ambulate in the parallel bars for 3 × 10 feet with an ankle-foot orthosis and minimal assist
C. Therapist will educate the patient and family regarding the use of an ankle-foot orthosis
D. Patient will performs it to stand transfer with contact guard

Q 67. An 86-year-old female is restricted to partial weight bearing on the left leg after a total hip replacement. Her upper extremity strength is 3+/5 and she resides alone. Which assistive device would be the most appropriate for the patient?

[Jayant Joshi/Repeat 2009/Pg. 208]

A. Lofstrand crutches
B. Axillary crutches
C. Large base quad cane
D. Walker

Q 68. A patient with a right radial head fracture is examined in physical therapy. The patient's involved elbow range of motion begins at 15 degrees of flexion and ends at 90 degrees of flexion. The therapist should record the patient's right elbow range of motion as:

[Orthopedic Physical Assessment/Magee/3rd Ed/Pg. 35]

A. 0-15-90
B. 15-0-90
C. 15-90
D. 0-90

Answer　　55 D　　56 A　　57 A　　58 A　　59 C　　60 A　　61 D　　62 A　　63 C　　64 C　　65 A　　66 A
　　　　　　　67 B　　68 C

Q 69. A therapist reviews the medical record of a patient with Broca's aphasia. This condition most often results from a VCA that affects the:
[Physical Rehabilitation/Saullivan/5th Ed./Pg. 711]
A. Anterior cerebral artery   B. Middle cerebral artery
C. Posterior cerebral artery   D. Basilar artery

Q 70. A 72-year-old female involved in a motor vehicle accident fractures the middle third of her femoral shaft. The patient's physician is concerned about the effects of prolonged bed rest and would like the patient to begin walking as soon as possible. Which form of treatment would facilitate early weight bearing through the involved extremity?
[Essential Orthopedics/Maheshwari/3rd Ed./Pg. 121]
A. Immobilization in a hip spica caste
B. Internal fixation with an intramedullary nail
C. External mobilization
D. Skeletal traction

Q 71. A 25-year-old female rehabilitating from a fractured tibia is cleared for 50 lbs. of weight bearing through the involved lower extremity. The patient has no other significant medical problems and is expected to progress to full weight bearing within three weeks. The most appropriate assistive device for the patient is:
[Hopbenfield/1st Ed/Pg. 375/]
A. Wooden axillary crutches
B. Walker
C. Cane
D. Lumminum Lofstrand crutches

Q 72. A therapist instructs a patient how to transfer to a wheelchair after ambulating 125 feet with a walker. The most appropriate instruction to assist the patient when beginning to sit is:
[Physical Rehabilitation/Saullivan/5th Ed./Pg. 533]
A. Let go of the walker and reach Backwards for the wheelchair while sitting down
B. Let go of the walker and reach backwards for the wheelchair before beginning to sit down
C. Maintain contact with the walker with both hands until seated in the wheelchair
D. Maintain contact with the walker with one hand and reach backwards for the wheelchair with the other while sitting down.

Q 73. A patient using a standard wheelchair discusses the design of her home with a therapist in preparation for discharge. The patient informs the therapist that the home is 150-years-old and has narrow doorways. If the patient is to safely propel the wheelchair through the doorway, the doorway width should be at least:
A. 20 inches   B. 26 inches
C. 32 inches   D. 38 inches.

Q 74. A therapist begins prosthetic training activities for a patient with a transtibial amputation. Which of the following is the most appropriate initial activity?
[Jayant Joshi/Pg. 245]

A. Ascending and descending stairs
B. Marching in place
C. Walking on even ground
D. Weight shifting in standing

Q 75. A thirteen-year-old girl discusses the possibility of anterior cruciate ligament reconstruction with her orthopedic surgeon. The girl injured her knee while playing soccer and is concerned about the future impact of the injury on her athletic career. Which of the following factors would have the greatest influence on her candidacy for surgery?
[Tidy's Physiotherapy/12th Ed./Pg. 49]
A. Anthropometric measurements
B. Hamstrings/quadriceps strength ratio
C. Skeletal maturity
D. Somatotype

Q 76. A 50-year-old rehabilitating from a recent stroke has good strength in the affected lower extremity except trace to poor strength n the right ankle joint. The patient's sensation is severely impaired for deep pressure, light touch and sharp stimuli. The patient also has severe fluctuating edema at the ankle. The most appropriate orthosis for this patient is:
[Essential Orthopedics/Maheshwari/3rd Ed/Pg. 282]
A. Metal upright ankle-foot orthosis
B. Polypropylene solid ankle-foot orthosis
C. Prefabricated posterior leaf orthosis
D. Metal upright knee-ankle-foot orthosis

Q 77. A therapist examines a patient referred to physical therapy with olecranon bursitis. During the initial examination the therapist identifies diffuse swelling in the elbow joint. Which of the following joints would be affected with swelling in the elbow complex?
[Jayant Joshi/Reprid 2004/Pg. 37]
A. Ulnohumeral joint
B. Ulnohumeral and radiohumeral joints
C. Radiohumeral and proximal radioulnar joints
D. Ulnohumeral radiohumeral, and proximal radioulnar joints.

Q 78. A patient status postmedical meniscus repair is referred to physical therapy. Which of the following would be the responsibility of the physician postoperatively?
[Joint Structure and Function/Norkin/3rd Ed/Pg. 336]
A. Specify the parameters for superficial modality application
B. Specify the frequency and duration of range of motion exercises
C. Determine weight bearing status
D. Select an appropriate resistive exercise program

Q 79. A therapist performs girth measurements on a patient rehabilitation from knee surgery. The therapist takes for measurements 5 cm and 10 cm above the superior pole of the patella with the patient in supine. The girth measurements are recorded as 32 cm and 37 cm on the right and 34 cm and 40 cm on the left. Which of the following conclusions can be made regarding the strength of the patient's quadriceps?
[Joint Structure and Function/Norkin/3rd Ed./Pg. 95]

Answer   69 B   70 B   71 B   72 A   73 B   74 D   75 B   76 C   77 A   78 C

A. The right quadriceps will be capable of producing a greater force than the left
B. The left quadriceps will be capable of producing a greater force than the right.
C. The right and left quadriceps will be capable of producing equal force.
D. Not enough information is given to form a conclusion

Q 80. A physical therapist recommends a wheelchair for a patient rehabilitating from a CVA with the goal of independent mobility. The left upper and lower extremities are flaccid and present with edema. There is normal strength on the right, however the patient's trunk is hypotonic. The patient is cognitively intact. The most appropriate wheelchair for the patient is:

[Physical Rehabilitation/Saullivan/5th Ed./Pg 1302]

A. Solid seat, solid back, elevating leg rests, and anti-tippers
B. Sling seat, sling beck, arm board, and elevating leg rests
C. Light weight, solid seat, solid back, arm board elevating leg rests
D. Light weight, solid seat, solid back, arm board, and standard footrests

Q 81. Movements of the temporomandibular joint result chiefly from the action of the temporalis, masseter, and medial and lateral pterygoids. Which muscle does not assist in elevating the mandible?

[Human Anatomy/B.D.Chaurasia/Vol. 3/4th Ed./Pg. 145]

A. Temporalis
B. Masseter
C. Lateral Pterygoid
D. Medial Pterygoid

Q 82. The majority of orthopedic surgeons use a posterior surgical approach during total hip replacement surgery. Why is this particularly important when designing a postoperative rehabilitation program?

[Jayant Joshi/Reprint 2004/Pg. 208]

A. The majority of dislocations occur anteriorly and when combined with a posterior surgical approach it is particularly important to limit motions which stress the anterior aspect of the hip. These motions include extension, adduction, and medial rotation
B. The majority of dislocations occur posteriorly and when combined with a posterior surgical approach it is particularly important to limit motion, which stresses the posterior aspect of the hip. These motions include flexion, adduction, and medial rotation
C. Orthopedic surgeons use a posterior surgical approach to avoid unnecessary anterior instability, which is the most common direction for dislocation at the hip.
D. This statement is false. The majority of orthopedic surgeons use an anterior approach for total hip replacement surgery

Q 83. A therapist determines that a patient rehabilitating from an anterior cruciate ligament reconstruction is not ready to return to athletic competition. Which of the following best supports the therapist's decision?

[Orthopedic Physical Assessment/Magee/3rd Ed./Pg. 535]

A. A 20 percent quadriceps peak torque deficit at 60 degrees per second
B. Trace effusion in the knee after a therapy session
C. A 5 degree limitation in knee flexion
D. Inability to complete a functional progression

Q 84. A person with an anterior cruciate ligament insufficiency, who elects not to have surgical reconstruction, could probably expect to reach which minimal functional level?

[Kisner/5th Ed./Pg. 734]

A. Able to participate in all sports
B. Able to participate in light recreational sports
C. Cannot play any type of sport
D. Problems with normal walking

Q 85. It is extremely important to thoroughly instruct patients about specific precautions before and after total hip replacement surgery. Patients that do not understand or choose to disregard this information often experience subluxation or dislocation. Which of the following would be considered good advice after total hip replacement surgery?

[Jayant Joshi/Reprint 2009/Pg. 208]

A. Use a raised toilet seat
B. Use an abduction pillow for one week postoperatively
C. Avoid sitting in high and hard chairs
D. Slowly bend forward when picking objects from the floor

Q 86. A 26-year-old female presents with a diagnosis of recurrent patella dislocation. Which direction does the patella most often dislocate:

[Kisner/5th Ed/Pg. 711]

A. Superior
B. Inferior
C. Medial
D. Lateral

Q 87. A therapist examines a patient referred to physical therapy diagnosed with a lateral collateral ligament sprain. Which nerve can be palpated immediately below the bead of the fibula.

[Human Anatomy/B.D. Chaurasia/Vol 2/4th Ed./Pg. 107]

A. Common peroneal
B. Tibial
C. Sural
D. Lateral plantar

Q 88. A physical therapist reviews the medical record of a patient who sustained brachial plexus injury. The record states that the medial cord of the brachial plexus was partially severed. Which nerve would you expect to be the most seriously affected by the injury?

[Human Anatomy/B.D. Chaurasia/Vol. 1/4th Ed./Pg. 52]

A. Axillary
B. Median
C. Musculocutaneous
D. Medial Pectoral

Q 89. Tenderness elicited through palpation on the floor of the anatomic snuffbox can often be indicative of a fracture. A fracture in this area would likely involve the:

[Jayant Joshi/Reprint 2009/Pg. 113]

A. Hamate
B. Lunate
C. Scaphoid
D. Pisiform

Answer   79 C   80 D   81 C   82 C   83 A   84 D   85 B   86 D   87 A   88 A   89 C

Q 90. A physical therapy treatment plan for a patient rehabilitating from an anterior shoulder dislocation includes progressive resistive exercises. Which muscle groups should be emphasized during rehabilitation?

[Jayant Joshi/Reprint 2009/Pg. 80]

A. Abductors, lateral rotators
B. Adductors, lateral rotators
C. Abductors, medial rotators
D. Adduction, medial rotators

Q 91. A therapist examines a patient rehabilitating from an injury to the temporomandibular joint and concludes that the patient is restricted in a capsular pattern. Which of the following would be the most likely clinical presentation?

[Orthopedic Physical Assessment/Magee/5th Ed./Pg. 203]

A. Protrusion is most restricted
B. Protrusion in most restricted
C. Mouth opening is most restricted
D. Mouth closing is most restricted

Q 92. A patient is referred to physical therapy after sustaining a complete tear of the anterior cruciate ligament. The patient's ligament injury is best described as a:

[Jayant Joshi/Reprint 2009/Pg. 31]

A. Grade I Sprain
C. Grade I Strain
B. Grade III Sprain
D. Grade III Strain

Q 93. A patient with a C6 spinal cord injury relies on tenodesis to assist with functional activities. Which condition will reduce the benefits of tenodesis?

[Physical Rehabilitation/Saullivan/5th Ed./Pg. 972]

A. Lengthening of the long finger flexors
B. Excessive hamstrings length
C. Insufficient hamstrings length
D. Transferring with the fingers flexed

Q 94. A patient is treated in physical therapy after injuring his hamstrings. The medical chart describes the injury as an avulsion fracture of the ischial tuberosity. This injury usually results from:

[Human Anatomy/B.D.Chaurasia/Vol.1/Pg. 311]

A. Forceful extension of the hip with an extended knee
B. Forceful extension of the hip with a flexed knee
C. Forceful flexion of the hip with an extended knee
D. Forceful flexion of the hip with a flexed knee

Q 95. A therapist instructs a 62-year-old female rehabilitating from an ankle sprain in the use of a straight cane. The patient is confused as to why it is necessary to use the cane in the left hand since it is her right ankle that is injured. The most appropriate explanation would be:

[Joint Structure and Function/Norkin/3rd.Ed./Pg. 318]

A. Using the cane in the left hand will increase your base of support
B. Using the cane in the left hand will improve your coordination and balance
C. Using the cane in the left hand will reduce the pressure over your injured ankle
D. Using the cane in the left hand will allow more weight bearing on your injured ankle
E. And will therefore accelerate your rehabilitation time

Answer   90 C   91 C   92 B   93 A   94 C   95 C

Model Question Papers

Model Question Paper - 1

Q 1. Which type of joint is 5th carpometacarpal?
A. Pivot
B. Plane
C. Ball socket
D. Saddle

Ans. (D) It has two degrees of freedom. Metacarpals produce a mobile transverse arch at the level of metacarpal head.

Q 2. MCP flexion range in index finger is:
A. 110°
B. 90°
C. 95°
D. 100°

Ans. (B) Range of MCP flexion increases ulnarly. For little finger flexion is 110°.

Q 3. The most common site of ivory ostema (compact osteoma) is:
A. Pelvis
B. Mandible
C. Skull
D. Vertebrae

Ans. (C) Osteomal are benign outgrowths of bone found mainly on the bones of the skull.

Q 4. Dupuytren's contracture is fibrosis of:
A. Palmar fascia
B. Sartorius
C. Forearm muscle
D. None of the above

Ans. (A) Dupuytren's contracture is shortening of the palmar fascia and underlying tendons which allow people to flex their fingers.

Q 5. All are predisposing factors of osteogenic sarcoma, except:
A. Paget's disease of bone
B. Radiation
C. Viral infection
D. Bone infarction

Ans. (C) Radiation, paget's disease of bone, bone infarction all are the risk factors of osteogenic sarcoma. Viral infection is not a risk factor.

Q 6. Adson's test is performed in:
A. Scalenus anticus syndrome
B. Cervical rib
C. Both of these
D. None of these

Ans. (A) Adson's test is a provocative test for thoracic outlet syndrome accompanied by compression of subclavian artery by a cervical rib or tightened anterior and middle scalene muscles.

Q 7. The primary defect in flat foot is the following:
A. Weakness of short palmar ligament
B. Collapse at lateral longitudinal arch
C. Collapse of medial longitudinal arch
D. Shortening of plantar aponeurosis.

Ans. (C) Medial longitudinal arch is higher than the lateral longitudinal arch. So the collapse of medial longitudinal arch cause pes planus (flat foot).

Q 8. Femoral retroversion leads to:
A. Toe-in gait
B. Toe-out gait
C. Circumduction gait
D. Genu recurvatum

Ans. (B) Femoral retroversion producs lateral rotation of the femur and thus alters the knee joint axis. This will lead to a 'toe-out' gait.

Q 9. During bilateral stance, shifting of the pelvis to the right side will result in:
A. Left side pelvis drop
B. Left side pelvic hike
C. Right pelvic drop
D. All the above

Ans. (A) Because, the right hip will adducted and the left hip will be abducted.

Q 10. All the following are causes of coxa-vara except:
A. Malunion of trochanteric fracture
B. Congenital
C. Rickets and osteomalacia
D. Dislocation of hip

Ans. (D) The normal neck shaft angle in a femur is 160° at birth decreasing to about 125° in adult life. An angle less than 120° is called coxa vara. Dislocation does not cause cause coxa vara.

Q 11. A building contractor suddenly complains of lower backache which increases on bending down he has:
A. Renal colic
B. Tuberculosis of spine
C. Disc prolapsed
D. Fibrositis

Ans. (C) During bending down there is more pressure exert on the back and compresses the nerve and pain get worsen when you make movement.

Q 12. Fat embolism is commonly due to:
A. Fracture femur
B. Fracture both bones of forearm
C. Fracture calcaneum
D. Crush injury of foot

Ans. (A) It is a complication of fracture in long bones, such as femur.

Q 13. The most common nerve involved in Volkamann's ischemia contracture of forearm includes:
A. Radial
B. Ulnar
C. Median
D. Posterior interosseous

Answer

1 D	2 B	3 C	4 A	5 C	6 A	7 C	8 B	9 A	10 D	11 C	12 A
13 C											

Ans. (C) Volkmann's ischemic contracture results from acute ischemia of muscles fibers of the flexor group of muscle of the forearm which nerve supply is median.

Q 14. Commonest type of shoulder dislocation:
A. Subcoracoid
B. Subglenoid
C. Posterior
D. Subclavicular

Ans. (B) Capsular ligament is least supported inferiorly where dislocation are common called subglenoid dislocation.

Q 15. Avascular necrosis of bone is most common in:
A. Scapula
B. Scaphoid
C. Calcaneus
D. Cervical spine

Ans. (B) Avascular necrosis is common complication of a scaphoid fracture. Since the scaphoid blood supply comes from two different vascular branches of the radial artery, fracture can limit access to blood supply.

Q 16. Tennis elbow is:
A. Olecranon bursitis
B. Pain over the medial epicondyle
C. Pain over the lateral epicondyle
D. Myositis ossificans

Ans. (C) Tennis elbow is also called lateral epicondylitis. It can be caused by repetitive wrist and arm motion which is usually seen in tennis players.

Q 17. Finkelstein's test is associated with:
A. De Quervain's disease
B. Dupytrein's contracture
C. Carpal tunnel syndrome
D. Any of the above

Ans. (A) This test is used to diagnose De Quervain's disease disease in people who have wrist pain.

Q 18. Coxa vara is found in:
A. Perthe's disease
B. Tuberculosis
C. Rickets
D. Rheumatoid arthritis

Ans. (A) Coxa vara is a deformity of the hip where the angle between the head and shaft of femur is reduced to less than 120° that usually seen in Perthe's disease which is a rare childhood condition that affected hip.

Q 19. The most common site at disc prolapse is:
A. L_2-L_3
B. L_3-L_4
C. L_4-L_5
D. L_5-S_1

Ans. (C) The majority of spinal disc herniation occurs in the lumbar spine at L_4-L_5.

Q 20. Which statement is false?
A. Bone density decreases about 2% after 50 years
B. Trabecular becomes thin after 50 years
C. Trauma leads to fracture of femus
D. Cartilage does not involve in osteoarthrosis

Ans. (D) In osteoarthrosis, there is deterioration of the articular cartilage and subsequent changes in the articular tissue.

Q 21. Patellofemoral joint is:
A. A least congruent joint
B. More congruent joint
C. Hinge joint
D. None of above

Ans. (A) The total articular surface of patella is much smaller than the femoral trochlear surface

Q 22. After I_4 – S_1, the next commonest site of intervertebral disc prolapse is:
A. C_6 – C_7
B. T_{12} – L_1
C. L_1 – L_2
D. L_2 – L_3

Ans. (A) Common site in lumbar region are L_4-S_1 which are most common and next commonest in cervical region is (C_6 – C_7).

Q 23. In which of the following conditions numerous white spots are seen on the X-rays of many bones.
A. Engelmann's disease
B. Nail patella syndrome
C. Osteolysis
D. Osteopokilosis

Ans. (D) Osteopokilosis is autosomal dominant disorder there may also be whitish spots on the skin (disseminated lenticular dermatofibrosis).

Q 24. The proximal tibiofibular joint is reinforced by:
A. Anterior tibiofibular ligament
B. Posterior tibiofibular ligament
C. Both A and B
D. None of the above.

Ans. (C) It is reinforced by both tibiofibular ligament and capsule.

Q 25. Which is the most congruent joint in the human body?
A. Tibiofibular
B. Talocalcaneonavicular
C. Talocrural
D. Subtalar

Ans. (C) The structural integrity is maintained through out the range of motion.

Q 26. During pronation twist, the calcaneum undergoes:
A. Supination
B. Pronation
C. Abduction
D. Adduction

Ans. (A) The hindfoot undergoes supinate to maintain this foot on ground and counteract.

Q 27. The capsule at the ankle joint is:
A. Weak anteriorly and posteriorly
B. Weak mediolaterally
C. Both A and B
D. None of above

Ans. (A) Although it is reinforced by crucial tibiofibular interosseous ligament, the anterior and posterior tibiofibular ligament and tibiofibular interosseous.

Q 28. Hallux valgus means:
A. Outward deviation of great toe
B. Inward deviation of great toe
C. Outward deviation of fifth toe
D. Inward deviation of fifth toe

Ans. (A) Bunion known as Hallux valgus, a bony bump that forms on the joint at base of great toe which shows outward deviation of great toe.

Q 29. The most common cause of acute sciatica is due to:
A. Trauma
B. Secondaries of spine

Answer	14 B	15 B	16 C	17 A	18 A	19 C	20 D	21 A	22 A	23 D	24 C	25 C
	26 A	27 A	28 A									

C. Acute prolapsed interveretebral disc
D. Tuberculosis of spine

Ans. (C) Sciatica is a certain type of nerve pain that can be cause by a heriniated lumbar disc compressing sciatic nerve.

Q 30. One of the features given below is essential in the diagnosis of a fracture of bone:
A. Deformity
B. A crepitus
C. A partial or complete loss of continuity of the bone
D. None of the above

Ans. (C) Fracture is a partial or complete break in the continuity of bone.

Q 31. Dislocations occur most frequently in the:
A. Shoulder joint   B. Elbow joint
C. Hip joint   D. Knee joint

Ans. (A) Shoulder joint dislocation occurs because shoulder joint is less stable than hip, elbow and knee joint and shoulders joint has high mobility than stability.

Q 32. Which of the following is not true about myositis ossificans?
A. Associated with muscle tendon rupture
B. Inflammation around the ruptured muscle deposition of hydroxyapatite crystal
C. Common in supracondylar fracture
D. Ossification of musculoperiosteal hematoma

Ans. (A) Myositis ossificans is a condition where bone tissue forms inside muscle or other soft tissue after any injury. It occurs in large muscle of arm and legs.

Q 33. The least common cause of brachial Neuralgia is:
A. Cervical spondylosis   B. Pancoast tumors
C. Cervical rib   D. Tietze syndrome

Ans. (D) Tietze's syndrome is a rare inflammatory disorder characterized by chest pain and swelling of the cartilage at costochondral junction.

Q 34. Phalen's test is positive in:
A. Carpal tunnel syndrome   B. De Quervain's disease
C. Tennis elbow   D. Ulnar burisitis

Ans. (A) This test used in the diagnosis of CTS. This occurs when the median nerve is compressed at the wrist as in carpal tunnel syndrome.

Q 35. The most common cause of scoliosis in children is:
A. Hemivertebrae   B. Unequal limb length
C. Postpoliomyelitis   D. Marfan syndrome

Ans. (C) Postpolio patients experience gradual weakening in muscles, pain from joint degeneration and increased skeletal deformity, such as scoliosis is common in children.

Q 36. In cervical spondylosis which part at vertebral badly involved:
A. Inferior articular facet   B. Pars interarticularis
C. Superior articular facet   D. All of the above

Ans. (A) Cervical spondylosis is the degeneration of vertebral column. It chiefly affect the vertebral bodies and inferior articular facet joint.

Q 37. In children, fracture neck of femur is best treated by:
A. Plaster in abduction
B. Closed reduction (internal fixation)
C. Plaster in adduction
D. Traction

Ans. (B) Treatment for displaced fracture is by closed reduction and internal fixation. It is more convenient method.

Q 38. The most common deformity in clubfoot is:
A. Equinus   B. Equinovalgus
C. Equinovarus   D. Calcaneovalgus

Ans. (C) Clubfoot also called talipes equinovarus. It is a birth defect where one or both feet are rotated inward and downward.

Q 39. Painful arc syndrome is due to:
A. Fracture at greater tubercle of humerus
B. Chronic supraspinatus tendonitis
C. Subacromial bursitis
D. All of the above

Ans. (D) When rotator cuff tendons become inflamed or worm cause painful arc syndrome.

Q 40. Trigger finger occurs in:
A. Rheumatoid arthrits   B. Trauma
C. Osteosarcoma   D. Osteoarithritis

Ans. (A) It is locking of a finger in a bent position caused by inflammation of a tendon in the finger. It is common among people with RA.

Q 41. Claw hand is seen in:
A. Ulnar nerve injury   B. Carpal tunnel syndrome
C. Syringomyelia   D. Cervical rib

Ans. (A) Claw hand is a deformity of hand that develops due to ulnar nerve damage causing paralysis of lumbricals.

Q 42. Carrying angle is decreased in:
A. Cubitus varus   B. Cubitus valgus
C. Genu valgum   D. Genu varum

Ans. (A) Any variation of the angle less than normal are called cubitus varus

Q 43. Consider the following statements about carpal tunnel syndrome.
1. **It may occur in acromegaly**
2. **It may occur in pregnancy**
3. **It causes delayed ulnar nerve conduction**
4. **It may be associated with wasting of abductor pollicis. Of these statements:**
A. 1, 2 and 3 are correct   B. 2, 3 and 4 are correct
C. 1, 2 and 4 are correct   D. 1, 3 and 4 are correct

Ans. (C) Carpal tunnel syndrome is due to median nerve compression. In acromegaly the edematous synovial tissue composes the median nerve because of oversecretion of growth

Answer	29 C	30 C	31 A	32 A	33 D	34 A	35 C	36 A	37 B	38 C	39 D	40 A
	41 A	42 A	43 C									

hormone. In pregnancy there is a build up of fluid (edema) in the tissue in the wrist.

Q 44. Dupuytren's contracture at the hand commonly starts in: *(BIHAR 1991)*

A. Thumb   B. Index finger
C. Middle finger   D. Ring finger
E. Little finger only

Ans. (D) The condition most often affects the 4th ring and 5th little fingers.

Q 45. Galeazzi fracture is:
A. Supracondylar fracture of the humerus
B. Fracture of the distal radius with inferior radioulnar joint dislocation
C. Fracture of radius in the proximal site and dislocation of the elbow.
D. Fracture of the radial head

Ans. (B) Galeazzi fracture is fracture is fracture at the distal radius with inferior radioulnar joint dislocation

Q 46. _______ displacement of scapula is prevented by tension in the coracoclavicular ligament.
A. Upward rotation
B. Downslide

C. Medial displacement
D. No movement

Ans. (B) In this position capsule twist and tighten by itself.

Q 47. The method of joint construction in diarthroidal joint differs from:
A. Cartilaginous joint   B. Synarthrodial joint
C. Synchondroses joint   D. Symphysis joint

Ans. (B) Because the movement in synarthrodial is less compare to diarthroidal is less compare to diarthrodial joint.

48. Crimp is the wavy configuration of:
A. Elastin   B. Collagen
C. Fibronectic   D. Proteoglycans

Ans. (B) Because collagen has more nonelastic fiber than elastic.

Q 49. Finger flexor work at least during:
A. Wrist extension   B. Wrist flexion
C. Wrist radial deviation   D. Ulnar deviation

Ans. (B) Because of active insufficiency.

Q 50. Patella ability to perform its function depends:
A. Stability   B. Mobility
C. Both A and B   D. None of the above

Ans. (B) It works without restricting knee motion.

Answer   44 D   45 B   46 B   47 B   48 B   50 B

Model Question Paper - 2

Q 1. Which of the following fracture are best managed by closed means?

(AIIMS May 2012)

A. Fracture both means forearm in adults
B. Colles fracture
C. Monteggia fracture
D. Galeazzi fracture

Ans. (B) Colles fracture all other fractures require open reduction and internal fixation for anatomical alignment and rigid in mobilization

Q 2. Avulsion fracture of the anterior inferior iliac spine is because of the violent contraction of the:

A. Psoas major
B. Straight head of rectus femoris
C. Sartorius
D. Pectineus

Ans. (B) The straight head of rectus femoris tendon takes its origin from the anterior inferior iliac spine. Sometimes due to violent contraction of this muscle, spine may be pulled off and the fracture unites quickly in 3 – 4 weeks.

Q 3. In which of the following injuries around the hip is there true lengthening of the concerned lower limb?

(AIIMS Nov 2010)

A. Extracapsular fracture femur
B. Lateral dislocation of hip
C. Anterior dislocation of hip
D. Intracapsular fracture femur

Ans. (C) Anterior dislocations of hip is a rare injury sustained when the lower limbs are forcibly abducted and externally rotated. Clinically the limb is in an attitude of external rotation. There may be true lengthening.

Q 4. Hypovolemia is a serious problem with long bone fracture. What is the average blood loss following fracture shaft of femur?

(AIPG 2012)

A. 1,000-1,500 mL
B. 500 mL
C. No blood loss at all
D. 3,000-3,500 mL

Ans. (A) Average blood loss in fracture of femur would be 1,000-1500 mL in fracture of pelvis the blood loss would be around 1,500-2,000 mL.

Q 5. Which of the following fracture in known as Rolando's fracture?

(AIIMS May 2010)

A. Fracture base of 5th metacarpal
B. Fracture of ulnar styloid
C. Comminuted intra-articular fracture of base of first metacarpal
D. Fracture neck of second metatarsal

Ans. (C) Rolando's fracture is the comminuted in the intra-articular fracture of base of first metacarpal.

Q 6. Pure dislocation does not occur in the lumbar spine because:

A. The bodies of the lumbar vertebrae are stout
B. The facets of the lumbar vertebrae are stout and vertically placed
C. The ligamentum flavum in the lumbar region is well developed
D. The disc in the lumbar regions is so thick it does not allow the bone

Ans. (B) Because the vertically placed facet prevent any horizontal movement.

Q 7. Joint between manubrium and body of sternum belongs to the variety of:

A. Syndesmosis
B. Synchondrosis
C. Symphysis
D. Plane synovial

Ans. (C) The joint between manubrium and body of sternum is in the median plane of the body and allows limited movements. It is secondary cartilaginous joint called symphysis.

Q 8. Bilateral genu valgum is:

A. Symmetrical postural deviation
B. Symmetrical asymmetrical
C. Asymmetrical postural deviation
D. None

Ans. (A) Bilateral genu valgum is symmetrical postural deviation.

Q 9. Dowager's hump is a kyphosis condition that is found most often in:

A. Children
B. Sedentary males
C. Young women
D. Post menopausal osteoporosis

Ans. (D) It is found most often in postmenopausal women who have osteoporosis. The anterior aspect of the bodies of series of urethral collapses and leads to an increase in the posterior convexity of thoracic arc (the hump).

Answer   1 B   2 B   3 C   4 A   5 C   6 B   7 C   8 A   9 D

Q 10. __________ muscle is described as flexors, stabilizers, and extensors of lumbar spine.
A. Rectus abdominis
B. Spinalis capitis
C. Longissimus
D. Psoas major

Ans. (D) When spine is in flexed position, the Psoas cross anterior to the axis of rotation of lumbar intervertebral joints. Muscle has flexors movement and concentric contraction produce flexors.

Q 11. The IR lamp is positioned at a distance of:
A. 20 cm
B. 100 cm
C. 45,050 cm
D. None of the above

Ans. (D) None of the above. The IR lamp is positioned at a distance of 50-75 cm.

Q 12. Which carpal bone fracture is more common?
A. Scaphoid
B. Lunate
C. Hammate
D. Pisiform

Ans. (A) Over 80% of carpal fracture involve the scaphoid The scaphoid is located most radially. The scaphoid links the two rows of carpals.

Q 13. The cause of gun stock deformity is: *(AIIMS Nov 2012)*
A. Supracondylar fracture
B. Fracture both bones forearm
C. Fracture surgical head of humerus
D. Fracture fibula

Ans. (A) The common cause of gun stock deformity is supracondylar fracture and the deformity is the result of malunion occurring as a complication of supracondylar fracture.

Q 14. Tardy ulnar nerve palsy occurs as a delay equele of:
A. Supracondylar fracture of humerus
B. Posterior dislocation of elbow
C. Fracture of lateral condyle of humerus in children
D. Fracture of olecranon

Ans. (C) Tardy ulnar nerve palsy occur as a delay consequence of nonunion of lateral condyle in child resulting in cubitus valgus deformity which ultimately is the cause of ulnar nerve palsy.

Q 15. A pilot fracture of tibia is:
(DNB Dec 2010)
A. Intra-articular fracture of distal tibia
B. Compound fracture of tibia
C. Comminuted fracture of upper tibia
D. Intra-articular fracture of upper tibia

Ans. (A) This fracture is also called the plafond fracture.

Q 16. Dislocation of the inferior radioulnar joint and fracture head of radius is known as
A. Monteggia fracture dislocation
B. Galeazzi fracture dislocation
C. Essex-Lopresti dislocation
D. Soprano's dislocation

Ans. (C) Comminuted fracture of the head of radius with dislocation of inferior radioulnar joint is known as Essex-Lopresti fracture dislocation

Q 17. All the following are techniques for reduction of a dislocation shoulder except:
(DNB June 2009)
A. Kocher's maneuver
B. Brygant's maneuver
C. Surgical reduction
D. Hippocratic maneuver

Ans. (B) Reduction can be surgical or by closed means. The technique followed now is the Kocher's method for closed reduction.

Q 18. Bimalleolar fracture is called:
A. Pott's fracture
B. Massonaives fracture
C. Choparts fracture
D. Jane's fracture

Ans. (A) Pott's fracture is the Bimalleolar ankle fracture.

Q 19. Clutton's joints refers to which of the following
A. Swollen joints of OA
B. Heme arthrosis
C. Joint with effusion in congenital syphilis
D. Gouty arthritis

Ans. (C) Late manifestation of congenital syphilis, Cluttons joints is a painless synovitis occurring at puberty. It most commonly affects the knee and elbow, mostly bilaterally.

Q 20. Earliest sign of Volkman's ischemic contracture is:
A. Pulselessness
B. Pain on passive extension of fingers
C. Pallor of distal extremity
D. Crepitus

Ans. (B) Pain occurs in the flexor aspect of the forearm when the fingers are extended passively.

Q 21. All the following are treatment modalities for fracture neck of femur except (intracapsular)
A. Moore's pin fixation
B. Hemiarthroplasty
C. Cancellous scan fixation
D. Pin traction

Ans. (D) Intracapsular fracture of hip is managed differently in various age group but pin traction alone is not a definitive treatment.

Q 22. Osteotomy done for malunited supracondylar fracture is:
(J & K 2001)
A. Frinch
B. Shanz's
C. MC Murry's
D. McAlister

Ans. (A) Frinch osteotomy prevent the loss of correction achieve and is the commonly accepted method for correction of malunited supracondylar fracture.

Q 23. Main risk in fracture scaphoid is:
A. Nonunion
B. Malunion
C. Delayed union
D. Avascular necrosis

Ans. (D) Fracture scaphoid tears the artery, the blood supply is lost and avascular necrosis occurs.

Q 24. Barton's fracture of the wrist.
A. Involves Radiocarpal subluxation
B. Is a severe form of a Colle's fracture
C. Is often treated by open reduction and internal fixation
D. All of the above

Ans. (A) Barton's fracture is on intra-articular fracture of distal radius with dislocation of radiocarpal joint.

Answer	10 A	11 D	12 A	13 A	14 C	15 A	16 C	17 B	18 A	19 C	20 B	21 D
	22 A	23 D	24 A									

Q 25. Pulled elbow is:
A. A sprain of extensor tendons
B. Dislocation of head of radius
C. Fracture of lateral condyle of humerus
D. Dislocation of elbow

Ans. (B) Pulled elbow is dislocation of head of radius of its normal position at the elbow. It is caused by a sudden pull on a child's lower arm or wrist.   *(ANDHRA 1998).*

Q 26. Galeazzi fracture is a fracture of:
A. Upper end of ulna   B. Lower end of ulna
C. Upper end of radius   D. Lower end of radius

Ans. (D) Galeazzi fracture is at the distal head of the radius with dislocation of distal radioulnar joint.

Q 27. The characteristic feature of a frontal lobe tumor.
(DNB Dec 2010)
A. Abnormal gait   B. Aphasia
C. Distractibility   D. Antisocial behavior

Ans. (D) Antisocial behavior is one of the important fracture of frontal lobe tumor.

Q 28. Akinetic mutism is seen in lesion of which of the following lobes?
A. Parietal   B. Temporal
C. Occipital   D. Frontal

Ans. (D) Akinectic mutism is a medical term describing patients tending neither to move nor speak. It is the result of severe frontal lobe injury in which the pattern of inhibitory control is one of increasing passivity and gradually discussing speech and motion.

Q 29. If Wernicke's area is damaged in the dominant hemisphere it will result in?
(AIIMS May 2010)
A. Irrelevant and rapid speech
B. No effect of speech
C. Speech with difficulty in articulation
D. Incomprehension of written language

Ans. (A) Wernicke's area is the sensory speech area. It lies at temporoparietal junction. It is concerned with speech and understanding.

Q 30. Which of the following is a pain sensitive structure?
A. Dura   B. Arachnoid
C. Pia   D. All

Ans. (A) Basic physiology—pain sensitive structures in the brain: 1. Dura, 2. V nerve, 3 IX nerve, 4. X nerve, 5. Blood vessels.

Q 31. During supinators twist, the talus undergoes:
A. Supinators   B. Pronation
C. Abduction   D. Adduction

Ans. (B) During pronators, the foot undergoes adduction of talus and eversion of calcaneum to maintain contact.

Q 32. Tectorial membrane is the continuation of:
A. ALL   B. PLL
C. Ligament of flavum   D. Capsule

Ans. (B) PLL runs from 2nd cervical to sacrum, from C2 and above called as tectorial membrane.

Q 33. Hand to knee gait is also called:
A. Gluteus maximus gait   B. Dorsiflexor gait
C. Scissoring gait   D. Quadriceps gait

Ans. (D) Help the individual to extend the knee passively.

Q 34. Rectus femoris, vastus lateralis and medial gastrocnemius work ______ and ______ during ascending and descending stairs.
A. Eccentric and concentric   B. Both isometric
C. Concentric and eccentric   D. Eccentric and isometric

Ans. (C) Ascending stairs need positive work, descending stairs work as a energy absorber.

Q 35. MCP flexors range in index finger is:
A. 110°   B. 90°
C. 95°   D. 100°

Ans. (B) Range of MCP flexion increases ulnarly. For little finger function is 110°.

Q 36. Fairbank's triangle is seen in:
A. Infantile coxa vara
B. Congenital dislocation of hip
C. Pycnodysostosis
D. Arthrogryposis

Ans. (A) This is a X-ray finding. The epiphyseal plate may be too vertical. There may be a separate triangle of bone in the inferior portion of the metaphysis called the Fairbank's triangle.

Q 37. Trethowan's sign is used in the radiological diagnosis of:
(AIIMS Nov 2010)
A. Slipped capital femoral epiphysis
B. Perthe's disease
C. Tuberculosis of hip
D. Osteochondral fracture in hip joint

Ans. (A) Normally on AP view of hip a line drawn along the superior surface of the neck of femur passes through a third of head, whereas in slipped epiphysis the line passing superior to the head.

Q 38. Klippel-Feil triad does not include:
A. High scapula
B. Low post hairline
C. Restricted neck movements
D. Critical vertebral fusion

Ans. (A) Klippel-Feil syndrome is a congenital fusion of the critical vertebrae that may involve two segments a congenital block vertebrae or this entire cervical spine.

Q 39. In which of the following conditions, numerous white spots are seen on the X-rays of many bones.
A. Engelmann's disease   B. Nail patella syndrome
C. Osterolysis   D. Osteopoikilosis

Ans. (D) This is a autosomal dominant disorder, there may also be white spots on the skin.

Answer	25 B	26 D	27 D	28 D	29 A	30 A	31 B	32 B	33 D	34 C	35 B	36 A
	37 A	38 A	39 D									

Q 40. Which of the following is not a feature of Larsen's disease ?

AIMS Nov 2012

A. Marked joint laxity
B. Dislocation of hip
C. Vascular fragility
D. Instability of knees

Ans. (C) Vascular fragility giving rise to spontaneous breathing is not a feature of Larsen's disease. Other feature include subluxation of radial head, equinovarus deformities of the fact and disc face appearance.

Q 41. Clubfoot is common among:

A. Males
B. Binovular twins
C. Females
D. Uniovular twins

Ans. (A) In clubfoot, males are twice as likely as females to be brain with clubfoot.

Q 42. Which of the following statement is wrong in tendon transfer?

A. Contracture should be released priorly
B. Synergistic muscles are used to tendon transfer
C. Adequate tendon should be mobilized to gain length
D. All of the above

Ans. (B) In tendon transfer, the insertion of tendon is moved but the origin remain same.

Q 43. Upper motor neuron type of paralysis is seen in:

A. Poliomyelitis
B. Peripheral neuropathy
C. Cerebral palsy
D. Muscular dystrophy

Ans. (C) Spasticity a known impairment following an UMN lesion, such as in cerebral palsy. In CP, spasticity is regarded as the most common impairment.

Q 44. The nerve involved in carpal tunnel syndrome is:

A. Ulnar
B. Radial
C. Median
D. Anterior cutaneous nerve

Ans. (C) Carpal tunnel syndrome occurs only when there is increased pressure on median nerve.

Q 45. The level of the constricting nodule in case of Trigger finger is at:

A. Neck of the corresponding metacarpal bone
B. Metacarpophalangeal joint

C. Proximal interphalangeal joint
D. Distal interphalangeal joint

Ans. (B) A finger becomes locked in a bent position when tendon at metacarpophalangeal joint that flex the finger becomes inflamed and swollen.

Q 46. True about duputyrens contracture:

A. Slight preponderance in males
B. Slight preponderance in females
C. Much more common in males
D. Much more common in females

Ans. (C) It is a condition in which one or more finger become permanently bent in a flexed position. Gradual onset in males over so.

Q 47. Cervical spondylosis is more common at:

A. $C_1 - C_2$
B. $C_2 - C_3$
C. $C_6 - C_7$
D. $C_4 - C_5$

Ans. (C) It is usually occur at the $C_5 - C_7$ levels.

Q 48. All are causes of genu varum except:

A. Balint's disease
B. Rickets
C. Malunited fractures
D. Recurrent dislocation of patella

Ans. (D) Genu varum or bow legs a common condition in children below 4 year of age and the causes include A,B and C.

Q 49. Candle drip appearance on X-ray is a feature of:

A. Alzheimer's disease
B. Apert's syndrome
C. Ehlers–Danlos syndromes
D. Melorheostosis

Ans. (D) Patients presents with pain and stiffness confined to one limb. X-ray show irregular patches of sclerosis usually distributed in linear fashion through the limb, the appearance reminiscent way that congeals on the side of burning candle.

Q 50. Congenital muscular torticollis is caused by fibromatosis within the __________ muscle.

A. Trapezius
B. Splenius capitis
C. Sternocleidomastoid
D. Pectoralis major

Ans. (C) It may involve the muscle diffusely but more often is localized near the clavicular attachment of muscle

---

Model Question Paper - 3

Q 1. March fracture affects:
A. Neck of second metatarsal
B. Neck of the first metatarsal
C. Body of second metatarsal
D. None of these

Ans. (A) Because of recurrent stress on neck of second metatarsal.

Q 2. Which of the following muscles are stance phase muscles?
A. Quadriceps
B. Hamstring
C. Peroneus longus
D. Soleus gastrocnemius

Ans. (A) During stance, hip is in extension and quadriceps are chief extensor muscles of knee.

Q 3. A physiotherapist instructs a patient to move her lower teeth forward in relaxation to the upper teeth. This motion is termed as:
A. Protrusion
B. Retrusion
C. Lateral deviation
D. Occlusal position

Ans. (A) Protrusion, this is where the upper teeth protrude outward compared to the lower front teeth.

Q 4. Internal fixation is done in which fractures:
A. Compound fracture
B. Multiple fracture
C. Elderly person
D. All of these

Ans. (D) Internal fixation—it helps to stabilization of bone and also reduce nonunion and malunion of bones.

Q 5. Waddling gait is due to:
A. Gluteus muscles weakness
B. Paravertebral muscle weakness
C. Obturator nerve palsy
D. Adductor muscle weakness

Ans. (A) The waddling is due to weakness of the proximal muscles of the pelvic girdle. The patient uses circumduction to compensate for gluteal weakness.

Q 6. Conduction of nerve impulse is a factor in myelinated nerves because of:
A. Uninterrupted flow of impulse
B. Saltatory conduction
C. Circular current flow
D. Quick reversal of current flow

Ans. (B) Saltatory conduction is the propagation of action potential along myelinated axon potentials from one node of Ranvier to the next node.

Q 7. One of the function of basal ganglion is to:
A. Increase the muscle tone
B. Produce small jerky movements
C. Inhibit stretch reflex
D. Control auditory function

Ans. (A) Basal ganglia are associated with a variety of functions, including control of voluntary motor movement, movement increase muscle tone, eye involvement and emotion.

Q 8. Myositis ossificans is commonly seen at?
A. Elbow
B. Hip
C. Knee
D. Shoulder

Ans. (A) Myositis ossification usually occurs where a person has experienced a single traumatic injury, most common seen in elbow.

Q 9. Which of the following is seen in bilateral congenital dislocation of hip?
A. Waddling gait
B. Allies test positive
C. Shenton's line is broken
D. Trendelenburg test positive

Ans. (C) Stenton's line is line between neck of the femur to pubic symphysis which is break in bilateral congenital dislocation of hip.

Q 10. A patient reports pain radiating down her posterior leg in to the foot. She also exhibits weakness in planter flexion and absent Achilles reflex. Which spinal level would you expect to be involved?
A. L_2
B. L_3
C. L_5
D. S_2

Ans. (D) S_2 supply occur at posterior aspect of leg.

Q 11. Following structures are related posterior to head of pancreas, except:
A. Inferior vena cava
B. Terminal part of renal veins
C. Superior mesenteric artery
D. Right crus of diaphragm

Ans. (C) Aorta with the origin of superior mesenteric artery is related posterior to the body of pancreas and not the head of pancreas.

Q 12. All the following are useful in diagnosis of congenital dislocation of the hip except:
A. Ortolani test
B. Barlow's test
C. Slocum test
D. Galleazi or Alli's test

Ans. (C) Slocum test is used for testing anterolateral instability of knee.

Answer   1 A   2 A   3 A   4 D   5 A   6 B   7 A   8 A   9 C   10 D   11 C   12 C

Q 13. Lisfranc dislocation is:
A. Tarsometatarsal dislocation
B. Lunate
C. Scaphoid
D. Posterior dislocation of hip

Ans. (A) Tarsometatarsal dislocation is an injury of foot in which one or more of the metatarsal bone are displaced from the tarsus.

Q 14. Following form the posterior relation of the neck of pancreas:
A. Superior mesenteric and portal veins
B. Gastroduodenal artery
C. Inferior vena cava
D. Common bile duct

Ans. (A) Immediate posterior relation of neck of pancreas is formed by the superior mesenteric vein with the beginning of portal vein.

Q 15. Pseudo-orthosis can be due to all except:
A. Congenital
B. Post inflammatory
C. Traumatic
D. None of these

Ans. (B) Pseudo-orthosis can be by congenital and traumatic.

Q 16. The squat test is a clinical test used for the diagnosis of which of the following condition at the knee:
A. TB knee
B. Lateral collateral ligament tear
C. Menisci tear
D. GCT lower end of the femur

Ans. (C) Menisci tear. The squat test consist of several repetitions of a full squat with the feet and legs alternately fully internally and externally rotated as the squat is performed.

Q 17. The therapist examines a patient with C_6 spinal cord injury. Which muscle would not be innervated based the patient level of injury?
A. Biceps
B. Deltoid
C. Triceps
D. Diaphragm

Ans. (C) Triceps supply is C_7 so, triceps a muscle which is not involve is C_6 spinal injury.

Q 18. An almost even distribution of pressure occurred in:
A. Initial flexion
B. Mid flexion
C. Late flexion
D. Full extension

Ans. (B) Elastic tension increases with knee flexion.

Q 19. Following are the branches of posterior cord of branchial plexus except:
A. Thoracodorsal nerve
B. Dorsal scapular nerve
C. Axillary nerve
D. Radial nerve

Ans. (B) Dorsal scapular nerve is the nerve to rhomboids which crises from C5 root of brachial plexus.

Q 20. Commonest site of fracture scaphoid is:
A. Wrist
B. Proximal 1/3rd
C. Distal fracture
D. None of these

Ans. (A) A scaphoid fracture is a break of the scaphoid bone which is present in the wrist.

Q 21. In pes planus weight is borne on:
A. Metatarsal
B. Toes
C. Hindfoot
D. Midfoot

Ans. (D) This cause increase energy expenditure during walking.

Q 22. The McMurry's test is used in evaluation of:
A. Meniscal injuries
B. Fracture of hip
C. A joint following replacement arthroplasty
D. An orthopedic implant

Ans. (A) The McMurry's test evaluate a meniscal injury with the patient lying on the couch the surgeon standing on the side firmly grasps the foot in one hand and the knee with the other.

Q 23. Sequestrum is:
A. A piece of infected bone
B. A piece of dead bone
C. Organized inflammatory exudates
D. Segregated marrow tissue

Ans. (B) A piece of dead bone tissue formed with is a diseased or injured bone, typically in chronic osteomyelitis.

Q 24. Yellow elastic cartilage is present in:
A. Intervertebral disc
B. Epiglottis
C. Articular ends of long bones
D. Trachea

Ans. (B) Epiglottis contains elastic type of cartilage. It is made up of numerous cells inside the lacunae a network of elastic fibers pervading the matrix in between the cells.

Q 25. Cozen's test is a clinical test for diagnosis of:
A. De Quervain's tenosynovitis
B. Lateral epicondylitis
C. Carpal tunnel syndrome
D. Myasthenia gravis

Ans. (B) Lateral epicondylitis—Cozen's test is used for the diagnosis of tennis elbow, here pain at the lateral epicondyle can be reproduced by active dorsiflexion of the wrist against resistance with the elbow straight.

Q 26. At what level is it realistic for a patient having spinal cord injury to functionally ambulate?
A. C_7
B. T_1
C. T_6
D. L_1

Ans. (D) L_1 is a supply of inguinal ligament.

Q 27. Middle mediastinum contains the following structure except:
A. Azygos vein
B. Phrenic nerve
C. Pulmonary trunk
D. Ascending aorta

Ans. (A) Azygos vein is a content of posterior mediastinum and not the middle mediastinum.

Q 28. Following structure is situated retroperitoneally:
A. Cecum
B. Appendix
C. Head of the pancreas
D. Tail of the pancreas

Answer	13 A	14 A	15 B	16 C	17 C	18 B	19 B	20 A	21 D	22 A	23 B	24 B
	25 B	26 D	27 A									

Ans. (C) Head of pancreas is covered only anteriorly by peritoneum and remains as a retroperitoneal structure.

Q 29. The most preferred treatment of fracture neck femur in a young person is:
A. Hemiarthroplasty
B. THR
C. Conservative treatment
D. Closed reduction and internal fixation

Ans. (D) Closed reduction is performed and internal fixation is applied usually in the form of k wires to stabilize the fracture.

Q 30. Most common case of pathological fracture in a child is:
A. Malignancy
B. Bone cyst
C. Fibrous dysplasia
D. Juvenile Paget disease

Ans. (D) Juvenile Paget disease a rare genetic disorder characterized by markedly accelerated bone twin over, present in early childhood.

Q 31. Which of the following is a diagnostic test for acute hematogenous osteomyelitis?
A. Plain X-ray
B. Blood culture
C. CT scan
D. Clinical examination

Ans. (B) Blood culture should always be obtained when osteomyelitis is suspected, though they are often negative except in case of hematogenous osteomyelitis.

Q 32. Osteophytes developing at the joint, characteristically compresses spinal nerves at:
A. Intervertebral foramen
B. Anterior part of body
C. Posterior part of the body
D. Paradural area

Ans. (A) Spinal nerve passes through intervertebral foramen of vertebral disc, which compressed by developing osteophytes.

Q 33. Mandibular condyles protrudes ______ mm from ramus.
A. 10 mm
B. 20 mm
C. 30 mm
D. 11 mm

Ans. (B) Approximately 15–20 mm, condyles are palpated just in front of the external auditory meatus of ear.

Q 34. In pes cavus the subtalar joint goes ______ for position.
A. Pronated
B. Supinated
C. Everted
D. Varus

Ans. (B) Because of the unusual high medial longitudinal arch, the subtalar and transverse tarsal joints tend to near.

Q 35. Forward continuant constitutes ______ % of gait cycle.
A. 14-32%
B. 32-64%
C. 64%
D. 24%

Ans. (B) Occurs midstance to toe off.

Q 36. Prostate surgery or after delivery cause damage to:
A. Levator scapulae
B. Iliococcygeus
C. Levator ani
D. Coccygeus

Ans. (C) Coccygeus muscles assist with levator ani in supporting the pelvic viscera and maintaining intra abdominal pressure

Q 37. Hand to knee joint is seen in:
A. Athetoid cerebral palsy
B. Parkinsonism
C. Polio condition
D. Osteoarthritis

Ans. (C) Polio has weakness of quadriceps, so the patients walk with this gait.

Q 38. Brachioradialis muscle is paralyzed in radial nerve injuries of all the followings level except:
A. Axilla
B. Middle of the arm
C. Proximal to elbow
D. Distal to elbow

Ans. (D) Distal to elbow nerve supply to articular branch of dorsal ulnar nerve.

Q 39. Posterior tilting of the pelvis, upward movement of symphysis pubis and movement of sacrum close to the pelvis produces ______ at hip.
A. Flexion
B. Extension
C. Abduction
D. Adduction

Ans. (B) This brings the posterior aspect of the pelvis closure to the femur and thus produces hip extension.

Q 40. Loading response occurs until:
A. Leading limb strikes the ground
B. Initial contact of the opposite limb
C. Opposite limb lifts off the ground
D. Leading limb leaves the ground

Ans. (C) Loading response also called as flat foot that occurs immediately following initial contact continues lifts the contralateral extremity lifts off the ground.

Q 41. The motion occurs greater in the cervical region is:
A. Lateral flexion
B. Rotation
C. Flexion
D. Both A and B

Ans. (D) Lateral flexion and rotation are coupled motion.

Q 42. The strongest ligament of talocalcaneum is:
A. Interosseous talocalcaneal ligament
B. Cervical
C. Deltoid
D. Spring

Ans. (B) It lies anterior to the sinus tarsi and attaches in the neck of both calcaneum and talus.

Q 43. Tardy ulnar nerve palsy is seen in:
A. Cubitus valgus
B. Dislocation of elbow
C. Fracture scaphoid
D. Supracondylar fracture of humerus

Ans. (A) Typically tardy ulnar nerve palsy occur is as a consequences of nonunion of lateral condyle in child resulting in cubitus valgus deformity.

Q 44. Albers-Schönberg disease is:
A. Osteopetrosis
B. Osteoparosis
C. Cartilage
D. Collagen

Ans. (A) Osteopetrosis is 'stone bone' also known marble bone disease or Albers-Schönberg disease is an extremely rare inherited disorder whereby the bones harden becoming denser.

Q 45. Ulnar nerve injury at elbow would involve all of the following except:

Answer	28 C	29 D	30 D	31 B	32 A	33 B	34 B	35 B	36 C	37 C	38 D	39 B
	40 C	41 D	42 B	43 A	44 A							

A. Flexor carpi ulnaris
B. Hypothenar muscles
C. Flexor digitorum profundus
D. Interossei

Ans. (C) Flexor digitorum profundus is a hybrid muscle which have dual nerve supply, one is ulnar nerve and one is anterior interosseous nerve.

Q 46. Earliest symptoms of Volkmann ischemia is:
A. Pain in flexor muscles
B. Absence of pulse
C. Pain on passive extension
D. Cyanosis of limb

Ans. (B) Lack of blood flow to the forearm. This usually occurs when there is increased pressure due to swelling.

Q 47. Multiple bone fracture are seen in:
A. Rickets
B. Osteomalacia
C. Scurvy
D. Osteogenesis

Ans. (D) Osteogenesis imperfecta is a genetic disorder that prevents the body from building strong bones which cause multiple fracture in bone.

Q 48. If the axillary nerve was severed, what muscle could laterally rotate the humerus?
A. Teres major
B. Subscapularis
C. Infraspinatus
D. Teres minor

Ans. (C) Nerve supply of infraspinatus muscle is supra-scapular nerve.

Q 49. The lesion in Klumpkes paralysis is at:
A. Cervical plexus
B. Lower brachial
C. Upper brachial
D. Sacral plexus

Ans. (B) Klumpkes paralysis is a variety of partial palsy of the lower roots of the brachial plexus.

Q 50. Pivot test is done for:
A. ACL
B. PCL
C. Medial meniscus
D. Lateral meniscus

Ans. (B) This test is tests for assessing anterior cruciate injury. An important determinant as to how knee will function.

Model Question Paper - 4

Q 1. Normal 'Q' angle is:
A. 5°–10°
B. 10°–15°
C. 15°–20°
D. 26°–32°

Ans. (B) The 'Q' angle is the line connecting between axis to midpoint at patella and tibial tubercle to midpoint of patella (which is 10°–15°).

Q 2. The distal articular surface of the ankle joint is made up of:
A. Body of calcaneum
B. Body of talus
C. Medial malleolus
D. Lateral malleolus

Ans. (B) It has 3 articular surfaces, medially with tibia. Laterally by fibula and superiorly from the malleolus.

Q 3. The MCL is otherwise called as:
A. Deltoid
B. Spring
C. Bifurcate ligament
D. None at above

Ans. (A) Because of its shape, more stable ligament and it tears during tibial malleolus fracture.

Q 4. The point at initial contact in stair gait is located on:
A. Stance middle portion
B. Heels
C. Lateral portion
D. Anterior

Ans. (D) The point at the initial contact at the foot is on anterior portion of the foot in stairs. It travels posteriorly to the middle at the foot as weight accepted.

Q 5. A typical BOS in walking is about:
A. 2–4 inches
B. 1–2 inches
C. 3–6 inches
D. None of these

Ans. (A) BOS is less in walking. BOS stands for base of support.

Q 6. The basic pathology in myositis ossificans progressive is in:
A. Muscle fibers
B. Serum chemistry
C. Body collagen
D. None of the above

Ans. (A) Myositis ossificans progressive involves only tendon, fascia, aponeurosis and muscle.

Q 7. Trigger finger is:
A. A feature at carpal tunnel syndrome
B. Injury to fingers while operating a gun
C. Stenosis tenovaginitis of flexor tendon or affected finger
D. Any of the above

Ans. (C) Trigger finger is also known as stenosis tenovaginitis that affect tendons of hand, making it difficult to bend the affected finger.

Q 8. Cervical spondylosis:
A. Most frequently results from an incidence of acute trauma.
B. Causes compression of nerve roots to produce an upper motor neuro lesion in the lower limbs.
C. Produces pain and paresthesia over the lateral aspect at the forearm and thumb when affecting the 6th cervical nerve.
D. Most frequently affects the upper cervical vertebral

Ans. (C) Cervical spondylosis usually affect C_5-C_7 so C_6 injury produces pain and paresthesia over the lateral aspect of the forearm and thumb.

Q 9. Dupuytren's contracture is seen in:
A. Colle's fracture
B. Thickening of palmar fascia
C. Radial nerve palsy
D. Supracondylar fracture of humerus

Ans. (B) Dupuytrens contracture is thickening at palmar fascia

Q 10. True dislocations of spine are most common in the:
A. Lumbosacral junction
B. Mid lumbar region
C. Cervical region
D. Dorsolumbar junction

Ans. (B) It is because most of weight is transfer from lumbar region and it caused by car accidents, sport collision and injuries falls.

Q 11. Reisser's turn buckle cast is applied for correction of:
(AIIMS 2009)
A. CDH
B. Scoliosis
C. Colles fractures
D. Clubfoot

Ans. (B) This is a body cast with a twin buckle in between. The tightening at the twin buckle stretches the concave side of the curve thus correcting the deformity.

Q 12. Approx. 40% at patients with congenital pseudoarthrosis of tibia present with lesion typical of:
(AIIMS 2012)
A. Hansen's disease
B. Tetralogy of Fallot
C. Alzheimer's disease
D. Von Recklinghausen's disease

Ans. (D) Approx. 40% of patients present with lesions typical at neurofibromatosis or Von Recklinghausens disease, e.g. cafe au lait spots, cutaneous fibromas which is inherited as an autosomal dominant trait.

Q 13. Oblique view is required to diagnose fracture of:
A. Capitate
B. Scaphoid
C. Navicular
D. Hammate

Answer   1 B   2 B   3 A   4 C   5 A   6 A   7 C   8 C   9 B   10 B   11 B   12 D

Ans. (B) Oblique view is external oblique projection examines the radiocarpal and distal radiocarpal joint along with distal radius and ulna. Scaphoid fracture result of tooth injuries and have a bad prognosis. It is not seen on plain film.

Q 14. The rotator cuff is composed of four of the following muscles except:
A. Teres minor
B. Supraspinatus
C. Infraspinatus
D. Teres major

Ans. (C) Rotator cuff muscle, such as supraspinatus, infraspinatus, subscapularis and teres minor.

Q 15. Fracture of clavicle is most common at:
A. Junction of medial 1/3rd and lateral 2/3rd
B. Junction of medial 2/3rd and lateral 1/3rd
C. Midpoint
D. Scapular end

Ans. (B) Fracture of clavicle is at junction at medial 2/3rd and lateral 1/3rd.

Q 16. Common injury to baby is:
A. Fracture humerus
B. Fracture clavicle
C. Fracture tibia
D. Fracture femur

Ans. (B) Clavicle is the only horizontal bone in body so during delivery the most common fracture is clavicle due to trauma and clavicle is skeletally immature.

Q 17. Which of the following is true about fat embolism?
A. Usually ensures after fracture of the lower limb
B. Uncommon complication of fracture
C. Spontaneously reversible process
D. All of the above

Ans. (A) Fat embolism is the complication of the fracture in long bones.

Q 18. In pad to side, the thumb is:
A. More adducted and less rotated
B. More abducted no rotation
C. Less adduction and more rotation
D. More adduction and less rotated

Ans. (A) It also known as key grip, because key is placed between thumb and side of index. FPB act more than OP.

Q 19. Wartenberg's sign is:
A. Abduction of little finger with loss of intrinsics
B. Adduction of little finger with loss of intrinsics
C. Abduction of ring finger with loss of intrinsics
D. Abduction of little finger without loss of intrinsics

Ans. (A) Ulnar nerve injuries can cause deficient because of unbalance pull from extensor digiti minimi.

Q 20. The MCL resist valgus stresses effectively in the:
A. Fully flexed
B. Extended
C. Semi flexed
D. None of above

Ans. (B) In this position valgus test is done to find out MCL injury.

Q 21. Which of the following statement regarding greenstick fracture is correct?
A. Fracture only occurs in rickety children
B. Any fracture in a child
C. Is generally in complete
D. None at above

Ans. (C) It is a fracture in young and soft bone of children. It occurs when a bone bends and cracks, instead at breaking completely into separate pieces.

Q 22. Which of the following is regarded as a definite sign of fracture?
A. Tenderness
B. Local body irregularity
C. Crepitus
D. Swelling

Ans. (C) Crepitus is a common sign of bone fracture. Crepitus can easily be created and observed by exerting a small amount of force on a joint, thus 'cracking it'.

Q 23. The strongest and the most important ligaments of the distal tibiofibular joint is the:
A. Crucial tibiofibular ligament
B. Anterior tibiofibular ligament
C. Posterior tibiofibular ligament
D. None of above

Ans. (A) It is a oblique fibular veins for a short distance between tibia and fibular.

Q 24. Thickness of intervertebral disc in the lumbar region is:
A. 3 mm
B. 3 cm
C. 9 mm
D. 13 mm

Ans. (C) In cervical it is 3 mm.

Q 25. The fluid content of nucleus at the disc in the newborn is:
A. 66%
B. 77%
C. 80%
D. 99%

Ans. (C) Depends on the age, the fluid content changes. It is 88% in newborn.

Q 26. In supracondylar fracture of humerus, the distal segment is often displaced to:
A. Inferiorly
B. Laterally
C. Posteriorly
D. Medially

Ans. (C) Supracondylar fracture are divided into two types-
1. Flexion type (rare)—distal segment displaced anteriorly
2. Extension type (98%)—distal segment is displaced posteriorly

Q 27. Lower branch of brachial plexus injury leads to:
A. Erb's palsy
B. Klumpke's palsy
C. Bell's palsy
D. Wrist drop

Ans. (B) Klumpke's paralysis is a form of paralysis involving the muscle of forearm and hand resulting from a brachial plexus injury in which C_8 and T_1 are injured.

Q 28. Which tendons get involved in Colle's fracture?
A. Abductor pollicis longus
B. Extensors pollicis brevis
C. Extensor pollicis longus
D. All of the above

Ans. (C) Fracture of the lower end of radius within inches of the distal articular surface of radius which involves extensor pollicis longus.

Q 29. Dinner fork deformity present in case of:
A. Smith's fracture
B. Student's elbow
C. Colle's fracture
D. All of these

Answer	13 B	14 C	15 B	16 B	17 A	18 A	19 A	20 B	21 C	22 C	23 A	24 C
	25 C	26 C	27 B	28 C								

Ans. (C) The distal fragment is displaced and tilted dorsally which gives the hand and wrist a typical deformity called dinner fork deformity in Colles' fracture.

Q 30. TENS is a:
A. Low frequency type of current
B. Microcurrent
C. High frequency type of current
D. Medium frequency current

Ans. (A) Low frequency—TENS, HVPGS. High frequency—SWD, MWD and medium frequency—IFT, Russian.

Q 31. Which muscle increases concavity of palmar arch?
A. Flexor carpi ulnaris
B. Flexor carpi radialis
C. Flexor carpi radialis brevis
D. External carpi ulnaris

Ans. (A) Intrinsic muscles form palmar arch.

Q 32. Regarding bursa all are true, except:
A. Contain synovial like fluid
B. Minimize functional force
C. End just distal to the volar crease
D. End just distal to palmar crease

Ans. (C) Two bursa present in wrist: Radial and ulnar bursa.

Q 33. Cocking phase of pitching a ball with result in________ glide of humeral head on fossa.
A. Anterior
B. Posterior
C. Inferior
D. Superior

Ans. (B) Acceleration phase there is anterior gliding of fossa occurs.

Q 34. In 180 of maximum range of elevation the initial 60 is continued by:
A. ST joint
B. GH joint
C. AC joint
D. SC joint

Ans. (A) 120° from glenohumeral joint.

Q 35. Which the muscle prevent the humerus head posteriorly?
A. Subscapularis
B. Infraspinatus
C. Deltoid
D. Rhomboids

Ans. (A) Posterior dislocation of head of humerus is prevented.

Q 36. The articulation of the scapular with the thorax depend on:
A. Acromioclavicular and sternoclavicular joint
B. Acromioclavicular and glenohumeral joint
C. Sternoclavicular and glenohumeral joint
D. Scapulothoracic joint and acromioclavicular joint

Ans. (A) Sternoclavicular and acromioclavicular joint are interdependent with scapulothoracic joint because of its attachment by its acromion process to the lateral end of clavicle.

Q 37. The depth of penetration of MWD is:
A. 0.5 cm
B. 3 cm
C. 1.3 cm
D. 9 cm

Ans. (B) MWD penetrate up to 3 cm.

Q 38. Which of the following conditions presents as primary amenorrhea and hypogonadism leading to early osteoporosis?
A. Down syndrome
B. Turner syndrome
C. Kleinfelter syndrome
D. Apert's syndrome

Ans. (B) Turner syndrome is a genetic disorder with a defect in one of the X-chromosome. Those affected are phenotypically female with a normal vagina and uterus but the ovaries are markedly hypoplastic or absent.

Q 39. Rissers localizer cast is used in the conservative management of

(AIIMS May 2012)

A. Dorsolumbar scoliosis
B. Idiopathic scoliosis
C. Kyphosis
D. Spondylolisthesis grade

Ans. (B) Risser localizer cast is used in the idiopathic variety of scoliosis most common in the dorsal spine > dorsolumbar scoliosis.

Q 40. Nursemaid's elbow is:
A. Elbow dislocation
B. Radial head subluxation
C. Radial head fracture
D. Lateral epicondylitis

Ans. (B) Common in children usually 2-4 years. Usually following child being pulled or swelling by the hand are the forearm, annular ligament structures and there is tenderness over the radial head.

Q 41. Cincinnati incision is generally used for correction of clubfoot this is a:
A. Curved posteromedial incision
B. Posterior longitudinal midline incision
C. Transverse circumferential incision
D. Midline incision over calcaneum

Ans. (C) The incision begins on the medial aspect of the foot in the regions of naviculocuneiform joint and extends posteriorly continuing over the Achilles tendon, lateral malleolus and over the sinus tarsi.

Q 42. Treatment of choice in Acute myositis ossificans is:
(Tamil Nadu 1991)
A. Immobilization of elbow
B. Short wave diathermy
C. Passive movements of arm
D. Active exercises

Ans. (A) Movement may aggravate the myositis ossificans so immobilization of elbow is best treatment.

Q 43. Volkmann's ischemic contracture is due to:
(BIHAR 1991)
A. Injury to ulnar and median nerve
B. Injury to median nerve
C. Contracture of palmar fascia
D. Ischemic vascular injury to the muscle

Ans. (D) Volkmann's ischemic contracture occurs when there is a lack of blood flow to the forearm muscle.

Q 44. The most common cause of pathological fracture is:
A. Delayed union
B. Malunion
C. Nonunion
D. Secondary deposits

Answer	29 C	30 A	31 A	32 C	33 B	34 A	35 A	36 A	37 B	38 B	39 B	40 B
	41 C	42 A	43 D									

Ans. (D) Pathological fractures is a bone fracture caused by disease including secondary malignant bone tumors, osteoporosis, secondary deposits, cyst, etc.

Q 45. Fracture shaft of femur in adult unites by:
A. 3–4 weeks
B. 3–4 months
C. 4–6 months
D. None of these

Ans. (B) Most femoral shaft fracture take between 3 to 6 months to completely heal.

Q 46. Rocker bottom foot occurs in:
A. Hallux valgus
B. Hallux rigidus
C. Congenital vertical talus
D. Congenital clubfoot

Ans. (C) Also known as congenital vertical talus is an anomaly of foot.

Q 47. Management in case of rupture of disc at L_5, S_1 is:
A. Emergency removal of disc
B. Joint effusion
C. Immobilization for 2 weeks with spinal back
D. Traction

Ans. (C) This helps the spinal nerve inflammation to decrease.

Q 48. The frequency of infrasonic waves lie between:
A. Below 20 Hz
B. 1–5 kHz
C. 10–20 kHz
D. 1–3 MHz

Ans. (A) The frequency of infrasonic waves is under 20 Hz.

Q 49. Interferential therapy is not used for:
A. Muscle stimulation
B. Pain relief
C. Muscle re-education
D. Wound healing

Ans. (D) Ultrasound is used for wound healing.

Q 50. Continuous passive motion apparatus is used to:
A. Increase range of motion
B. Maintain range of motion
C. Strengthen knee muscle
D. All of the above

Ans. (A) CPM apparatus instantly moves the joint through a controlled ROM and in most cases ROM is increased overtime.

Answer   44 D   45 B   46 C   47 C   48 A   49 A   50 A

Model Question Paper - 5

Q 1. In spondylolisthesis, there is fracture of vertebra in:
A. Spinous process
B. Pars interarticularis of the neural arch
C. Transverse process
D. Body

Ans. (B) In spondylolisthesis occurs when the vertebrae shifts forward due to instability from the pars fracture.

Q 2. Cobb's angle is measured for:
A. Lordosis
B. Lateral flexion
C. Kyphosis
D. Scoliosis

Ans. (D) Cobb's angle is used as a standard measurement to determine and track the progression of scoliosis.

Q 3. Which one of the following statement regarding bow leg is correct?

(ANDHRA 1998)

A. Physiologically corrected
B. Surgery is required as early as possible
C. It is a progressive deformity
D. Idiopathic variety is request type

Ans. (A) In most cases, bowed legs will naturally begin to straighten as the child grows up to 3 years.

Q 4. Hallux valgus is associated with all except:
A. An exostosis on the medial side at the head at the first metatarsal
B. A bunion
C. Osteoarthritis at the metatarsophalangeal joint
D. Over-riding or under-riding of the second toe by the third

Ans. (A) Hallux valgus also known as bunion—a bunion is formed when the big toe pushes against the next top. Tight shoes, foot, steers and arthritis are causes.

Q 5. The most important single special investigation in lumbar disc prolapse is:
A. Epidurography
B. Myelography
C. MRI
D. Discography

Ans. (C) MRI investigation of choice over the other investigation for herniated disc and become a gold standard to diagnose herniated disc. MRI represent a tool for morphologic and biochemical abnormalities analysis of disc disease.

Q 6. Idiopathic scoliosis is:
A. A lateral curvature of the spine
B. Rotation of the spine
C. Lateral curvature with rotation of the spine
D. Flexion deformity of the spine

Ans. (A) It is a type of spinal deformity in which a lateral, sideway curvature of the spine occurs.

Q 7. Regarding carrying angle, which is correct?
A. It is about 10° in male
B. It is about 20° in female
C. The carrying angle in male is always greater than female
D. Only A and B

Ans. (D) Carrying angle is 5–15° normal. But in female it is greater because of wider pelvis.

Q 8. Trigger finger due to:
A. Tenovaginitis
B. Synovitis
C. Bursitis
D. Fibrositis

Ans. (A) Trigger finger is due to inflammation of tendon in the finger known as tenovaginitis.

Q 9. If the osteoclast works faster than the osteoblast then you have:
A. Osteoporosis
B. Osteoarthritis
C. Osteosarcoma
D. Tendinosis

Ans. (A) Bone density will be less.

Q 10. Replacement of calcified articular cartilage by bone occurs by:
A. Epichondral ossification
B. Suprachondral ossification
C. Subchondral ossification
D. Endochondral ossification

Ans. (D) It helps in bone formation and growth.

Q 11. Which is having the large physiological cross-sectional level?
A. Brachialis
B. Biceps brachi
C. Brachioradialis
D. Pronator teres

Ans. (A) Biceps, brachioradialis, have small physiologic cross-sectional area.

Q 12. Nursemaid's elbow commonly occur in:
A. Nurses
B. Maids
C. Children
D. Sweepers

Ans. (C) Lifting a child up into the air by one or both hands or yanking a child by the hand cause dislocation.

Q 13. Weakness of elbow flexors may lead to_____ of elbow.
A. Extension
B. Hyperextension
C. Hyperflexion
D. Pronation

Ans. (B) Unable to produce counter force and it decreases stability.

Answer	1 B	2 D	3 A	4 A	5 C	6 A	7 D	8 A	9 A	10 D	11 A	12 C
	13 B											

Q 14. The function of costoclavicular ligament is checking of _________ movement.
A. Anterior
B. Posterior
C. Rotation
D. Elevation

Ans. (D) It is a strong ligament found between clavicle and first rib which cause elevation movement.

Q 15. The structure attach to the periphery of the glenoid cavity is called as _______.
A. Labrum
B. Cup
C. Cavity
D. All the above

Ans. (A) Labrum is lined by synovial fluid and it helps to increase curvature of the glenoid, prevent dislocation of shoulder.

Q 16. Which joint might consider the base of operation at scapula?
A. Scapulothoracic joint
B. Acromioclavicular joint
C. Sternoclavicular joint
D. Glenohumeral joint

Ans. (C) It is because of clavicle, since it is only structure attach to the scapula.

Q 17. Dynamic for distal radioulnar joint is provided by:
A. Superficial head of pronator quadratus
B. Deep head of pronator quadratus
C. Humeral head of pronator teres
D. Ulnar head of pronator quadratus

Ans. (B) Ulnar head of pronator teres depress during pronation.

Q 18. The ligament that extends from the inferior edge of ulnar's radial notch to insert in the neck at radius is:
A. Annular ligament
B. Quadrate ligament
C. Oblique cord
D. None of above

Ans. (B) Quadrate ligament reinforce the inferior aspect at joint capsule and helps to maintain the radial head in apposition of radial notch.

Q 19. During supination and pronation _______ acts as a stabilizers of elbow.
A. Triceps
B. Anconeus
C. Flexors
D. Extensors

Ans. (B) Anconeus assist in elbow extension.

Q 20. Cubital tunnel syndrome can be caused by repetitive contraction of:
A. FCR
B. FCU
C. Palmaris longus
D. Supinator

Ans. (B) Ulnar nerve injury cause numbers of the 4th and 5th metacarpal

Q 21. Froment's sign assesses the strength of:
A. Abductor pollicis longus
B. Flexor pollicis longus
C. Adductor pollicis
D. Opponent pollicis

Ans. (C) Used to detect ulnar nerve lesion.

Q 22. Common carpal bone get fracture is:
A. Lunate
B. Capitate
C. Scaphoid
D. Trapezium

Ans. (C) Lunate is the common bone gets dislocation and scaphoid is most radially so its higher chances to get fracture.

Q 23. Which of the following does not have the blood supply?
A. Capsule
B. Menisci
C. Cartilage
D. Muscle

Ans. (C) It is the structure gets degenerate early following immobilization.

Q 24. After L_4–L_5 or L_5–S_1 the next most common site of intervertebral disc prolapse is:
A. $C_7 - T_1$
B. T_{12}, L_1
C. L_1, L_2
D. C_5–C_6

Ans. (D) In cervical region $C_5 - C_6$ and $C_6 - C_7$ are the next most common.

Q 25. The best treatment for Dupuytrens contracture is:
A. Fasciotomy
B. Fasciectomy
C. Incision and release
D. Fasciectomy + skin transplantation

Ans. (C) Incise the Dupuytren's band and nodule. Release of contracture following excision of band. This is most convenient.

Q 26. Which of the following movement are restricted in frozen shoulder?
A. Abduction and internal rotation
B. Abduction and external rotation
C. All range of movements
D. Only abduction

Ans. (B) The movement involved in frozen shoulder are abduction and external rotation which get restricted to a greater extent.

Q 27. In de Quervain disease the following tendons are involved:
A. Abductor pollicis longus + extensor pollicis brevis
B. Abductor pollicis brevis + extensor pollicis longus
C. Adductor pollicis brevis + extensor pollicis longus
D. Extensor pollicis longus + flexor pollicis longus

Ans. (A) The disease affects the tendon of APL and EPB as they pass from the forearm into hand via fibro-osseous tunnel.

Q 28. In carpal tunnel syndrome, features are of:
A. Compression of ulnar nerve
B. Anesthesia over thenar eminence
C. Atrophy of hypothenar muscle
D. All of the above

Ans. (B) In thenar eminence there is no sensory loss during carpal tunnel syndrome.

Q 29. Gradual painful limitation of shoulders movements in an elderly suggest that the most priobable diagnosis is:
A. Arthritis
B. Osteoarthritis
C. Periarthritis
D. Myositis ossificans

Ans. (C) Periarthritis is the inflammation of soft tissue around the shoulder joint. It is more common in females and in people aged over so and it may occurs due to overuse of the shoulder joint.

Q 30. Known factors for idiopathic scoliosis is:
A. Unknown
B. Polio
C. Postural
D. Congenital

Ans. (A) Idiopathic scoliosis is unknown, the cause is unknown.

Answer	14 D	15 A	16 C	17 B	18 B	19 B	20 B	21 C	22 C	23 C	24 D	25 C
	26 B	27 A	28 B	29 C	30 A							

Q 31. Volkmann's Ischemic contracture is due to:
A. Arterial injury
B. Venous injury
C. Nerve injury
D. Increase of compartment pressure in the limb

Ans. (D) Volkmann's Ischemic contracture (VIC) occurs when there is increased pressure due to swelling, a condition called compartment syndrome.

Q 32. The most important factor in fracture healing is:
A. Good alignment
B. Organization to blood clot
C. Accurate reduction and 100% opposition of fractured fragments
D. Immobilization

Ans. (D) Immobilization restricted motion to allow the injured area to heal naturally.

Q 33. Last step in fracture healing is:
A. Hematoma
B. Callus formation
C. Remodelling
D. Consolidation

Ans. (C) Last step of fracture is healing is remodelling.

Q 34. Which of the following statement pertaining to greenstick fracture is true?
A. Any fracture in a child
B. Fracture only in rickety children
C. Only if there is no deformity
D. All of the above

Ans. (C) It is a fracture in young and soft bone of children. It occurs when a bone bends and cracks, instead of breaking completely into separate pieces.

Q 35. In recurrent anterior dislocation of shoulder, the movements that causes dislocation is:
A. Flexion and internal rotation
B. Abduction and external rotation
C. Abduction and internal rotation
D. Extension

Ans. (B) Anterior dislocation of shoulder is due to abduction and external rotation of shoulder associated with traumatic injury, such as fall, sport injury and it is slack inferiorly.

Q 36. Pulled elbow is:
A. Disarticulation of elbow
B. Subluxation of distal radioulnar joint
C. Subluxation of proximal radioulnar joint
D. None of the above

Ans. (C) Pulled elbow is subluxation of proximal radioulnar joint in children.

Q 37. Which of the following is the most common accessory bone of the foot?
A. Accessory calcaneum
B. OS vesalis
C. OS trigonum
D. Accessory navicular

Ans. (D) Accessory navicular also called prehallux. Os tibiale externum and navicular secundarium, is the most common accessory bone of the foot.

Q 38. Destruction and flattening of the head of femur is called:
A. Gout
B. Perthes disease
C. Reiters disease
D. Stills disease

Ans. (B) Perthes disease is a congenital dislocation at hip due to destruction and flattening of the head at femur.

Q 39. Loading response occurs until:
A. Leading limb strikes the ground
B. Initial contact of the opposite limb
C. Opposite limb lifts off the ground
D. Leading limb leaves the ground

Ans. (C) Loading response also called as flatfoot that occurs immediately following initial contact continues lifts the contralateral extremity lifts off the ground.

Q 40. Weights acceptances, pull up and forward continuance are the subdivisions of:
A. Stance phase
B. Swing phase
C. Midswing
D. None of above

Ans. (A) Swing phase classified as foot clearance (FCO), foot placement (Fp).

Q 41. In running, gastrocnemius activity begins at:
A. Double support
B. Float period
C. Heel strike
D. None of above

Ans. (C) Heal strike continues 15% of gait cycle.

Q 42. The coracoacromial arch prevents the dislocation of the humerus:
A. Superior
B. Inferior
C. Anterior
D. Posterior

Ans. (A) Superior dislocation because of an unopposed upward translating force on humerus.

Q 43. Clavicular depression is checked by:
A. Sternoclavicular ligament
B. Costoclavicular ligament
C. Interclavicular ligament
D. None of above

Ans. (C) It protects the structure below it like subclavian artery and brachial plexus.

Q 44. A thin area of capsule between superior and middle glenohumeral ligament is:
A. Foramen of Weitbrecht
B. Foramen of clovis
C. Zone of weakness
D. All of the above

Ans. (A) It is a point at weakness.

Q 45. Steerers are the muscle which steers the humerus head posteriorly is:
A. Subscapularis
B. Infraspinatus
C. Deltoid
D. Rhomboids

Ans. (A) Posterior dislocation of head of humerus is prevented by subscapularis.

Q 46. Lubrication created when nonparallel opposing surfaces slide on one another:
A. Squeeze film lubrication
B. Boundary lubrication

Answer	31 D	32 D	33 C	34 C	35 B	36 C	37 D	38 B	39 C	40 A	41 C	42 A
	43 C	44 A	45 A									

C. Hydrodynamic lubrication
D. Weeping lubrication

Ans. (C) Hydrodynamic lubrication resulting in lifting pressure and the fluid viscosity separates the joint surface.

Q 47. Uniaxial diarthrodial joints are joints in which the bony components are free to move in:
A. Two plane 3 axis
B. Two plane 1 axis
C. Two plane 2 axis
D. Three plane 3 axis

Ans. (C) It has two degree of movements.

Q 48. Tearing of the bony attachment at the tendon or ligament is called:
A. Failure
B. Rupture
C. Avulsion
D. Fracture

Ans. (C) Avulsion commonly olecranon, greater tuberosity of humerus and patella.

Q 49. Young's modulus is:
A. $\Delta L/Lo/F/A$
B. $\Delta/Lo/F/A$
C. $F/A/\Delta LILo$
D. $\Delta L/Lo/F$

Ans. (C) YM = stress/strain, stress = F/A, strain = $\Delta L/Lo$

Model Question Paper - 6

Q 1. Treatment of acute myositis ossification is:
A. Active mobilization
B. Passive mobilization
C. Immobilization
D. All of these

Ans. (C) Myositis ossification usually resolves on it's own. Immobilization is primary treatment of acute myositis ossificans.

Q 2. The most common source of bone and joint infection is:
A. Direct spread
B. Percutaneous
C. Lymphatic
D. Hematogenous

Ans. (D) Hematogenous—originating in or carried by the blood. Blood is most common source of infections.

Q 3. The lesion is Klumpke's paralysis is at:
A. Cervical plexus
B. Lower brachial
C. Upper brachial
D. Sacral plexus

Ans (B) Klumpke's paralysis is a variety of partial palsy of the lower roots of the brachial plexus.

Q 4. Treatment of fracture clavicle in an infant is best treated by:
A. Cuff sling
B. Figure of 8 bandage
C. Open reduction
D. Shoulder cast

Ans. (B) Immobilize the bone and stop the blood flow to provide safeguard against contamination.

Q 5. Tom Smith arthritis is due to:
A. Pyogenic infections in infancy
B. TB
C. RA
D. DA

Ans. (A) Tom Smith arthritis is due to septic arthritis.

Q 6. Muscles involved in Volkmann's ischemic contracture?
A. Flexor pollicis longus
B. Flexor profundus
C. Flexor sublimis
D. All of the above

Ans. (D) Volkmann's contracture is a permanent shortening of forearm muscles. Above given all muscles are forearm muscle which involves in Volkmann's contracture.

Q 7. Multiple bone fracture in a newborn is seen in:
A. Scurvy
B. Syphilis
C. Osteogenesis imperfecta
D. All of these

Ans. (C) Osteogenesis imperfecta a group of inherited disorder characterized by fragile bone that break easily.

Q 8. TB of spine start in:
A. Vertebral body
B. Nucleus pulposus
C. Annulus fibrosus
D. Paravertebral fascia

Ans. (D) TB of spine starts in paravertebral fascia.

Q 9. True flexor of the elbow joint are:
A. Biceps
B. Brachialis
C. Brachioradialis
D. Teres minor

Ans. (A) Biceps is a chief flexor muscle of elbow flexion.

Q 10. The dorsum of the middle finger is supplied by:
A. Radial nerve
B. Median
C. Ulnar
D. Radial and median

Ans. (D) Dorsum of the middle finger is supplied by radial and median nerve.

Q 11. Cock-up splint is used in:
A. Ulnar nerve palsy
B. Brachial plexus palsy
C. Radial nerve palsy
D. Both 'A' and 'C'

Ans. (C) Cock-up splint provides foam padding to keep wrist in extension and comfort.

Q 12. Regarding bursa all are true except:
A. Contain a synovial like fluid
B. Minimize frictional force
C. End just distal to the volar crease
D. End just distal to the palmar crease

Ans. (C) Two bursa present in wrist: Radial and ulnar bursa.

Q 13. Commonest site of TB spine:
A. Dorsolumbar
B. Thoracic
C. Lumbar
D. Sacral

Ans. (A) Spinal TB is one of the most common site of dangerous form of skeletal TB. Most common site is dorsolumbar.

Q 14. Thompson squeeze test is performed for the clinical diagnosis of a:
A. Fracture shaft of the femur
B. Ruptures tendo-Achilles
C. Myositis ossificans
D. Compartment syndrome

Ans. (B) The test is positive for complete rupture when there is no plantar flexion of the ankle. Also called Simmond test.

Q 15. Pott's spine is most common in which segment:
A. Cervical
B. Thoracic
C. Lumbar
D. Sacral

| **Answer** | 1. C | 2. D | 3. B | 4. B | 5. A | 6. D | 7. C | 8. D | 9. A | 10. D | 11. C | 12. C |
| | 13. A | 14. B | | | | | | | | | | |

Ans. (B) Pott's disease is the most common as well as one of the dangerous form of skeletal TB. Mostly occur at thoracic spine.

Q 16. The abduction contracture at the hip joint is evaluated by:
A. Thomas test
B. Gerhardt's test
C. Ober's test
D. Ely's test

Ans. (C) Ober's test determines the tightness of the iliotibial band or in other words is used to determine abduction contracture of the hip.

Q 17. Earliest feature of spine TB is:
A. Gibbus
B. Muscle spasm
C. Pain
D. Psoas abscess

Ans. (C) Pain is earliest feature of spine, characteristic clinical features of spinal tuberculosis is pain, local tenderness, a cold abscess.

Q 18. Illi's ligament is known as
A. Superior intracapsular ligament
B. Superior pubic ligament
C. Inferior intracapsular ligament
D. Iliofemoral ligament

Ans. (A) First described by Illi. It is dense fibrous connective tissue that attaches from ilium to sacrum.

Q 19. Audible click occurs during opening and closing of mouth is called:
A. Reciprocal click
B. Click
C. Normal click
D. None of the above

Ans. (D) Limit mouth opening, pain around the jaw, liping seen around the articular surfaces.

Q 20. Anterior cruciate ligament has connections with:
A. Lateral meniscus
B. Medial meniscus
C. Tibial condyles
D. All of the above

Ans. (C) It is the strong stabilizer on anterior translocation of knee.

Q 21. Forward flexion of trunk in erect standing is done by:
A. Rectus abdominis
B. Oblique abdominis
C. Hip flexor
D. No muscle activity only by gravity

Ans. (D) Gravity plays a major role in producing flexion during standing.

Q 22. The ligament that connects the axis and occipital bone of the skull is:
A. Alar
B. Ligamentum nuchae
C. Apical
D. All of the above

Ans. (C) It is like a fan shape attaches in upper cervical spine.

Q 23. The LCL composed of:
A. Anteroposterior talofibular
B. Calcaneofibular
C. Posterior talofibular
D. Both A and B

Ans. (C) In LCL the anterior talofibular ligament is weakest and LCL more prone for injury. It resist various stress.

Q 24. _______ is also called as joint compressors.
A. Lumbricals
B. Interossei
C. Flexors
D. Extensors

Ans. (B) Interossei are effective stabilizers.

Q 25. Major muscle work in hook grip is:
A. FDP
B. FDS
C. FCR
D. Both A and B

Ans. (D) Carrying a briefcase or book is a best example.

Q 26. The lateral calcenonavicular ligament is:
A. Bifurcate ligament
B. Spring ligament
C. Plantar calcaneonavicular ligament
D. Deltoid ligament

Ans. (B) Joins laterally with the medial bands of the bifurcate ligament

Q 27 Rotation and fixation (lateral) to the same side are functions of:
A. Multifidus
B. Rotators
C. Iliocostalis
D. Iliopsoas

Ans. (C) Other muscles like longissimus, spinalis, quadratus lumborum and serratus posterior produce the same.

Q 28. The linear distance between two successive point of contact of opposite limbs is:
A. Stride length
B. Step length
C. Width of BOS
D. None of above

Ans. (B) Heel strike of one extremity to other.

Q 29. Cold abscess is commonly due to infection of:
A. Skull
B. Ribs
C. Spine
D. Sternum

Ans. (C) Cold abscess is characteristics clinical feature of spine TB.

Q 30. The glenohumeral joint capsule is:
A. Anterior and inferiorly
B. Posteriorly
C. Superiorly and laterally
D. None of the above

Ans. (A) Joint capsule is twice size of humeral head.

Q 31. Treatment of CTEV should begin:
A. Soon after birth
B. After discharge from hospital
C. After 1 month
D. After 2 years

Ans. (A) CTEV is congenital talipes equinovarus. A birth defect is which the foot is twisted out of the shape or position.

Q 32. All muscle work in tip to tip prehension, except:
A. FPL
B. APL
C. FDP
D. Interossei

Ans. (B) These also assist in pad to pad prehension.

Q 33. MCP joint is a _____ type of joint.
A. Saddle
B. Ellipsoidal
C. Condyloid
D. Plane

Ans. (C) It has 2° of freedom.

Answer	15. B	16. C	17. C	18. A	19. D	20. C	21. D	22. C	23. C	24. B	25. D	26. B
	27. C	28. B	29. C	30. A	31. A	32. B	33. C					

Q 34. _______ muscle has attachment from muscle alone.
A. Interossei
B. Lumbricals
C. Palmaris longus
D. FCR
Ans. (B) Lumbricals are short extensors of IP.

Q 35. Most common dislocation of the hip is:
A. Posterior
B. Anterior
C. Central
D. None
Ans. (A) The acetabulum is directed anteriorly, inferiorly, externally so the posterior dirt is least protected by the bony pelvis. Capsule at back of the joint is weaker.

Q 36. Chvostek's sign is positive in:
A. Hypoparathyroidism
B. Euthyroidism
C. Megaloblastic anemia
D. Hypercortisolism
Ans. (A) On tapping over the branches of the fascial nerve at the angle of the jaw there will be twitching at the corner of the mouth.

Q 37. Patient comes with RR 30/min, HR 120/min, quadrparesis, sensory level at sternum, where does the injury lie?
A. C1 – C2
B. C5 – C6
C. T1 – T2
D. T3 – T4
Ans. (B) Sensory level of sternum is upper thoracic and the vertebral level corresponding to this would be lower cervical and thoracic.

Q 38. Lift off test is done for:
A. Supraspinatus
B. Infraspinatus
C. Teres minor
D. Subscapularis
Ans. (D) Lift test is tests for shoulder.

Q 39. The following is true in the treatment of posterior dislocation:
A. Closed reduction under anesthesia
B. Open reduction
C. Skeletal traction
D. Soft tissue
Ans. (A) Closed reduction is initial method for treatment and usually occur in emergency department. Posterior dislocation of hip require emergency treatment and condition is too painful, so anesthesia require for treatment.

Q 40. All are causes of pathological fracture except:
A. Anemia
B. Osteoporosis
C. Radiation
D. Osteomalacia
Ans. (A) Anemia is not the pathological fracture of bone. Osteoporosis, osteomalacia and radiation causes weakening of the bone and leads to fracture.

Q 41. The most common bone fractured during birth:
A. Clavicle
B. Scapula
C. Radius
D. Humerus
Ans. (A) Due to outstretched fall and trauma it occur as result of a difficult delivery or trauma at birth.

Q 42. In posterior compartment syndrome which passive movement cause pain:
A. Dorsiflexion of foot
B. Foot inversion
C. Toe dorsiflexion
D. Toe flexion
Ans. (C) In posterior compartment syndrome pain is elicited on.

Q 43. Bohler's angle is measured in the fractures involving:
A. Calcaneum
B. Talus
C. Navicular
D. Cuboid
Ans. (A) Angle subtended between posterior subtalar articular surface and the upper surface of the body posterior to the joint.

Q 44. The most common complication of extracapsular fracture of neck of femur is:
A. Avascular necrosis
B. Nonunion
C. Malunion
D. Myositis ossificans
Ans. (C) Malunion is a clinical term used to indicate that a fracture has healed, but that it has healed in less than an optimal position.

Q 45. The most common complications of intracapsular fracture neck of femur is:
A. Malunion
B. Osteoarthritis
C. Nonunion
D. Shortening
Ans. (C) Nonunion is permanent failure of healing which is common complication of fracture of neck of femur.

Q 46. All of the following names are associated with test operations around the hip joint except:
A. Bryant
B. Shenton
C. McMurray
D. Salter
Ans. (D) A Salter–Harris fracture or growth plate fracture is fracture that involves the epiphyseal plate or growth plate of a bone.

Q 47. Flexion, abduction and external rotation with limb length discrepancy is seen in:
A. Posterior dislocation of hip
B. Central dislocation of hip
C. Anterior dislocation of hip
D. Fracture neck of femur
Ans. (C) Flexion, adduction and external rotation of limb occurring anterior dislocation of hip.

Q 48. Medial epicondyle fracture results in injury to:
A. Radial
B. Median
C. Ulnar
D. Axillary
Ans. (C) Ulnar nerve which is reported between 10 – 16%

Q 49. Increased intercondylar distance is seen in fracture of all except:
A. Olecranon
B. Medial epicondyle
C. Lateral epicondyle
D. Lateral condyle
Ans. (A) In olecranon fracture, intercondylar distance is maintained and there is no disturbance in intercondylar distance.

Answer 34. B   35. A   36. A   37. B   38. D   39. A   40. A   41. A   42. C   43. A   44. C   45. C
46. D   47. C   48. C   49. A

Q 1. Measurement of axillary crutches:
A. 5 cm below posterior axillary and 15 cm laterally with patient in supine lying
B. 7 cm below anterior axilla and 10 cm laterally with patient in standing position
C. 4 cm below anterior axilla and 10 cm medially with patient supine lying
D. 5 cm below postaxilla and 12 cm laterally with patient standing

Ans. (A) Axillary crutches can be measured 5 cm below posterior axillary and 15 cm laterally with patient in supine lying

Q 2. Microwave diathermy is contraindicated in all of the following except:
A. Infection
B. Pregnancy
C. Tumorous conditions
D. Sprain

Ans. (D) Microwave diathermy (MWD) accelerate the healing of sprain.

Q 3. The rate at which laser energy produced or absorbed is measured in:
A. Joules
B. J/s
C. J/m^2
D. J/cm^2

Ans. (C) Rate of laser energy production is measured in J/m^2.

Q 4. Group of fiber bundles enclosed by a loose connective tissue sheath is called:
A. Epitenon
B. Peritenon
C. Einthesis
D. Endotenon

Ans. (D) Endotendon cover the fibers, nerves, blood vessels, lymphatic, collagen Type I + II and forms fascicle.

Q 5. The method of joint construction in diarthrodial joint differs from:
A. Cartilaginous joint
B. Synarthrodial joint
C. Synchondroses joint
D. Symphysis joint

Ans. (B) Because the movement in synarthrodial is less compare to diarthrodial joint.

Q 6. Stress strain curve of a bone demonstrates that cortical bone is stiffer than:
A. Cortical bone
B. Soft bone
C. Cancellous bone
D. Others

Ans. (C) According to Young's modulus cortical bone can withstand more stress than cancellous.

Q 7. The isometric tension in a muscle fiber is greater at its:
A. Optimal sarcomere length
B. Tensile state
C. Structured state
D. No change

Ans. (A) Muscles have a diminished ability to produce or maintain isometric contraction at extreme range of joint.

Q 8. The restriction of GH abduction at medial rotation of the clavicle is due to the impingement of _____ on arch.
A. Lesser tubercle
B. Acromion process
C. Greater tubercle
D. Neck of humerus

Ans. (A) Greater tubercle impact on acromion in lateral rotation and abduction of GH joint.

Q 9. Treatment of choice for old nonunited fracture of shaft of femur:

(AIMS 94)

A. Compression plating
B. Bone grafting
C. Nailing
D. Compression plating with bone grafting

Ans. (D) In old, internal fixation is required for proper positioning of bone and bone grafting is also request for replacing the missing bone in the case of nonunited fracture of shaft of femur.

Q 10. Flexion, adduction and internal rotation are characteristic posture in:
A. Anterior dislocation of hip joint
B. Posterior dislocation of hip joint
C. Fracture of femoral head
D. Fracture shaft of femur

Ans. (B) Posterior dislocation occur when the femur is adducted, flexed and internally rotated.

Q 11. Dashboard injury results in:
A. Anterior dislocation of hip
B. Posterior dislocation of hip
C. Central dislocation of hip
D. Fracture neck femur

Ans. (B) A dashboard injury occurs when drivers bent knee slams against the dashboard, pushing in the shin bone just below the knee and causing PCL tear and posterior dislocation of hip.

Q 12. Telescopic test is useful to diagnose:
A. Perthes disease
B. Intracapsular fracture neck of femur
C. Malunited trochanteric fracture
D. Ankylosis of hip joint

Ans. (B) Intracapsular fracture neck of femur is one clinical test to check stability of hip.

Answer 1 A 2 D 3 C 4 D 5 B 6 C 7 A 8 A 9 D 10 B 11 B 12 B

Q 13. What would be ideal during positioning of SWD electrode relative to the tissue?
A. Placing at an angle to each other
B. Placing parallel to skin
C. Placing parallel to each other
D. None of the above

Ans. (C) Because the density of electric field is greatest when electrodes are placed parallel to the skin.

Q 14. SWD is used for all of the following except:
A. Back pain
B. Hempohilliac joint
C. Osteoarthritis
D. Sprain

Ans. (B) People with hemophilia can bleed into the joint space after an injury after an injury and it can causes significant pain and can lead to chronic swelling and deformity.

Q 15. The number of layers of towel between the moist pack and skin should have at least:
A. 4 layers
B. 16 layers
C. 8 layers
D. 6 layers

Ans. (A) Moist hot packs are usually wrapped in 6 layers of towels in order to prevent burning.

Q 16. The contraplanar capacitor field method of SWD is used for the treatment of:
A. Superficial lesion of skin
B. Subcutaneous injuries
C. Deeply placed structures
D. Superficial muscle of spine

Ans. (C) In contraplanar method, deeper tissues are heated while in coplanar, superficial tissues are heated.

Q 17. Gamekeeper's thumb is:
A. Tear in the ulnar collateral ligament of thumb
B. Malunited Benitt's fracture
C. Ruptured flexor pollicis longus tendons
D. Ankylosis of first MCP joint

Ans. (A) Because it can be the result of gradual injury due to repetitive trauma to the thumb.

Q 18. Which of the following method is best to treat a comminuted fracture of distal pole of patella?
A. Patellectomy
B. Manipulation and POP casting
C. Wiring and attachment of fragments and POP again
D. Excision of the fragments and reattachment of the ligament to the proximal fragment

Ans. (C) In this situation it is imperative that as much patella as possible be pressured for a stable extensor apparatus at the knee.

Q 19. Abnormal functioning of cerebellum results in:
A. Parkinson's disease
B. Ataxic gait
C. Trendelenburg gait
D. All of the above

Ans. (B) It results in disturbance of normal mechanics results in loss of balance control.

Q 20. In pes cavus the subtalar joint goes for _______ position.
A. Pronated
B. Supinated
C. Everted
D. Varus

Ans. (B) Because of the unusual high medial longitudinal arch the subtalar and transverse tarsals joints tend to near or at the locked supinated position.

Q 21. A disturbance in kinesthetic sense about the ankle and foot following ankle sprains may lead to all, except:
A. Poor balance
B. Loss of stability
C. Bad posture
D. Good posture

Ans. (D) After an ankle sprain, it is less stable in the standing posture than before their injury due to loss of proprioceptors.

Q 22. The postural response in altered conditions is called as synergies. An example for fixed support synergy is:
A. Ankle synergy
B. Stepping
C. Grasping
D. None of the above

Ans. (A) Ankle synergy consists of discrete bursts of muscle activity on either the anterior or posterior aspects of the body that occur in a distal to proximal pattern in response to forward or backward movement of supporting platform.

Q 23. Common deformity seen in lateral view is:
A. Claw toes
B. Hallux valgus
C. Flatfoot
D. Scoliosis

Ans. (A) Claw toes are the deviation of optimal alignment of the toes and it will be seen in the lateral view. Other deformities will be best seen in AP view.

Q 24. Shear force is more at L_4/L_5 in _______ lift.
A. Squat lift
B. Stoop lift
C. Both
D. None of the above

Ans. (A) Squat lift produce more force than stoop lift.

Q 25. All muscle attach to measure transverse process of vertebral except:
A. Multifidus
B. Humbarium
C. Spinalis capitis
D. Semispinalis capitis

Ans. (C) Attach to spinous process, articular process of the vertebra.

Q 26. In the lower part of thoracic region the range of flexion and extension is greater than upper region, because:
A. Zygapophyseal facet lie in the frontal plane
B. Zygapophyseal facet lie in sagittal plane
C. Zygapophyseal facet lie in transverse plane
D. None of the above

Ans. (B) Upper thoracic region is less motion because of rigid ribcage

Q 27. Posterior facets of the talus moves _________ as the bone moves.
A. Opposite
B. Simultaneous
C. Both A and B
D. None of the above

Ans. (B) Posterior facet moves in the same directions where anterior and middle facets moves in opposite direction.

Q 28. Motion of talus is a complex twisting _______ like motion.
A. Screw
B. Translatory
C. Wedge
D. Linear

Ans. (A) It is because of anterior, middle and posterior can no longer accommodates.

Answer	13 C	14 B	15 A	16 C	17 A	18 C	19 B	20 B	21 D	22 A	23 A	24 A
	25 C	26 B	27 B	28 A								

Q 29. Sit ups are often performed in a bent knee position to reduce lumbar load and activity of:
A. Pelvis
B. Lumbar spine
C. Hip
D. Knee

Ans. (B) High compression force involved in sit ups, that is why sit up is not used in exercise.

Q 30. During promotion of foot, the metatarsal joint undergoes:
A. Pronation twist
B. Supination twist
C. Both A and B
D. None of the above

Ans. (B) The entire forefoot undergoes on inversion rotation around hypothetical axis at second ray.

Q 31. Lumbar pelvic rhythm can increase ROM available by adding the range from:
A. Hip joint
B. Lumbar spine
C. Thoracic spine
D. Knee

Ans. (B) Flexion of lumbar spine well increase ROM of forward flexion and thus increase the lumbar pelvic rhythm.

Q 32. Intramedullary fixation is ideal in case of fracture of shaft of femur when there is:
A. A transverse fracture
B. A compound fracture
C. Soft tissue interposition between fractured ends
D. Such a fracture in child

Ans. (A) Intramedullary rod is forced into the medullary cavity of bone and is used to treat fracture of long bones of the body.

Q 33. Stellate ganglion block is mainly used for:
A. Compound palmar ganglions
B. De Quervains synovitis
C. Sudecks dystrophy
D. OA of carpometacarpal joint

Ans. (C) Stellate ganglion block is used to treat or diagnose reflex sympathetic dystrophy are Sudick's dystrophy.

Q 34. Most common cause of scoliosis is:
A. Idiopathic
B. Traumatic
C. Congenital
D. TB

Ans. (A) The cause of scoliosis is unknown.

Q 35. Abnormally high patella is associated with
(UP 199)
A. Nail patella syndrome
B. Rupture of quadriceps tendon
C. Recurrent dislocation
D. Fracture through patella

Ans. (C) High patella (abnormal) is a positional faults as the superior displacement of the patella within the trochlear groove of the femur due to recurrent patellofemoral dislocation.

Q 36. In per rectal examination, femoral head is palpable in:
A. Anterior dislocation of lip
B. Posterior dislocation of hip
C. Central dislocation of hip
D. Lateral dislocation of hip

Ans. (C) When a central hip dislocation occurs, the femoral head is forced downwards or inferior out of a joint which is easily palpable.

Q 37. Prosthetic replacement of femoral head is indicated for one of the following sites of fractures:
A. Intertrochanteric fracture of femoral neck
B. Subcapita fracture neck femur
C. Transtrochanteric fracture femur
D. Basal fracture of femoral neck

Ans. (B) In subcapital fracture, the fracture line extends through the function of the head and neck of femur in which arthroplasty is require treatment.

Q 38. Behcet's syndrome is most common in:
A. Ankle
B. Wrist
C. Knee
D. Hip

Ans. (C) Joint dwelling and pain often affect the knee in people with Behcet's disease.

Q 39. Traumatic dislocation of hip is characterized by:
A. Adduction internal rotation deformity
B. Abduction external rotation deformity
C. Adduction external rotation deformity
D. Abduction internal rotation deformity

Ans. (A) Traumatic dislocation of hip are of two types—posterior and anterior and nine out of ten dislocation are posterior and the affected limb will be in a position of flexion adduction and internally rotated.

Q 40. Monteggia fracture is a fracture of:
A. Lower 1/3rd of radius
B. Upper 1/3rd of radius
C. Lower 1/3rd of ulna
D. Upper 1/3rd of ulna

Ans. (C) It is a fracture of proximal third of ulna with dislocation of proximal head of radius.

Q 41. In 65-year-old male with history of fracture neck of femur 6 weeks old, treatment of choice:
A. SP nailing
B. McMurray's osteotomy
C. Hemiarthroplasty
D. None

Ans. (C) McMurray's osteotomy and SP nailing is a procedure in which bone recovery is require. Hemiarthroplasty is half replacement of hip joint which is more convenient to older patient.

Q 42. The most common complication of transcervical fracture of femur is:
A. Avascular necrosis
B. Malunion
C. Nonunion
D. None

Ans. (C) It is known to cause many complications like non-union, AVN, etc. but the most common is nonunion.

Q 43. A side swipe injury is usual at the:
A. Knee
B. Elbow
C. Wrist
D. Spine

Ans. (B) This injury is seen in people sitting with their elbows outside the window of the vehicles in which they are travelling. When another vehicle coming in the opposite direction hits their elbows.

Q 44. Delayed union of tibia in the presence of an intact fibula is an indication for:
A. Internal fixation
B. Fibular segmental excision
C. Bone grafting
D. External fixation

Answer	29 B	30 B	31 B	32 A	33 C	34 A	35 C	36 C	37 B	38 C	39 A	40 C
	41 C	42 C	43 B									

Ans. (D) Delayed union of tibia prevent opposition of the tibial fragments in such situation it can only be achieved by external fixation.

Q 45. Von Rosen splint is used for treatment for:
A. Congenital dislocation of hip
B. Hail chest
C. Cervical spine injuries
D. Gunstock deformity

Ans. (D) von Rosen splint is a H-shaped splint, the crossbar of H being extended on each side and it is widely used for treatment of gunstock deformity.

Q 46. All the following are contraindications for skin traction except:

(AIIMS May 2012)

A. Laceration of the skin in the area to which the traction is applied
B. Impairment of circulation
C. Presence of fracture proximal to the traction site
D. Dermatitis

Ans. (C) In addition to A, B and D, the other contraindication to skin traction is marked shortening of bony fragments when the fracture weight required will be greater than that can be applied through skin.

Q 47. Fatigue or stress fractures occur from repeated stress. The fractures occur in the:

(AIIMS May 2009)

A. Ribs
B. Bones of skull
C. Metatarsals
D. Clavicle

Ans. (A) The metatarsals, fibula and the tibia in that order are the most common sites of fatigue fracture.

Q 48. A greenstick fracture is one in which:
A. There is a fracture of single cortex
B. There is a wound on the surface of skin
C. A fragment is lost externally
D. Fractured fragments are displaced perpendicularly

Ans. (C) It is one where one cortex is fractured and the other cortex is intact. Common in children.

Q 49. Which of the following tendons is ruptured frequently after fracture of lower end of radius?
A. Extensor pollicis longus
B. Abductor pollicis brevis
C. Anconeus
D. Palmaris longus

Ans. (B) The tear in tendon of EPL may be because of attribution rather than direct injury and should not be sutured end to end.

Q 50. The source of fat emboli is probably the:
A. Bone marrow
B. Brain
C. Liver
D. Muscle

Ans. (A) This condition is more common in patients with multiple closed fractures.

Answer   44 D   45 D   46 C   47 A   48 C   49 B.   50 A

Model Question Paper - 8

Q 1. The bony triangle is maintained in:
A. Supracondylar fracture of humerus
B. Posterior dislocation of elbow
C. Intercondylar fracture of humerus
D. Lateral condylar fracture of humerus
Ans. (A) The three bony point relationships of elbow is maintained in supracondylar fracture of humerus is normal.

Q 2. The most common deformity seen in supracondylar fracture of humerus is:
A. Inability to supinate and pronate
B. Varus
C. Valgus
D. None
Ans. (B) Cubitus varus deformity is the commonest deformity seen in supracondylar fracture of humerus.

Q 3. Prosthesis at head of femur applied in:
A. 40 years young male with head of femur
B. 40 years young male with neck of femur
C. 40 year young male with posterior dislocation of hip
D. 65 years old male with nonunited fracture neck of femur
Ans. (D) Hemiarthroplasty or total arthroplasty are more common treatment for older patient.

Q 4. In Colle's fracture not seen in:
A. Proximal impaction
B. Lateral rotation
C. Dorsal angulation
D. Medial rotation
Ans. (D) Medial rotation is not seen in Colle's fracture.

Q 5. The most common injury is a 7 years old child due to fall on outstretched head is:
A. Dislocation of shoulder
B. Colle's fracture
C. Fracture of clavicle
D. Supracondylar fracture of humerus
Ans. (D) Fall an outstretched hand causes supracondylar fracture of humerus.

Q 6. Fall on outstretched hand may lead to fracture of:
A. Shoulder
B. Clavicle
C. Scaphoid
D. Coronoid process
Ans. (C) Scaphoid fracture is a break in one of the small bones of wrist. This type of fracture occurs most often after a fall into an outstretched hand.

Q 7. Fracture femur in infants is best treated by:
A. Open reduction
B. Closed reduction
C. IM nailing
D. Gallow's splinting
Ans. (D) Gallow's splinting can be given to the children less than 2 years and applied for more than 4 weeks it is safe.

Q 8. Treatment of choice for old nonunited fracture of shaft of femur:
A. Compression plating
B. Bone grafting
C. Nailing
D. Compression plating with bone grafting
Ans. (D) In old nonunited fracture bone internal fixation is required for proper poisoning of bone and bone grafting is also require for replacing the missing bone.

Q 9. McMurray's osteotomy is based on the following principle:
A. Biological
B. Biomechanical
C. Biotechnical
D. Mechanical
Ans. (B) One of the principle of osteotomy is to restore biomechanical advantage.

Q 10. The femur is fractured at birth at:
A. Upper third of shaft
B. Middle third of shaft
C. Lower third of shaft
D. Neck region
Ans. (A) Mostly femur fracture is uncommon at birth. But sometime upper third of shaft fracture is occurred.

Q 11. Vascular sign of Narath is noticed in:
A. Fracture neck of femur
B. Perthes disease
C. Posterior dislocation of hip
D. All of the above
Ans. (C) If vascular sign of Narath is positive then the femoral head displaced from hip joint due to hip dislocation.

Q 12. The treatment of choice for a 4 week old femoral neck fracture in a 55-year-old man is:
A. Open reduction and internal fixation
B. McMurray's osteotomy
C. Hemi replacement with arthroplasty
D. THR
Ans. (C) Posterior dislocation of hip occur when the femur is adducted, flexed and internally rotated.

Q 13. Which is not heat therapy?
A. SWD
B. Infrared therapy
C. Ultrasound
D. Infer/interferential therapy
Ans. (B) Infrared therapy is not heat therapy in which surface heat present.

Answer	1 A	2 B	3 D	4 D	5 D	6 C	7 D	8 D	9 B	10 A	11 C	12 C
13 B												

Q 14. Reduce Bohler's angle is seen in:
A. Calcaneum
B. Talus
C. Navicular
D. Cuboid

Ans. (A) Bohler's angle is the angle between the superior articular surface and the upper surface of the tuber is 35 degree.

Q 15. Modified Allens test is for checking the proper arterial supply at the:
A. Arm
B. Forearm
C. Wrist
D. Elbow

Ans. (C) The hand is elevated and the patient is asked to make a fist for about 30 second wrist deformity observe.

Q 16. In posterior dislocation of shoulder Hill-Sachs lesion is seen in:
A. Anterior
B. Anteromedial
C. Posterior
D. Posteromedial

Ans. (B) Hill-Sachs fracture is a cortical depression in the posterior superior head of the humerus bone.

Q 17. The statement regarding posterior cruciate ligament is:
A. Attached to medial surface of lateral condyle
B. Intrasynovial
C. Prevent posterior dislocation of tibia
D. Relaxed during the flexion of knee

Ans. (C) Prevents posterior dislocation of tibia, taut during flexion of knee.

Q 18. The squat test is a clinical test used for the diagnosis of which of the following condition at the knee:
A. TB knee
B. Lateral collateral ligament tear
C. Menisci test
D. GCT lower end of the femur

Ans. (C) Squat test consist of several repetitions of a full squat with the feet and legs alternately fully internally and externally rotated as the squat is performed.

Q 19. A positive Yergason's test indicates:
A. Bicipital tendinitis
B. Acromioclavicular subluxation
C. Dislocation of the shoulder
D. Radial head fracture

Ans. (A) Resisted supination of the forearm with the elbow bent is Yergason's test.

Q 20. Biceps acts as an effective flexor at ________ degree of elbow flexion.
A. 0°
B. 45°
C. 90°
D. 110°

Ans. (C) Full extension muscle force is translatory.

Q 21. All the statement about volar plate are true, except:
A. It is a fibrocartilage
B. Restrict hyperextension
C. Blends with capsule
D. Plates are unilayered

Ans. (D) Plates are unilayered.

Q 22. During swing phase of gait, GRF is:
A. Increase
B. Does not exist
C. Decrease
D. Is constant

Ans. (B) Since foot is not contact with ground.

Q 23. Tracking down of patella is associated with:
A. Medial shift
B. Lateral shift
C. Tilting
D. None of above

Ans. (C) So called as patella tilt, tilt occurs due to asymmetry of femoral condyles.

Q 24. The distal articular surface of the ankle joint is made up of:
A. Body of calcaneum
B. Body of talus
C. Medial malleolus
D. Lateral malleolus

Ans. (B) It has three articular surfaces, medially with Tibia.

Q 25. The lateral calcaneonavicular ligament is:
A. Bifurcate ligament
B. Spring ligament
C. Plantar calcaneonavicular ligament
D. Deltoid ligament

Ans. (B) Joints laterally with the medial bands of the bifurcate ligament.

Q 26. The lamellar are arranged in ________ rings that totally enclose the nucleus.
A. Concentric
B. Eccentric
C. Circular
D. Triangular

Ans. (A) Encompass the nucleus inside.

Q 27. In toddlers COG is _____ than adults.
A. Higher
B. Lower
C. No change
D. Both A and B

Ans. (A) So large BOS is need to maintain stability.

Q 28. The dorsiflexion of the first ray is accompanied by:
A. Inversion, adduction
B. Inversion, abduction
C. Eversion, adduction
D. Eversion, abduction

Ans. (A) The axis is oblique.

Q 29. Functions of synovial fluid all except:
A. Nutrition supply
B. Lubrication
C. Stability
D. Shock absorber

Ans. (C) In the joint surface—rolling, gliding, spinning takes place.

Q 30. Which of the following does not have the blood supply?
A. Capsule
B. Menisci
C. Cartilage
D. Muscle

Ans. (C) It is the structure gets degenerated early following immobilization.

Q 31. ______ muscle prevents unwanted micturition and defecation.
A. Levator scapulae
B. Iliococcygeus
C. Levator ani
D. Coccygeus

Ans. (C) Also helps to constrict opening in pelvic floor.

Answer	14 A	15 C	16 B	17 C	18 C	19 A	20 C	21 D	22 B	23 C	24 B	25 B
	26 A	27 A	28 A	29 C	30 C	31 C						

Q 32. First dorsal interossei has no attachment:
A. Lateral
B. Medial
C. Distal
D. Proximal
Ans. (C) Other 3 has both proximal and distal wing tendon.

Q 33. Cartilaginous changes on the lateral face of patella is seen in:
A. Chondromalacia patella
B. Osteoarthrosis
C. Rheumatoid arthritis
D. All the above
Ans. (C) CMP means softening of cartilage. It occurs due to aging and stress.

Q 34. 50% of body weight is by:
A. Head
B. Arms
C. Trunk
D. Legs
Ans. (C) The HAT weight as 75%.

Q 35. Active extension of one finger leads to passive extension of adjacent finger is due to presence of:
A. Volar interossei
B. Volar end plate
C. Juxta tendinea
D. Dorsal interossei
Ans. (C) Fibrous connections produce active extension.

Q 36. Proximal wing tendon produce _____ effect in MCP joint Adduction.
A. Abduction
B. Adduction
C. Flexion
D. Both A and B
Ans. (D) It acts directly on proximal phalanx.

Q 37. IP extension is governed by:
A. Proximal wing tendon
B. Distal wing tendon
C. Caudal wing tendon
D. Distal to proximal wing tendon
Ans. (B) Assist by distal wing tendon of DI and VI.

Q 38. In thumb, how many sesamoid bones are attached to volar plate on its palmar surface?
A. 1
B. 2
C. 3
D. None of above
Ans. (B) 2 sesamoid bones are attached to volar plate on it's palmar surface.

Q 39. Strongest ligament in the hip is:
A. Iliofemoral
B. Ischiofemoral
C. Pubofemoral
D. Ligamentum teres
Ans. (A) The superior bond of the iliofemoral ligament to the strongest and thickest of the hip joint ligaments.

Q 40. Terminal 15 of knee extension is provided by:
A. Vastus lateralis
B. Vastus intermedius
C. Vastus medialis
D. Rectus femoris
Ans. (B) It is the first muscle to get weakened during prolonged immobilization.

Q 41. Odd facet divides:
A. Medial and lateral half
B. Medial and extreme medial edge
C. Superior and inferior surface
D. None of the above
Ans. (B) 30% patella have 2nd ridge called odd facet.

Q 42. Patella ability to perform its function depends:
A. Stability
B. Mobility
C. Both A and B
D. None of the above
Ans. (B) It works without restricting knee motion.

Q 43. At 135 flexion, which facet of patella is in contact with femur?
A. Lateral
B. Odd facet
C. Medial facet
D. Both A and B
Ans. (D) No contact of medial facet since it completely out of surface.

Q 44. The attitude of limb in traumatic dislocation of hip joint is:
A. Flexion, adduction, external rotation
B. Flexion, adduction, internal rotation
C. Flexion, adduction and external rotation
D. Flexion and adduction only
Ans. (B) Posterior dislocation of hip occur when femur is flexed, adducted and internally rotated.

Q 45. In anterior dislocation of hip, the posture of lower limb will be:
A. Abduction, externally rotated and extension
B. Abduction, externally rotated and flexion
C. Abducted, externally rotated and flexion
D. Adducted, internally rotated and flexion
Ans. (B) Anterior dislocation of hip occur when femur is in abduction externally rotated and flexion.

Q 46. The transverse stabilizers includes all except:
A. Medial extensor retinaculum
B. Lateral
C. Patellar tendon
D. Vastus medialis
Ans. (C) All others produce transverse stability.

Q 47. The lateral articular surface of the ankle joint is made up of:
A. Talofibular ligament
B. Body of talus
C. Medial malleolus
D. Lateral malleolus
Ans. (B) The anterior and posterior talofibular ligaments support the lateral side of joint.

Q 48. The term ankle specifically refers to:
A. Talocalcaneum joint
B. Talocrural joint
C. Tibiofibular joint
D. None of above
Ans. (B) The articulating surface are tibiotalar surface and talofibular surfaces.

49. Degree of toe out is:
A. 4°
B. 7°
C. 6°
D. 8°
Ans. (B) It decrease as the speed of walking increases, it increase in men.

Q 50. In pes cavus, weight-bearing is primarily on:
A. Hindfoot
B. Forefoot
C. Midfoot
D. Lateral border
Ans. (A) Metatarsal also bears weight.

Answer	32 C	33 C	34 C	35 C	36 C	37 B	38 B	39 A	40 B	41 B	42 B	43 D
	44 B	45 B	46 C	47 B	48 B	49 B	50 A					

Model Question Paper - 9

Q 1. The commonest complication of Colle's fracture is:
A. Malunion
B. Nonunion
C. Sudeck's osteodystrophy
D. Rupture of EPL tendon

Ans. (C) Colle's fracture- finger stiffness is the commonest complications. Next to finger stiffness is malunion and least common is non union.

Q 2. The resistance to passage of sound is called as :
A. Cavitation
B. Attenuation
C. Phonation
D. Acoustic impedance

Ans. (D) Acoustic impedance is a measure of ease with which a sound wave propagates through a particular medium.

Q 3. Avulsion of extensor tendon give rise to:
A. Mallet finger
B. Dupuytrens contracture
C. Trigger finger
D. Swan neck deformity

Ans. (A) Mallet finger is a common injury involving either an extensor tendon rupture at its insertion or an avulsion fracture involving insertion of terminal extensor tendon.

Q 4. Total claw hand is caused by injury to:
[All India 93]
A. Radial nerve
B. Ulnar and radial nerve
C. Ulnar and medial nerve
D. Radial and median nerve

Ans. (C) Total claw hand involving all digits and resulting from combined ulnar and median nerve palsy.

Q 5. Thoracic kyphosis in children is most often due to:
A. Traumatic
B. Pott's spine
C. Congenital
D. Normal

Ans. (C) It is the most common etiology of spinal cord compression due to spine deformity excluding TB and is considered to be congenital as it occurred prior to birth.

Q 6. The Milwaukee brace is used to for correction of:
A. Congenital dislocation of hip
B. Clubfoot
C. Scoliosis
D. Patella alta

Ans. (C) Milwaukee brace is an active corrective spinal orthosis used almost exclusively In the ambulant treatment of structural scoliosis.

Q 7. Which of the following prosthesis (cervical) movement best controlled at the cervical spine:
A. Soft collar
B. Somi brace
C. Halo body orthosis
D. None of these

Ans. (C) The halo body orthosis controls the movement at the cervical spine better than all other orthosis of the cervical spine.

Q 8. Depth of penetration of MWD is:
A. 0.5 cm
B. 3 cm
C. 1.3 cm
D. 9 cm

Ans. (B) MWD can penetrate up to 3 cm.

Q 9. Hill-Sachs lesion in recurrent shoulder dislocation is:
A. Injury to humeral head
B. Rupture of tendon supraspinatus muscle
C. Avulsion of glenoid labrum
D. None of the above

Ans. (A) Hill-Sachs lesion is a posteriolateral humeral head compression fracture typically secondary to recurrent anterior shoulder dislocation.

Q 10. Treatment of fracture clavicle in an infant is best treated by:
[JIPMER 87]
A. Cuff and sling
B. Figure of eight bandage
C. Open reduction
D. Shoulder cast

Ans. (B) Figure of eight bandage is used to limit joint movement of the clavicle and is tied to each axilla and cross between the scapulae in such a way that both Shoulders are braced up.

Q 11. After an operation of femur bone chest X-ray shows wide spread mottling throughout the lung field like a snow storm. It is a diagnostic of:
[CSE 1999]
A. Fat embolism
B. Shock lung
C. Bronchopneumonia
D. Atelectasis

Ans (A) During fracture of long bone, fat embolism occur. The dislodgement of emboli which block the blood supply and emboli may seen in lung field which is shown by X ray.

Q 12. All the following are "head at risk signs"(radiological) that correlate positively with a poor result in the outcome of Perthes disease except:
A. Lateral subluxation of the femoral head
B. Speckled calcification lateral to the capital epiphysis
C. Shallow acetabulum
D. Gage sign -a radiolucent "V" shaped defect in the lateral epiphysis and adjacent metaphysis

Ans. (C) Shallow acetabulum correlates poorly with outcome in congenital dislocation of hip. In addition to a band the other 'head at risk' signs are diffused metaphyseal reaction and horizontal physis.

Answer   1 C   2 D   3 A   4 C   5 C   6 C   7 C   8 B   9 A   10 B   11 A   12 C

Q 13. The proportion of solid wax to mineral oil in paraffin wax treatment should be:
A. 7:1
B. 5:1
C. 4:1
D. None of the above

Ans (A) Composition of wax: paraffin: mineral oil is 7:3:1.

Q 14. Tinel's sign is positive in:
A. Peripheral nerve regeneration
B. Tendon injury
C. Tenosynovitis
D. Rheumatoid arthritis

Ans. (A) The sign that a nerve is irritated. It is positive when lightly banging over the nerve elicits a sensation of tingling or pins and needles in the distribution of nerve.

Q 15. Foot drop is seen in:

[Delhi 1998]

A. Tibial nerve injury
B. Achilles tendon injury
C. Popliteal nerve injury
D. Common peroneal nerve injury

Ans. (D) Common peroneal nerve that controls the muscle involve in lifting the foot.

Q 16. Polio paralysis differs from paralysis due to other causes:

[Karnataka 94]

A. Weakness
B. Deformity of limb
C. No sensory loss
D. Full recover is possible

Ans. (C) Polio paralysis is a disease of anterior horn motor neurons of the spinal cord and brain stem. It is loss of motor neuron and denervation of associated skeletal muscle.

Q 17. The glenohumeral joint capsule is slack:
A. Anteriorly and inferiorly
B. Posteriorly
C. Superiorly and laterally
D. None of the above

Ans. (A) Joint capsule is twice size of humeral head.

Q 18. Elevation of clavicle result in ___ movement in sternum:
A. Up slide
B. Down slide
C. Rotation
D. Spin

Ans. (B) Scapular elevation articulate with clavicle elevation is not a pure motion but it is associated with concomitant upward rotation of scapula. It helps to increase elevation of arm.

Q 19. Ultrasound can be used to treat:
A. Osteomyelitis
B. Soft tissue injury
C. Open fracture
D. All of the above

Ans. (B) In soft tissue injuries therapeutic ultrasound can both manage pain and facilitate healing.

Q 20. Colle's fracture occur at:
A. Distal 1/3rd of radius
B. Proximal 1/3rd of radius
C. Olecranon process of ulna
D. Distal 1/3rd of ulna

Ans. (A) Colle's fracture is the fracture at the distal 1/3rd of radius at its corticocancellous junction.

Q 21. Plantar fasciitis:

[Jipmer 1989]

A. Is not associated with infection elsewhere in the body
B. Is caused by a bony spur on the plantar surface of the OS calcis
C. Can be relieved by supplying insoles
D. Is a type of Dupuytrens disease

Ans. (C) The insoles cushion protect your foot from the aggravating shock of each step and support your arch to prevent the plantar fascia from stretching further so it can heal.

Q 22. Common vertebral level of spondylolisthesis is:

[Bihar 1989]

A. L4-L5
B. L3-L4
C. T12-L1
D. L5-S1

Ans. (D) Spondylolisthesis is most common occur at the L5 -S1 level with anterior dislocation of the L5 vertebral body on the S1 vertebral body.

Q 23. Biceps brachii act as a:
A. Flexor of knee
B. Extensor of knee
C. Flexor of elbow
D. Extensor of knee

Ans. (C) Biceps brachii is a flexor muscle of elbow.

Q 24. The most common cause of pressure sore in the foot in India is:
A. Leprosy
B. Thorn prick
C. Diabetes
D. Syringomyelia

Ans. (C) When blood sugar levels are high or fluctuate regularly skin tissue that would normally heal may not properly repair itself because of nerve damage.

Q 25. The carpel tunnel syndrome usually occurs in:
A. Cushing's disease
B. Addison's disease
C. Acromegaly
D. All of the above

Ans. (C) Carpel tunnel syndrome in acromegaly is that edematous synovial tissue compress the median nerve because of oversecretion of growth hormone.

Q 26. Formula of dry Plaster of Paris is:
A. $CaSO_4 \cdot \frac{1}{2}H_2O$
B. $CaSO_4 \cdot 2H_2O$
C. $CaSO_4$ only
D. $CaSO_4 \cdot 5H_2O$

Ans. (A) The chemical name of POP is Calcium sulphate hemihydrate.

Q 27. The most common cause of nonunion is:
A. Infection
B. Inadequate immobilization
C. Ischemia
D. Soft tissue mobilization

Ans. (B) Movement restrict union.

Q 28. Shoulder dislocation is caused by vigorous:
A. Flexion with internal rotation
B. Flexion with external rotation
C. Abduction with external rotation
D. abduction with internal rotation

Ans. (C) Shoulder dislocation mechanism is usually due to vigorous abduction and external rotation.

Answer	13 A	14 A	15 D	16 C	17 A	18 B	19 B	20 A	21 C	22 D	23 B	24 C
	25 C	26 A	27 B	28 C								

Q 29. Poliomyelitis is caused by viral infection is:
A. Posterior horn cell
B. Anterior horn cell
C. Muscle
D. Peripheral nerves
Ans. (B) Polio virus enters the CNS and replicates in anterior horn cell of spinal cord.

Q 30. Degenerative bone disease is called as:
A. Osteoarthritis
B. Rheumatoid arthritis
C. Gouty arthritis
D. Synovitis
Ans. (A) Osteoarthritis is a degenerative bone and joint disease.

Q 31. When vasodilatation is not desired the duration of cryotherapy should be:
A. 30 minutes
B. More than 15 minutes
C. Less than 15 minutes
D. None of the above
Ans. (C) Maximum vasodilatation occurs in 20-30 minutes. Therefore when vasodilatation is not desired duration of cryotherapy should be less than 15 minutes.

Q 32. Common site of disc prolapse is:
A. C5-C6
B. T8-T9
C. L4-L5
D. L5-S1
Ans. (C) Majority of the spinal disc herniation occurs in lumbar spine (95%).

Q 33. Which movement of the shoulder gets restricted when supraspinatus torn?
A. Flexion
B. Adduction
C. Abduction
D. Rotation only
Ans. (C) Function of supraspinatus is abduction of arm.

Q 34. Which nerve is involved in carpel tunnel syndrome?
[Bihar 1991]
A. Ulnar nerve
B. Radial nerve
C. Median nerve
D. Posterior cutaneous nerve of the forearm
Ans. (C) Carpel tunnel syndrome is a common condition that causes pain. Numbness and tingling in hand and arm due to median nerve compression.

Q 35. A 40-year-old patient sustained left shoulder injury and developed anterior dislocation of shoulder joint causing sensory loss over lateral side of the arm. The nerve involve is:
A. Radial nerve
B. Axillary nerve
C. Musculocutaneous nerve
D. Ulnar nerve
Ans. (B) Due to anterior dislocation of shoulder joint, the axillary nerve will compress causing sensory loss over lateral side of forearm.

Q 36. Volkmann ischemic contracture is commonly due to:
A. Tight plaster
B. Tight splint
C. Both
D. None
Ans (C) Tight plaster n tight splint both block the flow of blood and cause ischemia in forearm muscle that give rise to claw like deformity.

Q 37. Which statement pertaining to green stick fracture is correct?
A. Any fracture in child
B. Is generally complete
C. Fracture only in rickety children
D. All of the above
Ans. (B) Fracture in a young soft bones bend and break into two separate pieces.

Q 38. Duga's test is helpful in:
A. Dislocation of hip
B. Scaphoid fracture
C. Fracture neck of femur
D. Anterior dislocation of shoulder
Ans. (D) A simple clinical test for dislocated shoulder.

Q 39. Luxatio erecta:
A. Tear of the glenoid labrum
B. Inferior dislocation of the shoulder
C. Anterior dislocation of the shoulder
D. Defect in the humeral head
Ans. (B) Luxatio erecta is a specific term for inferior dislocation of GH joint.

Q 40. Ideal treatment with fracture neck of humerus in a lady will be:
A. Triangular sling
B. Hemiarthoplasty
C. Chest arm bandage
D. Internal fixation
Ans. (A) triangular sling helps to support the elbow and restrict the movement which help to stabilize an injury. Immobilization help in healing. Triangular sling avoid gravitational force exerting any pull in the shoulder girdle and shoulder joint complex.

Q 41. In addition to therapeutic intervention, the therapist should also do:
A. Documentation
B. Counselling
C. Both a and b
D. None of the above
Ans. (C) documentation as well as counselling are important apart from therapeutic intervention.

Q 42. For immediate management of soft tissue injury acronym RICE stands for:
A. Rubbing, instant heat, clean and elevation
B. Reassurance, immunization, cold and electric stimulation
C. Rest, ice, compression and elevation
D. Resisted, isometric, contracted, bioelectric stimulation
Ans. (C) RICE stands for rest, ice, compression and elevation

Q 43. Recurrent dislocation is least common in:
A. Shoulder
B. Knee
C. Patella
D. None
Ans. (B) knee is most stable joint than shoulder and patella.

Q 44. Bankart's lesion involves:
A. Anterior aspect of head of humerus
B. Anterior aspect of glenoid labrum
C. Posterior aspect of glenoid labrum
D. Posterior aspect of head of humerus
Ans. (B) Bankart lesion is an injury of anterior glenoid labrum of the shoulder due to anterior dislocation.

Answer	29 B	30 A	31 C	32 C	33 C	34 C	35 B	36 C	37 B	38 D	39 B	40 A
	41 C	42 C	43 B	44 B								

Q 45. The most common bone fractured during birth:
A. Clavicle
B. Scapula
C. Radius
D. Humerus

Ans. (A) Clavicle due to outstretched fall and trauma. It occurs as result of a difficult delivery or trauma at birth.

Q 46. Brachioradialis muscle is supplied by:
A. Median nerve
B. Radial nerve
C. Anterior interosseous nerve
D. Posterior interosseous nerve

Ans. (B) Brachioradialis muscle is supplied by a branch from the radial nerve, given by the nerve in front of lateral intermuscular septum before its posterior interosseous branch arises.

Q 47. Ulnar nerve supplies following muscle in the forearm:
A. Flexor carpi radialis
B. Flexor carpi ulnaris
C. Extensor carpi ulnaris
D. Pronator teres

Ans. (B) Ulnar nerve supplies one and half muscle in the flexor compartment of the forearm: flexor carpi ulnaris and medial half of flexor digitorum profundus.

Q 48. In contrast bath the period of immersion in hot and cold bath is as:
A. Hot water—30 secs and cold water—10 secs
B. Hot water—10 secs and cold water—30 secs
C. Hot water—3-4 minutes and cold water—1 minute
D. Hot water—1 minute and cold water—3-4 minute

Ans. (C) Warm and cold contrast bath are with the ratio 3 minutes warm to 1 minute cold.

Q 49. Perthes disease affects the child commonly between:
[AIIMS 2010]
A. 1-4 year of age
B. 4-8 year of age
C. 10-15 year of age
D. Less than 1 year

Ans. (B) Perthes disease is an osteochondritis of the epiphysis of the femoral head. The disease occurs commonly in boys in the area group of 5-10 year. The child presents with the pain in the hip, often radiating to knee.

Q. 50. All of the following are a feature of a CTEV shoe that is a modification of a normal shoe except:
A. Straight inner border
B. Presence of metatarsal bar
C. Outer shoe rise
D. None of the above

Ans. (B) CTEV shoes are modified shoes used once the child states walking. Its feature are straight inner border to prevent fore foot adduction outer shoe rise to prevent inversion, no heel to prevent equinus.

Presence of a metatarsal bar is not a feature of CTEV Shoes.

Answer 45 A 46 B 47 B 48 C 49 B 50 B

Model Question Paper - 10

Q 1. Second order lever is the lever of:
[Joint Structure and Function/Norkins/4th Ed./Pg. 50]
A. Stability
B. Instability
c. Speed
D. Efficiency

Ans. (D) 2nd order lever is more efficient because its mechanical advantage is maximum and mechanical advantage is equal to effort arm upon weight arm. Hence second order lever mechanical advantage is always more than 1st and 3rd.

F________W________E

Q 2. Anterior pelvic tilt is produced by:
[Therapeutic Exercise Foundation/Kisner/ 5th Ed./Pg. 646]
A. Hip extensors and abdominals
B. Hip flexors and lumbar extensors
C. Hip adductors and trunk side flexors
D. None of the above

Ans. (B) Anterior pelvic tilt is produced by pull of the hip flexors anteriorly and contraction of lumbar extensors posteriorly.

Q 3. Choose the correct statement:
[Joint Structure and Function/Norkins/ 4th Ed./Pg. 165]
A. Physiological concentric muscle work is greater than eccentric
B. Physiological cost of static muscle work is greater than concentric
C. Physiological cost of eccentric muscle work is greater than concentric
D. Physiological cost of isometric is greater than eccentric

Ans. (A) Physiological concentric muscle work is greater than eccentric due to more recruitment of motor units. More the number of motor units more is the physiologic cost. Concentric is less efficient so need higher work to be done.

Q 4. Which of the following statements is true regarding the muscle strengthening?
[Therapeutic Exercise Foundation/Kisner/ 5th Ed./Pg. 642]
A. Increase and decrease in speed of movement is progression of concentric work
B. Increase in speed of movement is progression of eccentric muscle work
C. Decrease in speed of movement is a progression of static work
D. All of the above

Ans. (A) According to force velocity relationship increase and decrease in speed of movement is progression of concentric work.

Q 5. Trendelenburg's sign is said to be positive when:
[Orthopedic Physical Assessment/Magee/ 5th Ed./Pg. 7]
A. Sound side pelvis drop down while standing on affected side
B. Affected side pelvis drop down while standing on sound side
C. Sound side pelvis elevated while standing on affected side
D. None of the above

Ans. (A) Trendelenburg's sign is said to be positive when sound side pelvis drops down while standing on affected side because muscles of opposite side (hip abductors. become weak and hence can't control sound side pelvis drop.

Q 6. SCM tightness is characterized by:
[Therapeutic Exercise Foundation/Kisner/ 5th Ed./Pg.389]
A. Neck side flexion towards the affected side with rotation to the opposite
B. Neck side flexion towards the sound side with rotation to affected side
C. Neck side flexion and rotation towards the affected side
D. Neck side flexion and rotation towards the sound side

Ans. (A) Since the function of SCM is neck side flexion towards the same side with rotation to the opposite side it tends to attain that position when short/tight.

Q 7. What should be the temperature of water in hydrotherapy unit?
[Physical Agent & in Rehabilitation/2nd Ed./Pg.262]
A. 27 to 35 degree
B. 22 to 42 degree
C. 32 to 35 degree
D. None of the above

Ans. (A) The temperature of water is 27° to 35°.

Q 8. When there is a permanent deformation with a load of low magnitude and long duration in the elastic range it is known as:
[Physical Agent & in Rehabilitation/2nd Ed./Pg.123]
A. Fatigue Failure
B. Reaching elastic limit
C. Creep
D. Ultimate strength

Ans. (C) When there is a permanent deformation with a load of low magnitude and long duration in the elastic range it is known as creep. This is a property of elastic tissues.

Answer   1 D   2 B   3 A   4 A   5 A   6 A   7 A   8 C

Q 9. Cadence is the number of steps per minute, which is equal to _ in normal human locomotion.

[Joint Structure and Function/Norkin/4th Ed./Pg. 523]

A. 70 – 90
B. 90 – 110
C. 90 – 130
D. 70 – 130

Ans. (D) Cadence is 70 – 130 in normal human locomotion

Q 10. Which manipulation is used to obtain sensory stimulation?

[The Book of Massage Clair/Maxwell Hudson/ 1st Ed./Pg. 30]

A. Stroking
B. Effleurage
C. Kneading
D. Friction

Ans. (A) Stroking is used to obtain sensory stimulation as it stimulates peripheral superficial nerves innervating the skin.

Q 11. Negativity of resting membrane potential is due to:

[Physical Agent in Rehabilitation/2nd Ed./Pg.85]

A. Potassium is more permeable than sodium
B. Three sodium ejected for two potassium
C. Potassium is brought into the cell and sodium expelled out of the cell
D. All of the above

Ans. (D) negativity of resting membrane potential is due to all of the above.

+ + + + + + + + + + + + + + + + +

- - - - - - - - - - - - - - - - - - - -

Q 12. To prevent the occurrence of eddy current:

[Electrotherapy/Clayton's/9th Ed./Pg.22]

A. An insulator is used
B. A spherical conductor is used
C. A laminated conductor is used
D. None of the above

Ans. (C) A laminated conductor is used to prevent eddy currents. Since these currents occur in conductors and lamination reduces them.

Q 13. The name of the coil used to produce faradic current in past was:

[Clayton's/9th Ed./Pg.55]

A. Choke oil
B. Smart Bristow faradic coil
C. Induction coil
D. none of the above

Ans. (B) Smart Bristow faradic coil was used to produce faradic currents in the past.

Q 14. The technique to stretch adhesion in a muscle is called:

[Low and Reed/Butter Worth Heinmann/ 3rd Ed./pg 113]

A. Faradism under pressure
B. Faradic foot bath
C. faradism under tension
D. none of the above

Ans. (C) For removal of adhesion faradic foot bath is not sufficient hence giving faradic current in stretched position muscle tension. should be used to effectively remove the adhesions.

Q 15. Nonmyelinated fibers are:

[Textbook of Medical Physiology Vol -1/ A.K. Jain/3rd Ed./Pg.150]

A. Aa
B. Ab
C. Ac
D. C

Ans. (D) C fibers are nonmyelinated.

Q 16. Depolarization of nerve occurs when the current is beyond threshold value about:

[Electrotherapy Explained/Low and Read/ 3rd Ed./Pg. 10]

A. 1 mv
B. 10 mv
C. 100 mv
D. 1 mv

Ans. (B) When the current is beyond 10 mv depolarization of the nerve occurs.

Q 17. Which is better electrotherapy modality for stress incontinence?

[Cameroon/2nd Ed./Pg. 232]

A. TENS
B. Faradic stimulation
C. IFT
D. IDC

Ans. (C) IFT is a better modality for stress incontinence.

Q 18. EMG reveals action potential of:

[Sullivan/5th Ed./Pg. 274]

A. Muscle
B. Motor unit
C. Nerve fiber
D. None of the above

Ans. (B) EMG reveals action potential of motor units. Since action potential is produced in motor units of muscles and EMG reveals electrical property of muscles.

Q 19. The factors/factor important for penetration of ion in to tissues is/are:

[Physical Agent in Rehabilitation/2nd Ed./Pg. 235]

A. Specific conductivity
B. pH of solution
C. Prescription formed by ions
D. All of the above

Ans. (D) Specific conductivity, pH of solution and prescription formed by ions all effect penetration of ion into tissues. More is the specific conductivity more is the penetration of ions.

Q 20. At rest scapula makes an angle of about how much with frontal plane:

[Joint Structure and Function/Norkin/ 4th Ed./Pg. 242]

A. 15 degree
B. 30 degree
C. 45 degree
D. 60 degrees

Ans. (B) At rest scapula makes an angle of about 30° with frontal plane.

Q 21. By which structure we check the downward pull of gravity on arm by the side?

[Joint Structure and Function/Norkin /4th Ed./Pg. 249]

A. Superior joint capsule
B. Rotator cuff
C. Glenohumeral ligaments
D. Deltoid

Ans. (A) Superior joint capsule checks the downward pull of gravity of arm by the side.

Q 22. Tightness of oblique retinacular ligament is characterized by:

[Joint Structure and Function/Norkin/4th Ed./Pg. 330]

Answer	9 D	10 A	11 D	12 C	13 B	14 C	15 D	16 B	17 C	18 B	19 D	20 B
	21 A											

A. Decreased DIP joint flexion with PIP flexion than with PIP extension
B. Decreased DIP flexion with PIP extension than that PIP flexion
C. Decreased IP joint flexion with MCP joint flexion than that with MCP joint extension
D. Decreased IP joint flexion with wrist flexion than that with wrist extension

Ans. (B) bony collateral slips of extensor expansion maintains extension at DIP because of their rupture will lead to unopposed action of flexors and hence flexion at DIP which is called mallet finger.

Q 23. Mallet finger is due to:
[Orthopedic Physical Assessment/ Magee/5th Ed./Pg. 409]

A. Contracture of FDP
B. Rupture of collateral slip of extensor expansion
C. Rupture of central slip of extensor
D. Rupture of volar plate

Ans. (B) In mallet finger there is rupture of collateral slip of extensor expansion as the collateral slips join together to get insert on middle phalanx.

Q 24. Avascular necrosis of scaphoid fracture occurs at:
[Essentials of Orthopedics and Applied Physiotherapy/ Jayant Joshi/Pg. 114]

A. Proximal half
B. Distal half
C. Whole bones
D. None of the above

Ans. (A) Due to blood supply of Scaphoid

Q 25. In neutral standing position hip joint is weaker:
[Kinesiology of Musculoskeletal System/ Neumann/1st Ed./Pg. 396]

A. Anteriorly
B. Posteriorly
C. Inferiorly
D. Superiorly

Ans. (A) Due to absence of musculature anteriorly.

Q 26. Slipped capita femoral epiphysis occur at:
[Essential Orthopaedics/Maheshwari/ 3rd Ed./Pg. 274]

a. Birth
B. 5-10 year
c. 11–15 year
D. 16-20 year

Ans. (C) Because it happens during the age for 10 to 15 years.

Q 27. Medial meniscus is more prone to injury than lateral because:
[Essential Orthopedics/Maheshwari/3rd Ed./Pg. 129]

A. It is relatively more mobile
B. It is less mobile
C. Medial compartment bears more weight than lateral
D. None of the above

Ans. (B) It is less mobile because it is attached to tibial plateau firmly with help of various ligaments.

Q 28. Cyriax principal of management for spinal problems is:
[Orthopaedic Medicine/James Cyriax/Vol -1/8th Ed./Pg. 304]

A. Oscillatory rhythmic gliding
B. Traction and manipulation
C. Self treatment
D. DTFM and injection

Ans. (B) Because Cyriax explains manipulation along with traction.

Q 29. Facilitation of extensor tone against gravity occurs by:
[Physical Rehabilitation/Sullivan/5th Ed./Pg. 196]

A. Vestibulospinal tract
B. Rubrospinal tract
C. Reticulospinal tract
D. Corticospinal tract.

Ans. (A) During maintenance of posture most of the extensor muscle working against gravity, which is performed by vestibulospinal tract.

Q 30. Apraxia is a result of lesion in:
[Neurology and Neurosurgery Illustrated/ Lindsay/4th Ed./Pg. 109]

A. Frontal lobe
B. Parietal lobe
C. Occipital lobe
D. Temporal lobe

Ans. (A) Apraxia is a disorder of voluntary skilled learned movement characterized by inability to initiate and perform purposeful movement. Motor centers are located in frontal lobe, so lesion in frontal lobe result in apraxia.

Q 31. Arnold Chiari malformation is associated with:
[Neurology and Neurosurgery Illustrated/Lindsay/ 4th Ed./Pg.375]

A. Multiple Sclerosis
B. Spina bifida
C. Syringomyelia
D. B and C

Ans. (D) In Arnold Chiari malformation cerebellum comes out of foramen magnum causing damping up of CSF therefore neural tube defect occurs. Example – Spina bifida and Syringomyelia.

Q 32. Post-traumatic amnesia and retrograde amnesia are the feature of:
[Maria Slokes/2nd Ed./Pg.105]

A. Cerebral contusion
B. Concussion
C. Cerebral laceration
D. Cerebral compression

Ans. (B) During concussion there occur a widespread activity over cortex and this is temporary and transient. Usually the sufferer suffers retrograde amnesia during concussion. Same may also occurs during contusion but it may involve more severity and thus it is not specific.

Q 33. Crossed hemiplegic means:
[Textbook of Medical Physiology/A. K. Jain/ 2nd Ed./Pg. 364]

A. Lesion above the pontine
B. At the level of pontine
C. Below pontine
D. None of the above

Ans. (B) Decussation of motor neurons occur at level of pontine

Q 34. The blood supply of nerve fibers stop at of elongation:
[Electrotherapy Explained/Low and Read/3rd Ed./Pg.85]

A. 15%
B. 5%
C. 10%
D. None of the above

Answer   22 B   23 B   24 A   25 A   26 C   27 B   28 B   29 A   30 A   31 D   32 B   33 B

Ans. (B) Nerves are delicate structure and during stretching up to 5% its blood supply may be affected due to elongation of delicate microvasculature.

Q 35. C1 dermatome is not there because:
[Gray's Anatomy/2nd Ed./Pg.69]
A. Dorsal root absent in cervical region
B. Relation of spinal root with vertebral column
C. C1 nerve is absent
D. None of the above

Ans. (A) Dermatomal supply is provided by dorsal root C1 nerve root has no dorsal component.

Q 36. Drop of QRS complex is found in:
[Brannon, Foley/CPR/3rd Ed./Pg.216]
A. 1st degree heart block   B. 2nd degree heart block
C. 3rd degree heart block   D. Both a and b

Ans. (B) Because in 2nd degree heart block minimum regeneration occur.

Q 37. Which all are the movement strategies associated with inspiration?
[Brannon, Foley/CPR/3rd Ed./Pg. 40]
A. Shoulder flexion, abduction, external rotation
B. Shoulder flexion, trunk extension up to eye gaze
C. Shoulder flexion, abduction, external rotation, trunk extension, eye gaze
D. Trunk extension, shoulder flexion, abduction, external rotation

Ans. (C) These movement increase the perfusion of chest cavity to maximum hence used during the inspiration.

Q 38. Pulsus paradoxous can occur due to the following condition except:
[Physical Rehabilitation/5th Ed./Pg. 96]
A. Asthma   B. Pericardial effusion
C. Upper airway obstruction D. Pneumonia

Ans. (D) When the systolic BP falls more than 10 mm Hg during inspiration the pulse is referred to as pulses paradoxus the possibility is in airways obstruction, asthma and pericardial effusion so the answer is pneumonia.

Q 39. Croup is inflammation of:
[Principle and Practice of Medicine/Davidson/ 20th Ed./Pg. 688]
A. Pharynx and larynx   B. Glottis
C. Larynx and trachea   D. Trachea

Ans. (C) Croup is a abnormal sound crowning heard best during inspiration especially coughing, occur due to laryngeal wrong scheme opening obstruction and trachea.

Q 40. Goose neck deformity is found in:
A. ASD   B. VSD
C. AP window   D. PDA

Ans. (A) In Goose neck deformity neck is forwardly placed due to overactivity of accessory muscles of respiration to compensate the increased oxygen demand of the body.

Q 41. Minimal muscle force is required when the joints is on:
[Therapeutic Exercise Foundation/Kisner/5th Ed.]
A. Closed pack position
B. Loose pack position
C. In between close and loose pack
D. In extension

Ans. (A) Because in closed pack position there is maximal articulation between joint surface and ligaments are taut to support the joint.

Q 42. A small carrying angle means there is risk of:
[Joint Structure and Function/Norkin's/4th Ed.]
A. Inferior dislocation   B. Posterior dislocation
C. Superior dislocation   D. Anterior dislocation

Ans. (C) because decrease in carrying angle increases the chance of ulna moving superiorly by changing its orientation.

Q 43. 5 degree of genu varum increases the compressive force on medical meniscus to:
[Therapeutic Exercise/Hall and Brody/ 2nd Ed./Pg.442]
A. 25%   B. 50%
C. 75%   D. 10%

Ans. (B) For details refer to Neuman's biomechanics.

Q 44. A subtalar pronation will:
[Therapeutic Exercise/Hall and Brody/Pg. 478]
A. Increase the Q angle
b. Decrease the Q angle
C. Q angle will be unchanged
D. None

Ans. (A) Pronation results medial tibial torsion on lower end results lateral tibial torsion on upper end which results lateral shifting of tibial tuberosity hence increases the Q angle.

Q 45. The vertebral border of scapula is __ inches away from midline.
[Joint Structure and Function/Norkin/ 5th Ed./Pg. 242]
A. 2″   B. 3″
C. 3.5″   D. 2.5″

Ans. (C) at resting position medical border of scapula is 3.5 inch away from spine in ideal posture. This distance may increase in rounded shoulders.

Q 46. Which splint is prescribed for claw hand deformity?
[Therapeutic Exercise Fundation/Kisner/ 5th Ed./Pg. 597]
A. Cock-up   B. Knuckle bender
C. Pan cake   D. Short opponens

Ans. (B) In claw hand deformity, flexion at PIP and DIP along with extension at MCP joint thus Knuckle bender is used for claw hand deformity.

Q 47. In A K prosthesis the foot piece is positioned in:
[Physical Rehabilitation/Sullivan/ 5th Ed./Pg. 1260]
A. Inset   B. Outset
C. Neutral   D. None of the above

Ans. (A) During preparation of prosthesis the middle piece is rotated 5° internally whereas foot piece is 5° toward outwards,

Answer	34 B	35 A	36 B	37 C	38 D	39 C	40 A	41 A	42 C	43 B	44 A	45 C
	46 B	47 A										

this will maintain the normal biomechanics of foot and help in push off phase.

Q 48. Lateral wedging is given to correct:
[Essentials of Orthopedics and Applied Physiotherapy/ Jayant Joshi/Pg. 344]

A. Genu valgus
B. Genu varum
C. Flat foot
D. None of the above

Ans. (B) Because in genu varum excessive weight is on lateral border of foot hence to unweight we will give lateral wedging.

Q 49. Which of the following is important for medicolegal point of view?
[Physical Rehabilitation/Sullivan/5th Ed./Pg. 10]

A. Documentation
B. Written informed consent
C. Realization of responsibility
D. All of the above

Ans. (D) Documentation is required for reevaluation and prognostic purposes, Written informed consent for the readiness of the subject, Realization of responsibility means confidentiality of patient data so all three answers are correct.

Q 50. Thoracic outlet syndrome in pregnancy is due to:
[Therapeutic Exercise Foundation/Kisner/5th Ed./Pg. 807]

A. Rounded shoulders which reduces the valid size
B. Fluid retention
C. Elevation of first rib
D. All of the above

Ans. (D) During pregnancy COG shifts anteriorly results in alteration of posture like protracted shoulder.

Answer   48 B   49 D   50 D

Model Question Paper - 11

Q 1. The contraindication of hydrotherapy is:

[Physical Agents in Rehabilitation/Cameroon/ 2nd Ed./Pg. 28]

A. Convulsions
B. Respiratory disease
C. Incontinence of bowel and bladder.
D. All of above

Ans. (D) Contraindication is convulsion because during hydrotherapy there can be drowning, in respiratory disease compression on chest wall due to hydrolic pressure results in decreasing lung compliance and spread infection. For continence risk of contamination of tank. So answer is all of the above.

Q 2. Good posture __________

[Joint Structure and Function/Norkins/ 3rd Edition/Pg 412]

A. Saves energy
B. Looks aesthetically good
C. Prevent musculoskeletal complication
D. All of above

Ans. (D) In good posture minimal muscle work required, which is pleasing to the eye and maintain good muscle length tension relationship.

Q 3. The unit of capacitance is __________

[Claytons Electrotherapy/9th Ed./Pg. 34]

A. Ampere
B. Volt
C. Farad
D. None of the above

Ans. (C) Unit of capacitance is Farad.

Q 4. Which exercise are harmful for RA joint?

[Physical Therapy in Arthritis/Joan, M. Walker/Pg. 253]

A. Passive stretching
B. Passive mobilization
C. Active stretching
D. Active mobilization

Ans. (B) Passive mobilization are harmful for RA because of irritation in synovial fluid.

Q 5. Spondylosis is characterized by:

[Essential Orthopedics / Maheshwari/3rd Ed./Pg. 34]

A. Hypermobility
B. Stiff spine
C. Spinal instability
D. Locking

Ans. (B) It is degenerative disease of intervertebral joint. Movement causes impingement of nerve root and therefore pain. So to prevent pain, muscles is in spasm, by muscle guarding phenomenon resulting in stiff spine.

Q 6. Hyperextension injury of knee may result in tearing of __________

[Joint Structure and Function/Norkins/3rd Ed./Pg. 339]

A. ACL
B. PCL
C. Collateral ligament
D. Meniscus

Ans. (B) PCL restrict backward translation of tibia. In hyperextension, tibia is backwardly translated, so PCL is teared.

Q 7. Ape thumb deformity occurs due to the involvement of __________

[Essential Orthopedics/Maheshwari/3rd Ed./Pg. 51]

A. Ulnar nerve
B. Median nerve
C. Radial nerve
D. Musculocutaneous nerve

Ans. (B) Median nerve supplies muscles of thenar eminence (opponens pollicis). In ape thumb deformity, thumbs comes in plane of the wrist due to paralysis of opponens pollicis.

Q 8. Normal sensory action potential is:

[Guyton/Pg. 576]

A. Biphasic
B. Triphasic
C. Tetraphasic
D. Multiphasic

Ans. (B) For details kindly see the Cameroons electrotherapy or Sullivan electrodiagnosis.

Q 9. Loss of light touch sensation is:

[Human Physiology and Biochemistry/A.K Jain/ 1st Edition/Pg. 358]

A. Thigmanesthesia
B. Dysethesia
C. Anesthesia
D. Aptopogrosia

Ans. (A) Light touch **thigmanesthesia** is used as a screening test for touch. Both the spinothalamic and DCML systems serve this sensation so it is not specific for either one.

Q 10. Which is not a feature of myasthenia gravis?

[Neurology and Neurosurgery/Lindsay/4th Ed./Pg. 481]

A. Muscle weakness
B. Muscle wasting
C. Muscle fatigability
D. Fasciculation

Ans. (B) Myasthenia gravis is a neuromuscular disorder without involving muscle fiber.

Q 11. In case of G.B.S partial to complete recovery takes usually within __________ months

[Neurology and Neurosurgery/Lindsay/4th Ed./Pg. 436]

Answer   1 D   2 D   3 C   4 B   5 B   6 B   7 B   8 B   9 A   10 B

A. Up to 3

B. 3 – 6

C. 6 – 9

D. 9 – 12

Ans. (B) In GBS spontaneous recovery occurs and the most of such recovery occurs within 6 month period from the day of acute onset.

Q 12. Increase in torsion angle of femur is referred to as __________.

[Joint Structure and Function/Norkins/ 3rd Edition/Pg 323]

A. Coxa valga

B. Coxa vara

C. Anteversion

D. Retroversion

Ans. (C) Coxa valga and vara are terms related to neck-shaft angle, anteversion is increase torsion angle of femur while retroversion is decrease torsion angle of femur.

Q 13. Knee flexion in prone lying is an example of:

[Joint Structure and Function/Norkins/3rd Ed./Pg. 30]

A. 1st order lever

B. 2nd order lever

C. 3rd order lever

D. 4th order lever

Ans. (C) Axis(knee joint) is closer to the effort arm hamstring muscle attachment while compared to the distance of knee axis from resistance arm (the COG of leg between knee and ankle). Thus it is 3rd class lever.

Q 14. Muscle is most efficient in __________ range.

[Joint Structure and Function/Norkins/3rd Ed./Pg. 96]

A. Outer

B. Outer part of middle

C. Inner part of middle

D. Inner

Ans. (B) Optional length-tension relationship for maximum cross bridge formation occurs in the outer part of the middle range.

Q 15. To have effect on intracellular calcium system the ultrasound duty cycle should be.

[Claytons Electrotherapy/9th Ed./Pg. 178]

A. 10%

B. 20%

C. 30%

D. 40%

Ans. (B) For details kindly see the Cameroons electrotherapy.

Q 16. Lesion in one optic tract produce __________.

[Neurology and Neurosurgery/Lindsay/4th Ed./Pg. 137]

A. Central scotoma

B. Homonymous hemianopia

C. Bitemporal hemianopia

D. Blindness

Ans. (B) Lesion of optic tract results in same side temporal field loss and the opposite side nasal field loss.

Q 17. The rhythm of tremor observed in Parkinson's disease at rest is about __________.

[Neurology and Neurosurgery/Lindsay/4th Ed./Pg. 361]

A. 4 – 7 beats/second

B. 10 – 20 beats/second

C. 4 – 7 beats/minute

D. 10 – 20 beats/minute

Ans. (A) Tremor frequency in various conditions:- 2 – 4 Hz => cerebellar or rubral tremor, 4 – 8 Hz Parkinsonian tremor (rarely an essential tremor), 8 – 10 Hz essential tremor or physiologic tremor, Postural tremors 8 – 12Hz, Rest tremors 3 – 7 Hz, kinetic/intentional tremors 2 – 5 Hz

Tremor amplitude may also be a helpful clue:- fine tremor → parkinsonism or essential tremor; coarse tremor → cerebellar or rubral tremor; wing-beating tremor → Wilson's disease

Q 18. Segmental demyelination is the predominant pathology in __________.

[Neurology and Neurosurgery/Lindsay/4th Ed./Pg. 436]

A. Ischemic neuropathy

B. Nutritional neuropathy

C. Lead poisoning

D. Guillain-Barre syndrome

Ans. (D) In case of GBS the segmental demyelination occurs; In ischemic/nutritional and lead neuropathy non- specific and diffused demyelination occurs.

Q 19. At birth the shape of the chest is __________.

[Joint Structure and Function/Norkin/3rd Edition/Pg 181]

A. Barrel like

B. Circular

C. Elliptical

D. Triangular

Ans. (B) Anterior, posterior and mediolateral diameter of chest is equal thus chest shape is circular in shape.

Q 20. Maximum diaphragmatic movement is __________.

[Joint Structure and Function/Norkin/3rd Ed./Pg. 177]

A. 1 cm

B. 2 cm

C. 6 cm

D. 4 cm

Ans. (C) Normal Diaphragmatic excursion should be 3-5 cm, but can be increased in well conditioned persons to 7-8 cm. in normal individual higher ranges can be up to 6 cm.

Q 21. A subtalar pronation will __________.

[Joint Structure and Function/Norkin/3rd Ed./Pg. 379]

A. Increase the Q angle

B. Decrease the Q angle

C. Q angle will be unchanged

D. None

Ans. (A) Pronation leads to external rotation of tibia and leads for increase in Q angle.

Q 22. During forward reach __________ use lumbar spine movement earlier.

[Joint Structure and Function/Norkin/3rd Ed./Pg. 144]

A. Males

B. Females

C. Children

D. Male and female equal

Ans. (A) Females have slight more lordosis as compared to males. Thus during forward reach males starts with lumbar movement followed by pelvic movement.

Q 23. When was Indian association of Physiotherapists formed?

A. 1951

B. 1953

C. 1962

D. 1981

Ans. (B) Fact

Q 24. Functional limitation in Nagi model is similar to __________ in ICIDH.

A. Impairment

B. Disability

C. Handicap

D. None of the above

Ans. (B) Nagi's impairment model consists of impairment, functional impairment and disability. The ICIDH model of

Answer	11 B	12 C	13 C	14 B	15 B	16 B	17 A	18 D	19 B	20 C	21 A	22 A
	23 B	24 B										

disability consists of Impairment, disability and handicapped. Thus the functional impairment in Nagi model is equivalent to disability of ICIDH model.

Q 25. Increased frequency of micturition during pregnancy is due to __________.
[Essential of Medical Physiology/Sembulingam/3rd Ed./Pg. 405]
A. Dilatation of the ureter by the action of progesterone
B. Compression of uterus by gravid uterus
C. Elongated urethra
D. All

Ans. (A) The increased model of progesterone causes ureter dilation and the leads to increased urinary frequency.

Q 26. In a normal curve the mean, median and mode are __________.
[Research Methods for Clinical Therapist/Hicks/4th Ed./Pg. 61]
A. Scattered   B. In one line
C. In mid line   D. At one side of the curve

Ans. (C) This is a characteristics of a normal curve.

Q 27. Extension of elbow is associated with __________.
[Joint Structure and Function/Norkin/3rd Ed./Pg. 237]
A. Ulnar abduction and forearm pronation
B. Ulnar abduction and supination of forearm
C. Inferior glide of ulna
D. Superior glide of radius

Ans. (A) kindly refer to Kapandji's biomechanics

Q 28. The function of meniscus is __________.
[Joint Structure and Function/Norkin/3rd Ed./Pg. 329]
A. Shock absorber   B. Lubrication nutrition
C. Load distribution   D. All

Ans. (D) Knee joint is incongruent joint. Therefore fibrocartilaginous disc, menisci is present which increases congruency of jont. As knee joint is main weight bearing joint menisci absorbs 50 % of weight and evenly distribute it.

Q 29. Cyriax principle of management for peripheral joint problems is __________.
[Orthopaedics Medicine/James Cyriax/Vol. 1/8th Ed./Pg. 304]
A. Oscillatory rhythmic glides
B. Traction and manipulation
C. Self-treatment
D. DTFM and injection

Ans. (D) The Cyriax school of thought believe in DTFM + injection for peripheral joint pathology, for the spinal pathology the same school traction +manipulation.

Q 30. HLA B 27 is negative in __________.
[Essential Orthopedics/Maheshwari/3rd Ed./Pg. 248]
A. Ankylosing spondylitis   B. Reiter's syndrome
C. Psoriatic arthritis   D. SLE

Ans. (D) SLE is autoimmune disease and it is not found to be associated with HLA B27.

Q 31. All of the following are true concerning scoliosis except:
[Essential Orthopedics/Maheshwari/3rd Ed./Pg. 234]
A. A 15 degree to 20 degree curve is mild curve
B. Bracing is an effective treatment tool
C. Scoliosis is named by the direction of concavity
D. Early detection is essential

Ans. (C) Named according to the direction of convexity and not because of concavity.

Q 32. Wilson's disease is __________.
[Essential Orthopedics/Maheshwari/3rd Ed./Pg. 208]
A. Hepatolenticular degeneration
B. Caused by disturbance of copper metabolism
C. Frequently familial
D. All of the above

Ans. (D) Wilson disease is related to liver, due to disturbed copper metabolism.

Q 33. 1 liter of oxygen expanded is equivalent to how much calories?
[Guyton/Pg. 793]
A. 10 kcal   B. 10 cal
C. 5 cal   D. 5 kcal

Ans. (D) Energy equivalent for 1 L of O^2 = 4.84 kcal

Q 34. Transtibial prosthesis with thigh corset is indicated in case of the following except.
[Orthosis and Prosthesis in Rehabilitation/lusaroi/Pg. 445]
A. Ideal stump   B. Mediolateral knee instability
C. Genu recurvatum   D. Very short stump

Ans. (A) In Ideal stump the corset is not required and a Velcro strap may be sufficient to stabilize the prosthesis on thigh. In recurvatum, short stump or instability the additional support is needed in form of corset.

Q 35. Injury rate is higher in which of the following exercise training?
[Therapeutic Exercise Foundation/Kisner/4th Ed./Pg. 78]
A. Concentric   B. Eccentric
C. Plyometric   D. In all of the above

Ans. (C) Because plyometrics is high intensity, high velocity exercises.

Q 36. Nodding movement of head is the example of ________ order lever.
[Joint Structure and Function/Norkin/3rd Ed./Pg. 28]
A. 1st   B. 2nd
C. 3rd   D. 4th

Ans. (A) Because fulcrum is located in between the effort arm and resistance. In this case effort arm may be greater than, equal to or lesser than the resistance arm.

Q 37. The temperature of PWB is __________.
[Claytons Electrotherapy/9th Ed./Pg. 163]
A. $30 - 40\,°C$ B. $40 - 50\,°C$
C. $25 - 55\,°C$ D. None of the above

Ans. (B) It's a fact. Kindly consult Low and reed electrotherapy.

Answer 25 A   26 C   27 A   28 D   29 D   30 D   31 C   32 D   33 D   34 A   35 C   36 A
37 B

Q 38. Squatting and descending the stairs become difficult in case of __________.
[Joint Structure and Function/Norkin/3rd Ed./Pg. 339]

A. ACL injury
B. PCL injury
C. MCL injury
D. Meniscus injury

Ans. (B) Those with PCL disorders should refrain from squatting below 50 to 60 degrees until the injury is fully healed. ACL and PCL forces have been shown to diminish at high degrees of knee flexion. Peak ACL forces occur between 15 to 30 degrees of flexion, decreasing significantly at 60 degrees and leveling off thereafter at higher flexion angles. PCL forces rise consistently with every flexion angle beyond 30 degrees of knee flexion, peaking at approximately 90 degrees, and declining significantly thereafter. Beyond 120 degrees, PCL forces are minimal.

Q 39. What is the minimum time required for a nerve impulse to travel through a reflex arc?
[Electrotherapy Explained Low and Reed/3rd Ed./Pg. 155]

A. 20 ms
B. 5 ms
C. 30 ms
D. 25 ms

Ans. (C) Fact

Q 40. Commonest embolus originates from:
[Tidy's Physiotherapy/12th Ed./Pg 273]

A. DVT
B. Varicose veins
C. Fat
D. Air

Ans. (A) DVT leads to most common form of embolus.

Q 41. Ely's test is done to check length of __________
[Orthopaedic Physical Exam Reider/4th Ed./Pg. 373]

A. ITB
B. Hamstring
C. Rectus femoris
D. Hip adductors

Ans. (C) Ely's test is used to evaluate rectus femoris test in prone lying position when heel is gently pushed towards buttocks until resistance or excessive discomfort is felt. Pelvis should remain at rest with no flexion at hip. If hip flexes while knee is flexed a tightness of Rectus femoris is indicated. Knee should bend freely up to 135 degree or heel should touch buttock.

Q 42. Equal pressure point in low lung volume remains at:
[Physical Rehabilitation/Sullivan/5th Ed./Pg. 562]

A. Traction
B. Lobar bronchi
C. Alveoli
D. Segmental bronchi

Ans. (C) Kindly refer to Frownfelter cardiopulmonary rehabilitation.

Q 43. Stair climbing requires approximately knee flexion:
[Joint Structure and Function/Norkin/3rd Ed./Pg. 467]

A. 85 degrees
B. 95 degrees
C. 105 degrees
D. 115 degrees

Ans. (A) Approximately knee flexion during stair climbing is around 85 degrees.

Q 44. Medium speed in Maitland's mobilization is equal to __________
[Orthopaedic Physical Exam/Reider/1st Ed./Pg. 329]

A. ½ per sec
B. 1 per sec
C. 2 per sec
D. 3 per sec

Ans. (B) Frequency of 1 HZ allows the mechanoreceptors to fire to alleviated the pain associated with pathology.

Q 45. What is normal grading of reflex?
[Orthopaedic Physical Exam Reider/1st Ed./Pg 329]

A. +
B. ++
C. +++
D. –

Ans. (B) Fact. – indicates absence of reflex; + indicated hyporeflexia; ++ is normal reflex; +++ is hyperreflexia

Q 46. Lateral wedging is given to correct:
[Essential Orthopedics/Maheshwari/3rd Ed./Pg. 276]

A. Genu valgus
B. Genu varum
C. flat foot
D. None of the above

Ans. (B) Because it will prevent foot supination and reduces lateral stresses on the tibiofemoral joint.

Q 47. Population mean is:
[Research Methods for Clinical Therapist Hicks/4th Ed./Pg. 25]

A. Sample mean +/- 2SEM
B. Sample mean +/- 1SD
C. Sample mean +/- 1SEM
D. Sample mean +/- 2SD

Ans. (C) This is the formula of population mean.

Q 48. Which class is lever of power:
[Joint Structure and Function/Norkin/3rd Ed./Pg. 30]

A. 1st class
B. 2nd class
C. 3rd class
D. 2nd & 3rd class

Ans. (C)

Q 49. Normal birth weight of the child is __________
[Essential Pediatrics/O.P. Ghai/6th Ed./Pg. 4]

A. 2800 gm
B. 3000 gm
C. 3200 gm
D. 3400 gm

Ans. (B) It's a fact.

Q 50. Mean + 1.96 SD covers __________.
[Research Methods for Clinical Therapists/Hicks/4th Ed./Pg. 62]

A. 68 % of area
B. 76 % of area
C. 95 % of area
D. 98 % of area

Ans. (C) When the distribution of the observations is Normal, then 95% of all observations are located in the interval **mean – 1.96 SD** to mean + 1.96 SD.

Answer	38 B	39 C	40 A	41 C	42 C	43 A	44 B	45 B	46 B	47 C	48 C	49 B
	50 C											

Model Question Paper - 12

Q 1. Which ligament in our body contains more elastin fibers?
[Therapeutic Exercise Foundation/Kisner/3rd Ed./Pg. 507]
A. Longitudinal ligament   B. Interspinous ligament
C. Ligamentum nuchae   D. Ligamentum flavum
Ans. (B)

Q 2. The appropriate current to know tendon rupture _______.
[Clayton's/Electrotherapy/9th Ed./Pg. 66]
A. Faradic current   B. TENS
C. Galvanic current   D. None of the above
Ans. (D) If tendon is ruptured then bony lever will not move by the faradic current thus can be detected

Q 3. Infrared has a strong effect on _______.
[Low and Reed/Electrotherapy/9th Ed./Pg. 291]
A. Bone   B. Fat
C. Skin   D. None of the above
Ans. (B) Infrared can be easily penetrate skin, and due to fat can not be easily dissipate thus leads to local tissue temperature rise

Q 4. Knee extension is limited by _______.
[Therapeutic Exercise Foundation/Kisner/3rd Ed./Pg. 507]
A. Bony contact   B. Tension in hamstring
C. Tension of posterior skin   D. The tension of joint capsule
Ans. (D)

Q 5. Sjogren's syndrome and Felty's syndrome are not associated with _______.
A. SLE   B. Scleroderma
C. Rheumatoid arthritis   D. Psoriatic arthritis
Ans. (D) Chronic inflammatory and autoimmune disease in which the salivary and lacrimal glands undergo progressive destruction by lymphocytes and plasma cells resulting in decreased production of saliva and tears. The primary form, often called sicca syndrome, involves both KERATOCONJUNCTIVITIS SICCA and XEROSTOMIA. The secondary form includes, in addition, the presence of a connective tissue disease, usually rheumatoid arthritis. The presence of a connective tissue disease, usually rheumatoid arthritis but sometimes systemic lupus erythematosus, scleroderma, or polymyositis; an abnormal immune response has been implicated.

Q 6. Quadriceps to hamstrings strength ratio is __
[Joint Structure and Function/Norkin/3rd Ed./Pg. 349]
A. 2:1   B. 3:2
C. 5:3   D. 5:4

Ans. (B) Conventionally, the hamstring:quadriceps strength ratio is calculated by dividing the maximal knee flexor (hamstring) moment by the maximal knee extensor (quadriceps) moment measured at identical angular velocity and contraction mode. The agonist-antagonist strength relationship for knee extension and flexion may, however, be better described by the more functional ratios of eccentric hamstring to concentric quadriceps moments (extension), and concentric hamstring to eccentric quadriceps moments (flexion). We compared functional and conventional isokinetic hamstring:quadriceps strength ratios and examined their relation to knee joint angle and joint angular velocity. Peak and angle-specific ($50°$, $40°$, and $30°$ of knee flexion) moments were determined during maximal concentric and eccentric muscle contractions ($10°$ to $90°$ of motion; 30 and 240 deg/sec). Across movement speeds and contraction modes the functional ratios for different moments varied between 0.3 and 1.0 (peak and $50°$), 0.4 and 1.1 ($40°$), and 0.4 and 1.4 ($30°$). In contrast, conventional hamstring:quadriceps ratios were 0.5 to 0.6 based on peak and $50°$ moments, 0.6 to 0.7 based on $40°$ moment, and 0.6 to 0.8 based on $30°$ moment.

Q 7. In case of AK amputee prosthetic knee stabilization can be achieved by _______.
[Orthopaedics/Jayant Joshi/Pg. 238]
A. Action of gluteus maximus
B. Trochanteric knee alignment
C. Extension aid
D. All of the above
Ans. (D) These mechanisms are used to stabilize the stump in the socket.

Q 8. In case of MCL injury strengthening of _______ should be given.
A. Pes anserinus and semimembranosus
B. Hamstrings
C. Hip adductors
D. Quadriceps
Ans. (A) Pes anserinus and semimembranosus muscle help to support the action of the MCL to stabilize the knee joint.

Q 9. Broca's area of brain is for:
[Human Physiology/A.K. Jain/ 1st Ed./Pg. 409]
A. Speech   B. Hearing
C. Locomotion   D. Vision
Ans. (A) Fact

Answer   1 B   2 D   3 B   4 D   5 D   6 B   7 D   8 A   9 A

Q 10. Appreciation of localization of light touch is lost when there is injury of _______.
[Human Physiology/A. K. Jain/1st Ed./Pg. 358]

A. Thalamus
B. Brainstem
C. Sensory Cortex
D. Peripheral

Ans. (C) Sensory cortex is important to perceive the sensations

Q 11. Following cement TKR , patient weans from crutches by _______.
[Brotzman/2nd Ed./Pg. 469]

A. Stitch removal
B. 3 week
C. 6 week
D. 3 month

Ans. (A) In cemented TKR the full weight bearing to tolerance level is allowed. And the full weight bearing can be done after stitch removal if tolerated by patients of cemented TKR. In uncemented TKR the partial weight bearing is initiated after 6 weeks and the full weight bearing is allowed around 3 months (12 weeks).

Q 12. Horner's syndrome is associated with _______.
[Refer to Text]

A. Myositis
B. Anhidrosis
C. All of them
D. None of the them

Ans. (B) Horner syndrome consists of ptosis, meiosis and anhidrosis

Q 13. Diaphragm functioning is tested clinically:
[Refer to Text]

A. Maximum breathing capacity
B. Inspiratory strength measurement
C. Measuring VC in supine and sitting
D. Both a and b

Ans. (C) Difference in the VC in supine and then sitting helps to give a testing idea of the diaphragm functioning.

Q 14. Quadriceps femoris shows peak force at _______ range.
[Joint Structure of Function/Norkin/ 3rd Ed./Pg. 349]

A. Outer range
B. Inner range
C. Mid range
D. Throughout the range

Ans. (C) The maximum activity is needed in the middle range. In terminal range the anatomical pulley (patella) helps to aid its action and thus reduces the force of contraction needed.

Q 15. A subtalar pronation will _______.
[Joint Structure of Function/Norkin/3rd Ed./Pg. 360]

A. Increase the angle
B. Decrease the angle
C. Q angle will be unchanged
D. None

Ans. (A) Subtalar pronation causes increase in the Q angle. (Refer to Kapandji's physiology of joints)

Q 16. _____ splint is prescribed for a case of median nerve injury.
[Refer to Text]

A. Cock-up
B. Knuckle bender
C. Pan cake
D. Short opponens

Ans. (D) In median nerve injury the short opponens splint helps to maintain the position of the hand.

Q 17. Physiotherapy modality suitable for pelvic inflammatory disease is _______.
[Clayton Electrotherapy/10th Ed./Pg. 164]

A. US
B. SWD
C. IFT
D. LASER

Ans. (B) PID the infection is located in deeper region and this cavity is communicating with the exterior. To target this deeper region the SWD is treatment of choice.

Q 18. Stress incontinence is characterized by _______.
[Refer to Text]

A. Overflow of urine
B. Involuntary loss of urine
C. Continuous flow of urine
D. Urgency

Ans. (D) During stress incontinence urgency of urination occurs and the involuntary loss of urine occurs when intra-abdominal pressure rises like during coughing, sneezing, etc.

Q 19. α is directly related to _______.
[Kothari/2nd Ed./Pg. 237]

A. Z value
B. Standard deviation value
C. Standard error value
D. Number of subjects

Ans. (A) Refer to Hicks biostatistics.

Q 20. The most common measure of variability is _______.
[Kothari/2nd Ed./Pg. 197]

A. Variance
B. Standard deviation
C. Standard error
D. All of them

Ans. (B) Standard Deviation is most common measure of variability and is almost mentioned in the data/result presentation as ±SD.

Q 21. Relaxed passive movements is useful for _______.
[Therapeutic Exercise Foundation/Kisner/ 5th Ed./Pg. 44]

A. Muscle strengthening
B. Improving joint range of motion
C. Remembrance of pattern of movement
D. Improving coordination

Ans. (C) When patient cannot perform the active voluntary movement then the passive movements help the brain to remember the pattern of the movement.

Q 22. Which is not true for iontophoresis?
[Clayton Electrotherapy/10th Ed./Pg. 64]

A. Eliminates first pass metabolism
B. Uncontrolled drug delivery
C. Avoid pain that accompanies injection
D. Decrease risk of infection

Ans. (B) Iontophoresis causes controlled drug delivery specific to the affected region and specific drug.

Answer	10 C	11 A	12 B	13 C	14 C	15 A	16 D	17 B	18 D	19 A	20 B	21 C
	22 B											

Q 23. What can be the source for iontophoresis in hyperhydrosis?

[Clayton Electrotherapy/10th Ed./Pg. 64]

A. Iodine
B. Acetic acid
C. Zinc
D. Tap water

Ans. (D) Tap water is used in iontophoresis to reduce hyperhydrosis.

Q 24. Infrared of 1000 nm wavelength can penetrate up to __________.

[Clayton Electrotherapy/10th Ed./Pg. 146]

A. Epidermis
B. Dermis
C. Muscle
D. Bone

Ans. (B) Refer to Clayton's electrotherapy.

Q 25. ____is the closed pack position of shoulder joint.

[Kinesiology Neuman/1st Ed./Pg. 115]

A. Abduction and external rotation
B. Flexion and external rotation
C. Rotator cuff
D. Deltoid

Ans. (A) During Abduction and external rotation the shoulder capsule is maximally taut and thus this is its closed pack position.

Q 26. Loss of light touch sensation is:

[Human Physiology/A.K. Jain/1st Ed./Pg. 358]

A. Atothiguranethesia
B. Dysethesia
C. Anesthesia
D. Aptopogrosia

Ans. (A) Light touch (**thigmanesthesia**) is used as a screening test for touch. Both the spinothalamic and DCML systems serve this sensation so it is not specific for either one.

Q 27. Increase in torsion angle of femur is referred to as __________.

[Kinesiology Neumam/1st Ed./Pg. 392]

A. Coxa valga
B. Coxa vara
C. Anteversion
D. Retroversion

Ans. (C) Increased angle of femur torsion is called anteversion and the reduction in torsion is retroversion.

Q 28. You are studying diabetes mellitus and diabetes insipidus in your clinical pathology course. Which of the following statements is not true about diabetes mellitus, but best describes diabetes insipidus?

[Human Physiology/A. K. Jain/1st Ed./Pg. 258]

A. It is a disorder of carbohydrate metabolism
B. It results from insulin deficiency
C. It is associated with the pancreas
D. It is associated with the pituitary gland

Ans. (D) Diabetes mellitus occurs due to pancreatic insufficiency while the diabetes insipidus occurs due to pituitary insufficiency.

Q 29. The name of the coil used to produce faradic current in past was __________

[Clayton Electrotherapy/8th Ed./Pg. 40]

A. Choke coil
B. Smart Bristow Faradic coil
C. Induction coil
D. None of above

Ans. (B) See Clayton's Electrotherapy.

Q 30. The skin resistance can be reduced before applying electrical stimulator.

[Clayton Electrotherapy/10th Ed./Pg. 296]

A. Washing the skin by soap and warm water and cleaning by applying spirit.
B. Massage the part in elevation if edema is present.
C. Soak the part with normal saline
D. All of the above

Ans. (D) This is the part of patient preparation for electrotherapy.

Q 31. In clinical pathology class, the professor describes a pathological disease that involves the arteries and veins of the lower extremity. The symptoms are inflammation, venous thrombosis, and ischemia of the feet. Which of the following diseases is being described by the professor?

[Medicine/Davidson/20th Ed./Pg. 603]

A. Raynaud's disease
B. Thromboangiitis obliterans
C. Thrombophlebitis
D. Pitting edema

Ans. (B) Raynaud phenomenon involves digital arterioles; Thrombophlebilitis involves veins and not arteries.

Q 32. Drop arm test indicates __________.

[Clinical Orthopaedic Rehabilitation/Brotzman/2nd Ed./Pg. 317]

A. Weakness of deltoid
B. Rupture of supraspinatus
C. Positive painful arc
D. None

Ans. (B) Drop arm test is clinical test used to check rupture of supraspinatus tendon.

Q 33. In neutral standing position the hip joint is weaker __________.

[Kinesiology Neuman/1st Ed./Pg. 399]

A. Anteriorly
B. Posteriorly
C. Inferiorly
D. Superiorly

Ans. (A) The position and orientation of femoral head in acetabulum makes it weakest anteriorly.

Q 34. The resting position for the hip is __________.

[Kinesiology Neuman/1st Ed./Pg. 394]

A. Neutral extension, abduction and rotation
B. 30 degrees of flexion, 30 degrees of abduction and slight external rotation
C. Neutral extension, 30 degrees of abduction and slight internal rotation
D. 30 degrees of flexion, slight adduction and internal rotation

Ans. (B) This is the resting position and is used to mobilize the hip joint. See Therapeutic Exercise by Carolyn Kisner.

Q 35. You are evaluating a 26-year-old male patient status post arthroscopic surgery. The physician requests that you evaluate the muscles that insert into the pes anserinus. You have the patient flex the knee and medially rotate the leg while the knee is flexed. Of the muscles listed below, which are you not evaluating?

[Kinesiology Neuman/1st Ed./Pg. 463]

A. Gracilis
B. Sartorius
C. Semimembranosus
D. Semitendinosus

Ans. (C) Semimembranous does not insert on the pes anserinus

Answer	23 D	24 B	25 A	26 A	27 C	28 D	29 B	30 D	31 B	32 B	33 A	34 B
	35 C											

Q 36. Parietal cerebral tumor cause _________.
[Churchill/3rd Ed./Pg. 310]
A. Progressive dementia
B. Contralateral hemiplegia
C. Falling away of contralateral outstretched hand
D. Epilepsy with aphasia
Ans. (C)

Q 37. Which of the following is not a brain stem reflex?
[Sophei Levitt/4th Ed./Pg. 89]
A. STNR   B. ATNR
C. Positive supporting   D. Crossed extension
Ans. (D) Crossed extension is spinal reflex.

Q 38. Righting is _________ level reflex.
[Sophei Levitt/4th Ed./Pg. 89]
A. Midbrain   B. CPR
C. Cerebellar   D. None of the above
Ans. (B)

Q 39. You are providing consultation to a facility considering adding occupational therapy services to the already developed physical therapy services. Prior to adding occupational therapy services, which of the following is the most important aspect to evaluate in determining if the program will be successful?
[Physical Rehabilitation/Sullivan/5th Ed./Pg. 4]
A. Contact physicians to see if they have occupational therapy patients in the area
B. Determine reimbursement for occupational services
C. Interview the physical therapists to see if they will be supportive to occupational therapy services
D. Determine if any of the facilities around you have occupational therapy services that will compete with yours

Ans. (C) Sometime the already established physical therapy wing may not be supportive to the plan to set-up occupational therapy section thus it is important to know if these two services will be supportive or in rival.

Q 40. Kreb cycle takes place in:
[Harper's Biochemistry/Pg. 177]
A. Cytoplasm   B. Mitochondria
C. Outside cell   D. Ribosome
Ans. (B) Kreb cycle takes place in mitochondria.

Q 41. You are given the description of a type of electrical stimulation as follows: medium-frequency current, approximately 4000 Hz, and four electrodes in a crossed pattern on the patient. What type of electrical stimulation is most likely being described?
[Electrotherapy/Clayton/8th Ed./Pg. 107]
A. Low-volt electric stimulation
B. High-volt electric stimulation
C. Russian stimulation
D. Interferential current stimulation
Ans.(D) kindly refer Nelson therapeutic Electrotherapy.

Q 42. The force frequency relationship between tonic muscles is _________.
[Essentials of medical physiology/Sembulingam/3rd Ed./Pg. 134]
A. Linear   B. Ramp and plateau
C. Curvilinear   D. None of the above
Ans. (B) The F-T curve of tonic muscles include ramp when muscles start functioning and gradually increase its contraction and the curve gets plateau when the maximum force has reached.

Q 43. _________ incision is used for gastrectomy.
[Tidy's Physiotherapy/12th Ed./Pg. 378]
A. Left upper paramedian   B. Right upper paramedian
C. Left subcostal   D. Midline
Ans. (A) Left upper incision on the left side helps to access the stomach for the gastrectomy.

Q 44. The physician suggests that you start massage of a patient with back pain to reduce muscle spasms and assist in alleviating pain. The physician recommends that the massage you utilize consist of a series of brisk blows in alternating fashion. Of the following massages, which has the physician recommended?
[Tidy's Physiotherapy/12th Ed./Pg. 442–444]
A. Tapotement massage   B. Friction massage
C. Kneading massage   D. Vibration
Ans. (A) The mentioned features are characteristics of Tapotement.

Q 45. Human body is made-up of _________ natural elements.
[Joint Structure Foundation/Norkin/3rd Ed./Pg. 2]
A. 3   B. 4
C. 5   D. 7
Ans. (B)

Q 46. For skewed data which is measure of variability is useful
[Research Methods for Clinical Therapists/Hicks/4th Ed./Pg. 54]
A. Percentile   B. Range of the datas
C. Interquartile range   D. None of the above
Ans. (C) Refer to Hicks biostatistics.

Q 47. Pelvic inflammatory disease as the inflammation of _________
[Tidy's Massage and Remedial Exercise/Pg. 455]
A. Uterus   B. Cervix
C. Ovary   D. Fallopian tube
Ans. (D) PID involves fallopian tubes;

Q 48. Posterolateral disc prolapse in lumbar spine is common, why?
[Tidy's Physiotherapy/13th Ed./Pg. 104]
A. Disc lies more posteriorly
B. Load is more
C. Posterior longitudinal ligament is narrower
D. All of the above
Ans. (D) All of the mentioned factors lead to the PIVD

Answer	36 C	37 D	38 B	39 C	40 B	41 D	42 B	43 A	44 A	45 B	46 C	47 D
	48 D											

Q 49. Erythema is best provoked by _________.

[Electrotherapy/Sheila Kitchen/11th Ed./Pg. 193]

A. UVA
B. UVC
C. UVB
D. All provoke erythema to the same extent

Ans. (C) Refers to Sheila Kitchen electrotherapy.

Q 50. Which of the following modalities would be most appropriate to implement in a treatment program for back pain in the following patient? Patient is a 24-year-old female, 2 months into her pregnancy. Patient has a long-standing history of chronic back pain as a result of an automobile accident 6 years ago. Patient currently is reporting acute pain across the low back when sitting, standing for long periods of time, and driving.

[Electrotherapy Explained Low and Reed/3rd Ed./Pg. 232]

A. Rest in a side-lying position, supported with pillows between her knees
B. Moist heat for 20 minutes in a side-lying position
C. Ultrasound pulsed at 2.0 W/cm²
D. Alternate knee to chest exercises

Ans. (B) Moist heat is most preferred treatment for the pregnant lady; in pregnancy the US is contraindicated.

Model Question Paper - 13

Q 1. The force frequency relationship between tonic muscles is _______.

[Sembulingam/3rd Ed./Pg. 134]

A. Linear
B. Ramp and plateau
C. Curvilinear
D. None of the above

Ans. (B) The Force velocity relationship of tonic muscle is ramp and plateau shape. Tonic muscles are antigravity muscles which maintain posture against gravity. When body is at rest and fully supported then these muscles activity is zero. When body is maintained in standing then these muscles fire to increase activity, thus they ramp up. When body is maintained in specific posture then they work at constant level, thus show activity at plateau.

Q 2. Pelvic inflammatory disease as the inflammation of _______ .

[Tidy's Physiotherapy/11th Ed./Pg. 455]

A. Uterus
B. Cervix
C. Ovary
D. Fallopian tube

Ans. (D) Inflammation of fallopian tube is PID: that of uterus is metritis/hysteritis; inflammation of ovary is oophoritis.

Q 3. A patient comes to the clinic complaining of inflammation and pain. The physician diagnosed the patient as having bursitis and recommended iontophoresis for treatment. Which of the following is the most frequent location of bursitis?

[K.M. Varghese Company/Tidy's Physiotherapy/ 12th Ed./Pg. 71]

A. Subacromion area
B. Knee
C. Elbow
D. Ischial tuberosity

Ans. (A) This is due to narrow space of subacromial region.

Q 4. Tension sutures are used in _______

[K. M. Varghese Company/Tidy's Physiotherapy/ 12th Ed./Pg. 379]

A. Thoracotomy
B. Thoracoplasty
C. Pneumonectomy
D. Hernia repair

Ans. (D) Tension sutures are needed to secure heavy segments or body parts like abdomen.

Q 5. The commonest structures impinged is:

[Orthopaedic Physical Assessment/Magee/5th Ed./Pg. 293]

A. Infraspinatus
B. Supraspinatus
C. Long head of biceps
D. Subacromial bursa

Ans. (B) It is due to its location in suprahumeral space and the high chances of impingement due to pressure of humeral head.

Q 6. Essence of pathology in RA is _______.

[Orthopaedics and Applied Physiotherapy/Jayant Joshi/ 1st Ed./Pg. 304]

A. Persistence synovitis
B. Articular cartilage damage
C. Deformity in joints
D. Tendon rupture

Ans. (A) Consistent persistent synovitis is important feature of RA.

Q 7. The minimum duration of exercise program to improve strength should be at least:

[K. M. Varghese company/Tidy's Physiotherapy/ 12th Ed./Pg 423/478]

A. 3 weeks
B. 10 weeks
C. 6 weeks
D. 12 weeks

Ans. (C) before 6 week if any strength improvement occurs, is due to the neural adaptation and is usually very short persisting.

Q 8. Enthesopathy occurs in _______ .

[Apley]

A. Rheumatoid arthritis
B. Ankylosing spondylitis
C. Psoriatic arthritis
D. SLE

Ans. (B) Its inflammation of the connective tissue at its attachment with bone.

Q 9. Short term memory is mediated by _______.

[Textbook of Physiology/A.K.Jain/Vol. II/3rd Ed./Pg. 1053]

A. Limbic system
B. Frontal lobe
C. Hippo campus
D. Parietal lobe

Ans. (B) short term memory also called as working memory is mediated by frontal lobe.

Q 10. Commonest intracranial tumor _______.

[Neurology and Neurosurgery/Lindsay/4th Ed./Pg. 299]

A. Angiomas
B. Meningiomas
C. Gliomas
D. Neuromas

Ans. (C) Glioma are commonest intracranial tumors.

Q 11. Lumbar spine is not involved in _______ .

[Orthopaedics and Applied Physiotherapy/Jayant joshi/ 1st Ed./Pg. 305]

A. Rheumatoid arthritis
B. Osteoarthritis
C. Ankylosing spondylitis
D. None of the above

Ans. (A) RA involves the smaller and distal joints. The axial joints are usually spared.

Q 12. The value of correlation coefficient is always:

[Research Methods for Clinical Therapists/Hicks/ 4th Ed./Pg. 77 – 80]

Answer   1 B   2 D   3 A   4 D   5 B   6 A   7 C   8 B   9 B   10 C   11 A

A. 0
B. between +1 and – 1
C. > 1
D. < 1

Ans. (B) This is a fact. Refer to Hicks book of statistics.

Q 13. Which of the following spinal orthosis controls LS flexion-extension

[Physical Rehabilitation/Sullivan 5th Ed./Pg. 1321]

A. Taylor
B. Knight
C. Haris
D. Taylor- Knight

Ans. (B) Knight brace is specifically used to restrict the movement of the lumbosacral flexion and extension, so suitable answer is B.

Q 14. For the edema reduction the following ions is used ______

[Electrotherapy Explained/Low and Reed/3rd Ed./Pg. 45]

A. Acetate
B. Copper
C. Hyaluronidase
D. None of the above

Ans. (C)

Hyaluronidase is hyaluronan degrading enzyme which reduces the hyaluronic acid component of connective tissues à high viscosity property of hyaluronic acid is lessenedà diffusion improvesà inflammation reduces.

Q 15. Pain in the buttock is suggested of pain of ______.

[The Lumbar Spine Mechanica Diagnosis/ Tinerapy Mckenzie/1st Ed./Pg. 121]

A. Lumbar spine
B. Hip joint
C. Piriformis
D. Trochanteric

Ans. (A) Hip pain is mostly felt in groin' trochanteric pain on outer lateral aspect of thigh; piriformis pain as deep dull pain and sometime like sciatica; the lumbar spine pain could be easily manifested in buttock.

Q 16. Socket with soft lining is provided in cases of ______.

[Physical Rehabilitational/Sullivan 5th Ed./Pg. 1223]

A. Partial foot
B. Syme's
C. BK
D. AK

Ans. (D) Refer to Sullivan.

Q 17. Ability to interpret letter written on the palmar surface of one's hand is ______.

[Physical Rehabilitation/Sullivan 5th Ed./Pg. 147]

A. Stereognosia
B. Ahylognosia
C. Graphesthesia
D. None

Ans. (C) Graphesthesia is the condition in which the subject can not appreciate the letters or alphabets like movement over the skin of palm.

Q 18. Skin from uniovular twin having common placenta is also accepted, which is called?

[K.M. Varghese Company/Tidy's Physiotherapy/ 12th Ed./Pg. 310]

A. Autograft
B. Isograft
C. Homograft
D. Heterograft

Ans. (B) An **Isograft** is a graft of tissue between two individuals who are genetically identical (i.e. monozygotic twins. Transplant rejection between two such individuals virtually never occurs.

Q 19. The best indicator of disk prolapse is ______.

[Orthopaedic Physical Assessment Magee/ 5th Ed./Pg. 565]

A. Bowstring test
B. SLR affected side
C. Crossed SLR
D. Bilateral SLR

Ans. (C) The crossed SLR shows posterolateral nerve root herniation; the remaining tests from the given options can be false positive due to lumbar spine/SI joint pathology, etc.

Q 20. The physiological feedback is ______.

[Physical Rehabilitation/Sullivan 5th Ed./Pg. 472]

A. Knowledge of result
B. Intrinsic
C. Knowledge of performance
D. Open loop

Ans. (D) The kind of feedback in physiological system is open loop type which can be influenced by stimulus from within body or from the factors lying outside the body.

Q 21. Moderate hearing impairment (40–50%. is said to occur when the dB level is ______.

[Physical Rehabilitation/Sullivan/5th Ed./Pg. 427]

A. 26 – 40 dB
B. 41 – 60 dB
C. 61 – 70 dB
D. 71 – 90 dB

Ans. (B) Mild: for adults: between 25 and 40 dB, for children: between 20 and 40 dB Moderate: between 41 and 55 dB; Moderately severe: between 56 and 70 dB; Severe: between 71 and 90 dB; Profound: 90 dB or greater.

Q 22. For patient with generalized weakness which test is useful?

[Physiology/K. Smbulingam/3rd Ed./Pg. 320]

A. Thyroid function
B. Parathyroid function
C. Serum cryoglobulin
D. Serum complement levels

Ans. (A) Generalized weakness may be due to thyroid hyperactivity.

Q 23. Carpometacarpal joint of thumb has got ______ **degrees of freedom.**

[Joint Structure Foundation/Norkin/3rd Ed./Pg. 277]

A. 1
B. 2
C. 3
D. 4

Ans. (C) CMC of thumb has 3 degree of freedom for Flexion/ extension, abduction/adduction and the circumduction.

Q 24. In simple regression the dependent variable should be put in:

[Research Methods for Clinical Therapists/ Hicks/4th Ed./Pg. 70-75]

A. X - axis
B. Y - axis
C. X or Y - axis
D. Z - axis

Ans. (B) Refer to Hicks biostatistics.

Q 25. Range of glenohumeral abduction is about ______.

[Joint Structure and Function/Narkin/3rd Ed./Pg. 209]

A. 180°
B. 160°
C. 100°-110°
D. 90°

Ans. (C) Out of total 180 degree abduction the GH and ST joint movement occurs around in ratio of 2:1.

Answer	12 B	13 B	14 C	15 A	16 D	17 C	18 B	19 C	20 D	21 B	22 A	23 C
	24 B	25 C										

Q 26. Push up is an example of _______.
[Therapeutic Exercise Foundation/Kisner/
5th Ed./Pg. 175]

A. Close kinetic chain exercise
B. Active free weight bearing exercise
C. Both a and b
D. Resisted exercise

Ans. (C) push up is a resisted exercise which in closed kinetic chain required to lift body weight against gravity.

Q 27. It takes about _______ for the graft to establish its own blood flow.
[K.M. Varghese Company/Tidy's Physiotherapy/
12th Ed./Pg. 312]

A. 3 – 4 days
B. 7 – 10 days
C. 3 weeks
D. 6 weeks

Ans. (A) This is the time in which neovascularization starts occurring.

Q 28. Nerve accommodation can be avoided by _______.
[Electrotherapy/Clayton/9th Ed./Pg. 60]

A. Surging the current
B. Using varying current
C. Using a varying current that rises and falls suddenly
D. None of the above

Ans. (C) Sudden rising currents are better able to tackle the accommodation process.

Q 29. Positive Apley's grinding test with external rotation of tibia and compression indicates lesion of _______.
[Orthopaedic Physical Assessment Magee/5th Ed./Pg. 791]

A. MCL
B. Medical Meniscus
C. LCL
D. Lateral Meniscus

Ans. (B) Apley grinding test with tibial lateral rotation checks for medial menisci while the same test with tibia medial rotation checks for lateral menisci.

Q 30. Active stump exercises can be started after _______.
[K.M. Varghese Company/Tidy's Physiotherapy/
12th Ed./Pg. 264-266]

A. Removal of the drainage tube
B. Stitch removal
C. 3 weeks
D. 6 weeks

Ans. (A) The exercises for stump can be started immediately after the drainage tube is removed, if the wound conditions appears satisfactory and vitals of patient are stable.

Q 31. Foot wear modification for calcaneal spurs is _______.
[Pg. 559/33]

A. Heel wedge
B. Gouged out heel
C. Heel cuff
D. Soft heel padding

Ans. (B) Both soft heel pad and the gouged out heel can be used, but sometimes soft heel pad can reduce the space available within footwear, so the gouged out heel is more appropriate option.

Q 32. Thomas heel is given in case of _______.
[Tidy's Physiotherapy/K.M. Varghese Company/
12th Ed./Pg 95]

A. Equines foot
B. Cavus foot
C. Flat foot
D. CTEV

Ans. (C) It is a medial heel wedge tilts the heel into varus and may be helpful in treatment of symptomatic pes planus and plantar fasciitis, this heel should not be used if calcaneus is in a varus position. This heel should extend from mid portion of navicular bone the medial side to a line that intersects the longitudinal axis of the fibula on the lateral side.

Q 33. A subtalar pronation will _______.
[Joint Structure and Function/Norkin/3rd Ed./Pg. 379]

A. Increase the Q angle
B. Decrease the Q angle
C. Q angle will be unchanged
D. None

Ans. (A) There occurs a direct relation between forefoot pronation and the increase in Q angle.

Q 34. Drop of QRS complex is found in _______.
[Physical Rehabilitation/Sullivan/5th Ed./
Pg. 602-611]

A. 1st degree heart block
B. 2nd degree heart block
C. 3rd degree heart block
D. Both a and b

Ans. (B) For details refer to Davidson pathology.

Q 35. Resorption of the terminal phalanx is not seen in:
[Essential Pediatrics/O.P. Ghai/6th Ed./Pg. 621]

A. Hyperparathyroidism
B. Reiter's syndrome
C. Scleroderma
D. Psoriasis

Ans. (B) Kindly refer for details Apleys orthopedics.

Q 36. Jefferson's fracture occurs at:
[Hoppenfeld Lippincott/Williams and Wilkins/
1st Ed./Pg. 514]

A. C1
B. C2
C. C1, C2
D. C2, C3

Ans. (A) Jefferson fracture involves C1 vertebra and involves anterior and posterior arches of the vertebra. It may be two, three or four part fracture. This fracture results from the axial loading.

Q 37. All are seen in chronic osteomyelitis except:
[Orthopaedics and Applied Physiotherapy/Jayant Joshi/
1st Ed./Pg. 187]

A. Sequestrum
B. Amyloidosis
C. Myositis ossificans
D. Metastatic abscess

Ans. (C) Chronic osteomyelitis leads to weakness of bone architecture and it does not lead to myositis ossificans. Myositis ossificans means formation of bone like mass in the muscle itself.

Answer 26 C   27 A   28 C   29 B   30 A   31 B   32 C   33 A   34 B   35 B   36 A   37 C

Q 38. Avascular necrosis occurs due to fracture of:
[Hoppenfeld/Lippincott Williams and Wilkins/
1st Ed./Pg. 439]

A. Medial femoral epicondyle
B. Olecranon
C. Talus
D. Fibula

Ans. (C) Avascular necrosis can occur due to talus neck fracture as it cuts down the blood supply to its distal portion.

Q 39. Osteochondritis dessicans occurs at:
[Orthopaedics and Applied Physiotherapy/
Jayant Joshi/1st Ed./Pg. 549]

A. Lateral surface lateral condyle
B. Medial surface of lateral condyle
C. Medial surface medial condyle
D. Lateral surface medial condyle

Ans. (D) For details refer to Tureck's orthopedics.

Q 40. Which is not a feature of myasthenia gravis?
[Neurology and Neurosurgery Lindsay/
4th Ed./Pg. 479-484]

A. Muscle weakness   B. Muscle wasting
C. Muscle fatigability   D. Fasciculation

Ans. (B) Muscle atrophy does not occur in myasthenia gravis.

Q 41. Segmental demyelination is the predominant pathology in ______.
[Neurology and Neurosurgery Lindsay/4th Ed/Pg. 436]

A. Ischemic neuropathy   B. Nutritional neuropathy
C. Lead poisoning   D. Guillain-Barre syndrome

Ans. (D) GBS syndrome leads to segmental demyelination. Lead poisoning, ischemia, and nutritional neuropathy lead to nonspecific demyelination

Q 42. The center of gravity of HAT is at ______.
[Joint Structure and Function/Norkin/3rd Ed./Pg. 412]

A. T10   B. T11
C. L1   D. T9

Ans. (B) The HAT consists of head- arms and trunk portion. The concentration of the combined mass of this segments is localized over the T11, thus COG is located at T11 for the HAT segment.

Q 43. A small carrying angle means there is a risk of ______.
[Joint Structure and Function/Norkin/3rd Ed./Pg. 234]

A. Inferior dislocation   B. Posterior dislocation
C. Superior dislocation   D. Anterior dislocation

Ans. (C) In case of small carrying angle the radius head remains uncovered on its superior aspect thus has high-risk of subluxating in superior direction.

Q 44. Which muscle is the little helper of latissimus dorsi?
[Human Anatomy B. D. Chaurasia Vol-1/
4th Ed./Pg. 146]

A. Teres minor   B. Teres major
C. Posterior deltoid   D. Subscapularis

Ans. (B) The teres major and the latissimus dorsi are the medial rotators; the other mentioned muscles are lateral rotators of the humerus.

Q 45. The structure which gives restraint in the maximum directions is ______.
[Joint Structure and Function/Norkin/3rd Ed./Pg. 336]

A. LCL   B. ACL
C. MCL   D. PCL

Ans. (C) MCL provides knee stability in most of the directions for knee movement. For details kindly refer to Physiology of joints Kapandji.

Q 46. Which muscle may not be an extensor of wrist when the forearm is pronated?
[Joint Structure and Function/Norkin/3rd Ed./Pg. 257]

A. ECRL   B. Extensor digitorum
C. ECRB   D. ECU

Ans. (D) ECU act as a ulnar deviator in pronated forearm position.

Q 47. In hip joint osteoarthritis the hypomobility is particularly for ______ movement.
[Tidy's Physiotherapy/Varghese Company/12th Ed./Pg. 70]

A. Extension   B. Flexion
C. Abduction   D. Rotation

Ans. (B) During hip flexion the articular surfaces of hip joint come in close contact with each other. Thus during flexion the roughened articular surfaces cause restriction in the hip movement.

Q 48. House maid's knee refers to ______.
[Tidy's Physiotherapy/K. M. Varghese Company/
12th Ed./Pg. 70]

A. Infrapatellar bursitis   B. Prepatellar bursitis
C. Suprapatellar bursitis   D. Quadriceps bursitis

Ans. (B) Infrapatellar bursitis is Clergyman's bursitis; Prepatellar bursitis is housemaid's bursitis.

Q 49. Tibiofemoral compressive load increases with knee flexion because of ______.
[Joint Structure and Function/Norkin/3rd Ed./Pg. 344]

A. Increase in weight transfer
B. Increase in quadriceps contraction
C. Increasing incongruence
D. None

Ans. (C) With increase in knee flexion the tibiofemoral articular surface area in contact increases, this increases the joint congruency and improves the joint compressive forces.

Q 50. Serum uric acid level is higher in ______.
[K. M. Varghese Company/Tidy's Physiotherapy/
12th Ed.Pg. 144]

A. SLE   B. Stills disease
C. Gout   D. None of the above

Ans. (C) In case of gout the uric acid crystals get deposit in the joint cavities and synovial fluid sometime.

Answer	38 C	39 D	40 B	41 D	42 B	43 C	44 B	45 C	46 D	47 B	48 B	49 C
	50 C											

Model Question Paper - 14

Q 1. You are treating a patient secondary to a foot injury. The patient reports that his pediatrist thought the spring ligament was injured as a result of his fall. Which of the following best describes the spring ligament of the foot?

[Joint Structure and Function/Norkin/3rd Ed./Pg. 371]

A. It is also called the plantar calcaneocuboid ligament
B. It is called the short plantar ligament
C. It helps to maintain the medial arch of the foot by supporting the head of talipes
D. The spring ligament is not highly elastic

Ans. (C) The spring ligament of the foot supports the head of the talipes, which helps to maintain the medial arch of the foot. All other statements regarding the spring ligament are false. The long plantar ligament supports the lateral longitudinal arch.

Q 2. Bursae may be found in most of the locations within the body. In which of the following anatomical areas would the bursae most likely not be found?

[Essential Orthopaedic Jayant Joshi/1st Ed./Pg. 33]

A. Subtendinous   B. Intramuscular
C. Subcutaneous   D. Subfascial

Ans. (B) The bursae are not found in intramuscular locations. Bursae are most likely found where friction is possible, for example between tendons, ligaments, and bones.

Q 3. A patient is sent to physical therapy secondary to a lower extremity injury. Reading the patient's past medical history, you note that the superficial peroneal nerve has been severed. Which of the following muscles would be emphasized in your treatment program?

[Human Anatomy BD Chaurasia/4th Ed./Pg. 160]

A. Tibialis anterior   B. Peroneus tertius
C. Peroneus brevis   D. Extensor hallucis longus

Ans. (C) The superficial peroneal nerve innervates both the peroneus longus and peroneus brevis. The deep peroneal nerve innervates the tibialis anterior, peroneus tertius, extensor hallucis longus, extensor digitorum longus, and extensor digitorum brevis.

Q 4. You are studying the various types of arthritis, specifically rheumatoid arthritis versus osteoarthritis. Which of the following would best describe the etiology of osteoarthritis?

[Tidy's Physiotherapy/12th Ed./Pg. 107]

A. Trauma to a joint recently
B. Underweight
C. Degeneration caused by aging
D. Recent injury to the joint

Ans. (C) The etiology of arthritis is degeneration caused by ageing. It is a degenerative joint disease of articular cartilage. Gout is a form of arthritis in which sodium urate crystals are deposited near or in the joint. It is common in the great toe.

Q 5. The professor is presenting a lecture on the advantages and disadvantage of the following exercises: Isometric, isokinetic, isotonic, and eccentric contractions. The professor informs the class that some of the disadvantages of a particular exercise are that it loads muscle at the weakest point and the momentum factor in lifting. These disadvantages best describe which of the following classifications of exercise?

[Therapeutic Exercise Foundation/Kisner/4th Ed./Pg. 69]

A. Isometric   B. Isotonic
C. Isokinetic   D. Free weights

Ans. (B) Disadvantages of isotonic exercise: loads muscle at the weakest point, momentum factor in lifting, does not develop accuracy at functional speeds.

Q 6. The patient is a 26-year-old male, status postankle fracture. The physician orders mobilization to increase joint range of motion. Which of the following is the maximum loose-packed position of the ankle joint?

[Orthopaedic Physical Assessment Davis J. Magee/5th Ed.]

A. 10° plantar flexion   B. 5° plantar flexion
C. 0° plantar flexion   D. 15° plantar flexion

Ans. (A) Loose-packed position is when the joint is in a resting position where the joint's range of motion is under the least amount of stress. The maximum loose-packed position for the ankle joint would be 10° plantar flexion, midway between inversion and eversion.

Q 7. On the patient described above, you decide to measure normal expansion at the xiphoid process. Which of the following would be the normal value for expansion when measured at the xiphoid process?

[Joint Structure and Function/Norkin/3rd Ed./Pg. 172]

A. 5 to 10 cm   B. 5 to 10 cm
C. 0.5 to 1.0 cm   D. 0.5 to 1.0 cm

Ans. (A) Normal expansion at the xiphoid process should measure approximately 5 to 10 cm.

Q 8. During the swing phase, acceleration stage, which muscles remain active throughout the entire stage to help shorten the extremity so it can clear the ground by holding the ankle in a neutral position?

[Joint Structure and Function/Norkin/3rd Ed.]

A. Tibialis posterior, peroneus brevis
B. Tibialis anterior, peroneus tertius
C. Tibialis anterior, peroneus tertius, extensor hallucis longus
D. Tibialis posterior, peroneus tertius, extensor hallucis longus

Ans.(C) Tibialis anterior, peroneus tertius, and extensor hallucis longus are muscles that are active during the swing phase, acceleration stage. These muscles remain active throughout the entire stage to help shorten the extremity so it can clear the ground by holding the ankle in a neutral position.

Q 9. During the swing phase, deceleration stage, which muscles contract to slow down the swing phase just prior to heel strike, thus permitting the heel to strike quietly in a controlled manner?

[Joint Structure and Function/Norkin/3rd Ed.]
A. Gluteus medius
B. Gluteus maximus
C. Hamstring
D. Quadriceps

Ans. (C) During the swing phase, deceleration stage, the hamstring muscles contract to slow down the swing phase just prior to heel strike, thus permitting the heel to strike quietly in a controlled manner.

Q 10. The sinus node acts as the cardiac pacemaker in the heart. The sinus node is a group of cardiac cells that discharges an impulse. Where is the sinus node located in the heart?

[Human Anatomy B. D. Chaurasia/4th Ed./Pg. 245]
A. Right atrium
B. Left atrium
C. Right ventricle
D. Left ventricle

Ans. (A) The sinus node, an area of specialized heart tissue, is located in the right atrium of the heart.

Q 11. A butcher is responsible for processing meat packaging. In the process of carving the meat he injures the second and third digits of his hand. The hand surgeon reports that the nerves in the second and third digits have been permanently injured. Which nerve/nerves would be injured?

[Human Anatomy B. D. Chaurasia/4th Ed./Pg. 111]
A. Ulnar nerve
B. Median nerve
C. Radial nerve
D. Ulnar/median nerve

Ans. (B) The median nerve innervates the second and third digits of the hand. The ulnar nerve is responsible for the fourth and fifth digits.

Q 12. When studying upper motor neuron lesions in neuroanatomy, you determine that which of the following is not a characteristic typically seen with this type of lesion?

[Tidy's Physiotherapy K. M. Varghese/12th Ed./Pg. 241
A. Muscle atrophy
B. Spasticity
C. Hyperreflexia
D. Babinski sign possible

Ans. (A) A characteristic that is not typically seen with an upper motor neuron lesion is muscle atrophy. A patient with an upper motor neuron lesion typically has spasticity, hyperreflexia, and Babinski sign is possible.

Q 13. You have received a physician's order to discharge an inpatient that has been under your care for a total knee replacement. Which of the following personnel would you contact first to start planning discharge from the hospital to home? Select the most appropriate answer.

[Jayant Joshi/1st Ed./Pg. 214]

A. The physician
B. Social worker
C. Patient's family
D. Home health agency

Ans. (B) The social worker should be contacted to start discharge planning in cooperation with the patient, family, and physical therapist. The physician has already given you the order for discharge so it is not necessary to contact him or her first. The home health agency can be contacted later through the social worker.

Q 14. You are testing a pediatric patient for symmetrical tonic reflex. You provide the test stimulus by flexing the patient's head. Which of the following best describes a positive reaction to this test stimulus?

[Essential Paediatrics O.P Ghai/6th Ed./Pg. 146]
A. The arms will flex and the legs will extend
B. The arms will extend and the legs will flex
C. The arms will flex and the legs will flex
D. The arms will extend and the legs will extend

Ans. (A) When the stimulus is flexing the head, the positive reaction will result in arm flexion and leg extension. If the test stimulus had been extending the patient's head, the positive response would then have been arm extension and leg flexion.

Q 15. You are providing an education program to an industry where repetitive motion injuries are commonly seen. To assist in decreasing repetitive injuries within this company, which of the following would be the most important concept to emphasize first?

[Therapeutic Exercise Foundation/Kisner/3rd Ed./Pg. 58]
A. Instruct the employees in proper warm-up procedures
B. Instruct the employees in strengthening exercises
C. Provide the company with isokinetic testing and the results on each employee
D. Provide posters on proper body mechanics

Ans. (A) The first step in performing an educational program to a company with repetitive motion injuries is to instruct the personnel in proper warm-up and stretching exercises as a prevention technique.

Q 16. A 26-year-old patient status post spinal cord injury as a result of a diving accident presents the following functional outcomes: vital capacity is 60 to 80%, patient is independent in bed mobility, patient is independent with pressure relief and a manual wheel-chair, and patient can assist with independent transfers. Based on the above listed outcomes, what would be the most likely level of lesion in this patient?

[Physical Rehabilitation Sullivan/5th Ed./Pg. 939]
A. C4
B. C5
C. C6
D. C7, C8

Ans. (C) A patient with a C6 level of lesion would have functional outcomes of vital capacity of 60 to 80%, independent in bed mobility, independent with pressure relief, independent in a manual wheelchair, and able to assist with independent transfers. C4 level of lesion would have functional outcomes of vital capacity of 30 to 50%, able to direct bed mobility and give occasional minimal assist, able to direct pressure relief activities, independent using a motorized wheelchair without hand controls on level surfaces, and able to direct all transfers.

Answer 8 C   9 C   10 A   11 B   12 A   13 B   14 A   15 A   16 C

A C5 level of lesion would have functional outcomes of vital capacity of 40 to 60%, able to give minimal assist with bed mobility, able to assist in a manual wheelchair, independent utilizing a motorized wheelchair with hand controls and able to direct transfers. A C7-C8 level of lesion would have functional outcomes of vital capacity of 60 to 80%, independent in bed mobility and pressure relief (including wheelchair push-ups, able to give moderate assist with transfers, independent on level surface with wheelchair.

Q 17. You are treating a 63-year-old lawyer for back pain who is referred to an orthopedic surgeon 60 miles out of town. The orthopedic surgeon owns his private clinic and tells the patient he must have physical therapy at his clinic. The patient approaches you because driving 20 minutes or more increases pain. What should you tell the patient?

[Physical Rehabilitation Sullivan/5th Ed./Pg. 53]

A. The physician is a fraud who is trying to make more money for his own physical therapy practice.
B. The physician owns his clinic, which is illegal; find another physician.
C. Tell the patient he has the right to attend the clinic of his choice. If he has any concerns, he should talk to his family physician that originally referred him for physical therapy.
D. Since the patient is a lawyer and interested in the physical therapy profession, discuss the legal and ethical information with him.

Ans. (C) Tell the patient he has the right to attend the clinic of his choice. If he has any concerns, he should talk to his family physician that originally referred him for physical therapy. It is important when talking that you be honest and up front about the patient's options to choose where to go for physical therapy.

Q 18. You are working with a cerebral palsy child. You notice that the child has great difficulty reaching for an object with one hand. The child prefers to reach for an object with both hands. What age would be considered normal for a child to be able to reach for an object with one hand?

[Essential Pediatrics O.P.Ghai/6th Ed./Pg. 44]

A. 3 months
B. 6 months
C. 1 year
D. 9 months

Ans. (B) At 6 months, a child should be able to reach for an object utilizing only one hand.

Q 19. You are assessing a patient with complaints of hip pain beginning at the greater trochanter with radiating symptoms extending down below the knee. There are no physical signs of injury and the patient is slightly tender to palpation on the greater trochanter. You suspect the patient's problems may be a result of iliotibial tightness. To evaluate the iliotibial band, which of the following tests would be the most appropriate to utilize?

[Orthopaedic Physical Assessment David J. Magee/
4th Ed./Pg. 632]

A. Thomas test
B. Straight leg raise test
C. Trendelenburg's test
D. Ober's test

Ans. (D) Ober's test is used to test for ilioband tightness. Thomas test is used to test for hip flexor tightness or contracture. Straight leg raise test evaluates hamstring tightness. Trendelenburg's test evaluates the strength of the gluteus muscle.

Q 20. Ans 18-year-old basketball player comes to the clinic complaining of acute left ankle pain. He reports that while practicing a jump shot, he came down and twisted his ankle on the lateral aspect. Upon evaluation, you find acute swelling and edema without the loss of integrity of the joint. The patient can ambulate without assistance or a support brace. Based on this information, which of the following is the correct grade to classify this patient's ankle sprain?

[Tidy's Physiotherapy K. M. Varghese/12th Ed./Pg. 40]

A. Grade four
B. Grade three
C. Grade two
D. Grade one

Ans. (D) A grade one sprain results in edema with very minor tearing and no loss of integrity to the ligament. A grade two sprain results in loss of integrity of the joint, and weight bearing with support or brace. A grade three sprain results in partial or complete tearing of the ligaments, and the patient is nonweight bearing initially. Grade four does not exist.

Q 21. You are the administrator of a facility determining the policy on retention and preservation of clinical records. The clinical records pertaining to patients must be maintained for a length of time after they are discharged. of the following, which is not an example of a policy on retention and preservation of clinical records?

[Tidy's Physiotherapy/12th Ed./Pg. 3]

A. Clinical records will be maintained for a period of 5 years from the date of patient discharge.
B. Clinical records of a minor will be retained for a period of 3 years after the patient comes of age.
C. Clinical records will be contained within a fireproof file cabinet on the premises.
D. Access to clinical records is available to all personnel from 8 am to 5 pm.

Ans. (D) The hours that the records are available are not relevant in a policy on retention and preservation of clinical records. Access to clinical records should not be available to all personnel but limited to authorized individuals. The authorized individuals should sign the appropriate medical releases.

Q 22. A patient is sent to physical therapy with a prescription for gait training. The physician has advised you to use a three-point gait pattern with axillary crutch nonweight bearing on the left lower extremity. The patient will need to be measured for correct crutch fitting. Which of the following would be the degree of elbow flexion that would be most desirable for axillary crutches?

[Concise Exercise Therapy Roshan lal/
1st Ed./Pg. 78]

A. O to 20°
B. 20° to 30°
C. 30°
D. 35°

Ans. (B) For accurate crutch measurement, the patient should have approximately 20° to 30° of elbow flexion. This would be considered the one best answer. In a three-point gait pattern, weight is borne on the noninvolved leg, then on both crutches,

---

Answer   17 C   18 B   19 D   20 D   21 D   22 B

then on the non- involved leg. Touchdown and progression to full weight bearing on the involved leg are usual.

Q 23. A 32-year-old female enters the emergency room with a knife injury to the spinal cord. The patient is referred to physical therapy for a comprehensive evaluation of the spinal cord injury. Medical history determines that the knife has caused a hemisection of the spinal cord. Of the following, which syndrome may be seen after a knife-type injury to the spinal cord that results in hemisection?

[Physical Rehabilitation Sullivan/5th Ed./Pg. 9441]

A. Marfan's syndrome
B. Amyotrophic lateral syndrome
C. Cerebellar syndrome
D. Brown-Sequard's syndrome

Ans. (D) Brown-Sequard's syndrome is a traumatic neurologic disorder resulting from compression of one side of the spinal cord above the 10th thoracic vertebrae. Brown-Sequard's syndrome results in hemisection of the spinal cord. It is typically seen after a knife- type injury. This also is an incomplete lesion, which typically results in loss of motor function on the same side as the lesion and loss of pain and temperature on the opposite side.

Q 24. While on the cardiopulmonary floor, the physician asks you to consult on another case. You find a 36-year-old male whose breathing alternates between periods of deep breathing and apnea. Therefore, the pattern of breathing is hyperpnea and apnea, especially when sleeping. What is another term for this type of breathing or disorder of rate and rhythm?

[Physical Rehabilitation Sullivan/5th Ed./Pg. 107]

A. Ataxic breathing
B. Biot's respiration
C. Cheyne-Stokes respiration
D. Sighing respiration

Ans. (C) Cheyne-Stokes respiration is an abnormal pattern of respiration characterized by alternating periods of apnea and deep, rapid breathing. Ataxic breathing associated with a lesion in the medullary respiratory centers is characterized by a series of inspirations and expirations. Biot's respiration is an abnormal respiratory pattern characterized by irregular breathing, often accompanied with a sigh with periods of apnea. Sighing respiration is periodic deep forced inspiration compressed gas or air in controlled ventilation.

Q 25. A patient is evaluated in a nursing home for an ulcer in the greater trochanter. The wound destruction is described in the following way: it involves full thickness of the dermis and undermining of the deeper tissues, and the muscle is slightly involved. There is no bone destruction. Given this information, which of the following stages would best describe this ulcer?

[Tidy's Physiotherapy/12th Ed./Pg. 276]

A. Stage one   B. Stage two
C. Stage three   D. Stage four

Ans. (C) Stage three involves full thickness of dermis and undermining of the deeper tissues, and the muscle may be involved. Stage one is destruction limited to the epidermis;

redness may be noted. Stage two is involvement of the epidermis, dermis, and subcutaneous fat, redness, edema, blistering, and hardening of the tissue. With stage four, full thickness is involved, penetrating to the fascia with possible muscle involvement and there is usually bone destruction.

Q 26. Your last patient of the day in the burn unit has an anterior neck burn. This patient has already received treatment to emphasize decreasing chances of flexion and healing in the area. It is now your responsibility to place this patient in a position to minimize contractures. Which of the following would be the correct positioning?

[Tidy's Physiotherapy K.M. Varghese/12th Ed./Pg. 307]

A. Flexion   B. Rotation
C. Extension   D. Hyperextension

Ans. (D) The neck should be placed in hyperextension to best minimize the chances of having a neck flexion contracture. Neck flexion contracture would be typically seen in the anterior burn, as this would be a position of comfort for the patient.

Q 27. A patient is referred to physical therapy with a diagnosis of Erb-Duchenne palsy/paralysis. The physician recommends a treatment program that will emphasize maintaining range of motion and preventing contractures. Erb-Duchenne paralysis is a result of damage to which of the following nerve roots?

[Tidy's Physiotherapy K. M. Varghese/12th Ed./Pg. 471]

A. C4, C5   B. C5, C6
C. C7, Cs   D. T1, T2

Ans. (B) Erb's palsy is a result of damage to the C5, C6 nerve root; signs of Erb's palsy include loss of sensation in the arm and paralysis and atrophy of the deltoid, biceps, and brachialis muscles. The typical position commonly seen in the affected extremity is arm adducted, internally rotated, elbow extended, and forearm pronated. Treatment emphasizes preventing contractures and range of motion.

Q 28. You are performing physical therapy in a nursing home where orthostatic hypotension occasionally occurs in some of the elderly patients. Which of the following would not be true concerning orthostatic hypotension?

[Physical Rehabilitation Sullivan/5th Ed./Pg. 601-602]

A. It can occur as a result of a patient assuming an upright position
B. It is common after long periods of bedrest
C. It is common in elderly patients
D. It lasts for only 24 hours

Ans. (D) Orthostatic hypotension is an abnormally low blood pressure occurring when an individual assumes the standing posture. It can last for more than 24 hours.

Q 29. You are working with a patient in the pulmonary wing of the hospital. You are observing the patient bedside, noting a particular pattern of breathing. The patient appears to be gasping for breath, and on occasion her shoulders and thorax rise on inspiration and her abdominal wall is retracted. Which of the following would you most likely suspect given this patient's pattern of breathing?

[Physical Rehabilitation Sullivan/5th Ed./Pg. 565]

Answer   23 D   24 C   25 C   26 D   27 B   28 D

A. She suffers from barrel chest
B. She is a paradoxical breather
C. She is an upper-chest breather
D. She has had a lung removed

Ans. (C) The pattern of breathing for an upper chest breather would be for the patient to gasp for breath and, on occasion, her shoulder and thorax would rise and her abdominal wall retract. This is because the patient is primarily breathing with her upper chest. Barrel chest is a large, rounded thorax. This is considered normal in some stocky individuals and those who live in high-altitude areas and have developed increased vital capacities. Paradoxical breathing is a condition in which a part of the lung deflates during inspiration and inflates during expiration.

Q 30. You are in anatomy class studying motions of the wrist. It is known that the motion that the wrist produces is actually a combination of several motions at several different articulations. Which of the following would best describe the axis of motion for the radial and ulnar deviation?
        [Joint Structure and Function/Norkin/3rd Ed./Pg. 258]
A. It lies in the sagittal plane through the capitate
B. It lies in the sagittal plane through the trapezoid
C. It lies in the coronal plane through the lunate
D. It lies in the coronal plane through the capitate

Ans. (A) The axis motion that the radial and ulnar deviation lies in would be the sagittal plane through the capitate. All other answers are incorrect.

Q 31. You are instructed to perform mobilization on the glenohumeral joint of a patient 6 weeks postheart surgery. You wish to increase abduction of the shoulder for this patient. Which of the following would be the correct mobilization technique?
        [Therapeutic Exercise Kisner/4th Ed./Pg. 122]
A. Inferior glide
B. Posterior glide
C. Anterior glide
D. Posterior and anterior glide

Ans. (A) Inferior glide is the correct mobilization technique to perform to increase abduction of the glenohumeral joint. Posterior glide would increase flexion and anterior glide would increase extension.

Q 32. You are a physical therapist working in private practice and in charge of marketing a new work-conditioning program to the public and physicians. You are on a fixed budget and must determine the most appropriate marketing media for you to utilize. Which of the following would gain the most access to the public and maintain cost control?
        [Tidy's Physiotherapy/K. M. Varghese/12th Ed./Pg. 2]
A. An extensive color brochure with pictures to be mailed to all physicians and insurance companies
B. A direct mail campaign to members of the community and surrounding communities
C. Newspaper advertisement
D. Telephone calls to physicians' offices and insurance companies

Ans. (C) With a fixed budget, the most effective and inexpensive way to reach an audience and gain access to a large number of potential patients would be to utilize a newspaper advertisement. Colored brochures with pictures are typically very expensive to create early on. Direct mail can be expensive, as it involves not only postage but also the cost of the actual brochure. Telephone calls, while inexpensive, do not reach a large group of people in a short period of time.

Q 33. A patient reports to the clinic experiencing an acute episode of back pain. Upon entering the clinic the patient's knee buckles and he must be transported to the department via a wheelchair. The physician's order states "evaluate and treat appropriately," with no specific indication for the frequency of treatment. Which of the following would be the appropriate frequency of treatment for this Particular patient?
        [Physical Rehabilitation Sullivan/5th Ed./Pg. 14]
A. Patient should be seen two times a day, daily at the outpatient facility
B. Patient should be seen three times a week
C. Patient should be seen daily Monday through Friday
D. Patient should be seen two times a week

Ans. (C) In the acute stages, the patient should be seen daily, Monday through Friday. Seeing the patient two times a day, daily, may be considered overutilization by the insurance carrier. Seeing the patient two to three times a week would be nonaggressive treatment for a patient in severe pain. When the patient is over the acute stage, it would be appropriate to decrease the number of visits.

Q 34. A patient is sent to physical therapy with a burn on the posterior aspect of the elbow. The patient has a low pain tolerance and was admitted to the hospital in the early morning. It is afternoon and the patient is sent down for physical therapy. Which of the following would be the most appropriate treatment program?
        [Therapeutic Exercise Foundation/Kisner/3rd Ed./Pg. 47]
A. Active range of motion emphasizing flexion
B. Active range of motion emphasizing extension
C. Passive range of motion emphasizing extension and positioning of the elbow in full extension
D. Whirlpool

Ans. (C) The most appropriate immediate treatment for a burn patient is passive range of motion in extension, as well as emphasizing position of the elbow in full extension. This is done to prevent flexion contractures. Depending upon the extent of the burn, whirlpool may be ordered for debridement.

Q 35. Investigative procedure most commonly and preferably of head injury used for investigation of an unconfused patient brought to the emergency department of the hospital:
        [Human Anatomy B. D. Chaurasia/4th Ed./Pg. 245]
A. CT Scan   B. MRI
C. PET Scan   D. History taking

Ans. (A) CT Scan is quick, less time consuming and does not affect implants/pacemaker.

Q 36. You are an educational instructor of a physical therapist program. You explain to the class that scores on testing are

---

Answer   29 C   30 A   31 A   32 C   33 C   34 C   35 A going to be compared to standard deviation of the mean. What percentage of students taking your examination would you expect to score within plus and minus one standard deviation of the mean?

[Hicks/4th Ed./Pg. 55]

A. 68%
B. 70%
C. 72%
D. 50%

Ans. (A) Standard deviation of the mean plus or minus one is graded based on the score of 68% of the students.

Q 37. Your patient is a 44-year-old female with low back pain resulting from no apparent cause/reason. You decide to set her up in traction with a hold period of 40 seconds, rest period 10 seconds, for 20 minutes at 60 pounds. What type of traction does this best describe?

[Physical Agents in Rehabilitation Cameroon 2nd Ed./Pg. 324]

A. Autotraction
B. Gravity lumbar traction
C. Manual traction
D. Intermittent mechanical traction

Ans. (D) Intermittent mechanical traction is described as intermittent traction when there is typically a hold and rest period. Autotraction utilizes a special traction bench made-up of two sections that can be individually angled and rotated. The patient applies traction by pulling with his or her own arms. With gravity lumbar traction, the lower border and the circumference of the rib cage are anchored through a specially made vest secured to the top of the bed. The patient is placed on a bed that is tilted vertically, putting the patient in a position in which the free weight of the legs and hips exerts a traction force on the lumbar spine by gravity. With manual traction, the therapist grasps the patient and manually applies a traction force either for a few seconds or by a sudden, quick thrust.

Q 38. A patient is seen in physical therapy for a disturbance in his static equilibrium. When testing the patient, you have him stand perfectly still and instruct him to close his eyes. Upon doing this the patient wavers from side to side and starts to fall, but you catch him and help him sit back down on the mat. Which of the following tests has most likely been performed on this patient?

[Orthopedic Physical Assessment David J. Magee/ 4th Ed./Pg. 109]

A. Labyrinthine righting reflex
B. Romberg's sign
C. Babinski's sign
D. Chronic labyrinthine test

Ans. (B) The description in this question describes the Romberg's sign. Labyrinthine righting is one of the five basic neuromuscular reactions involved in a change of body positions. The change stimulates cells in the canals of the inner ear, causing neck muscles to respond and adjust the head to the new position. The Babinski's sign involves the hallucis longus muscle.

Q 39. You are a physical therapist who has been sent out to consult with a nursing home secondary to ulcers on the ischial tuberosities of several patients. Upon entering the nursing home, you begin to observe the patients. You notice redness, edema, blistering, and hardening of tissue. The inflammation has extended into the fat layer and there is superficial necrosis. Which of the following stages is characterized by such symptoms?

[Physiotherapy Tidy's/12th Ed./Pg. 276]

A. Stage one
B. Stage two
C. Stage three
D. Stage four

Ans. (B) Stage two is associated with redness, edema, blistering, and hardening of the tissue. In stage two, there would also be an inflammation that extends into the fat layer with superficial necrosis. Stage one is associated with destruction limited to the epidermis; redness may be noted. Stage three involves full thickness of dermis and undermining of the deeper tissues; also the muscle may be involved. Stage four involves full thickness penetrating to the fascia with possible muscle involvement, and there is usually bone destruction.

Q 40. A physical therapist works part-time at an inpatient treatment facility, as well as being a self-employed contractor to several group homes. Is it the responsibility of the physical therapist to obtain individual malpractice and liability insurance for the contracted work?

[Physical Rehabilitation Sullivan/5th Ed./Pg. 10 -13]

A. Yes, it is the responsibility of the physical therapist working as an independent contractor to carry individual liability coverage.
B. No, liability coverage from the physical therapist's primary work setting provides comprehensive coverage.
C. No, it is the responsibility of the group homes to carry liability insurance for their contracted service providers.
D. Yes, liability coverage from the inpatient setting is nullified if the physical therapist takes on private clients.

Ans. (A) It is the responsibility of the physical therapist working as an independent contractor to carry individual liability coverage. Liability coverage for a physical therapist working in any kind of treatment facility extends only to the patients/clients treated under the auspices of that facility.

Q 41. You are evaluating a 26-year-old male patient status postarthroscopic surgery. The physician requests that you evaluate the muscles that insert into the pes anserinus. You have the patient flex the knee and medially rotate the leg while the knee is flexed. of the muscles listed below, which are you not evaluating?

[Joint Structure and Function/Norkin/ 3rd Ed./Pg. 348]

A. Gracilis
B. Sartorius
C. Semimembranosus
D. Semitendinosus

Ans. (C) Semimembranosus is the muscle that you would not be evaluating, as it does not insert into the pes anserinus. However, the semimembranosus extends the thigh, and flexes and medially rotates the leg. The three muscles that insert into the pes anserinus are the gracilis, sartorius, and semitendinosus. The pes anserinus is located at the medial border of the tibial tuberosity. The gracilis adducts the thigh, and flexes and rotates the leg medially. The semitendinosus extends the thigh, flexes and medially rotates the leg.

Q 42. A patient who has a lesion of the inferior gluteal nerve is referred to the clinic. Which of the following motions would most likely be affected to the greatest extent secondary to an inferior gluteal nerve lesion?

[Human Anatomy B. D. Chaurasia/4th Ed./Pg. 73]

A. Hip abduction
B. Hip adduction
C. Hip flexion
D. Hip extension

Ans. (D) The correct answer is hip extension as the inferior gluteal nerve supplies the gluteus maximus muscle. The gluteus maximus muscle is the main extensor of the thigh. Therefore, hip extension would be the motion most likely to be affected to the greatest extent. The superior gluteal nerve supplies the gluteus medius, gluteus minimus, and tensor fasciae latae.

Q 43. When performing ultrasound on a patient it is important to be aware of contraindications for its utilization. One contraindication is performing ultrasound over the epiphyseal or growth plate of a child. Which of the following statements is not true concerning the growth plate?

[Low and Reed/3rd Ed./Pg. 200]

A. It serves as a site of progressive lengthening that is needed in the long bones
B. It lies between the epiphysis and diaphysis as a transverse disk
C. It is formed of cartilage
D. It is found in all bones

Ans. (D) It is not true that the epiphyseal or growth plate is found in all bones. The epiphyseal or growth plate may only be found in long bones after growth has been completed. It is then replaced by a dense calcified formation known as an epiphyseal line.

Q 44. In a class on clinical pathology, the professor asks you what lupus erythematosus, scleroderma and dermatomycosis have in common. They can best be grouped together as which of the following?

[K.M. Varghese/Tidy's Physiotherapy/12th Ed./Pg. 145]

A. Acute infections
B. Acute bacterial diseases
C. Collagen vascular diseases
D. Circulatory disorders

Ans. (C) These three pathologies together are best described as collagen vascular diseases.
Lupus erythematosus is a chronic inflammation disease of the connective tissue, affecting skin, joints, kidney, and nervous system. A butterfly rash is characteristic. Scleroderma is a chronic disease causing sclerosis of the skin and certain organs, e.g, lungs, heart, and kidney. Skin is taut, edematous, firmly bound to subcutaneous tissue, and leathery. Dermatomycosis is a skin infection caused by certain fungi.

Q 45. You are treating a patient who is complaining of right shoulder pain. The patient has been diagnosed with a frozen adhesive capsulated shoulder. Which of the following would describe the capsular pattern of the glenohumeral joint?

[Orthopedic Physical Assessment David J. Magee/5th Ed./Pg. 208]

A. External rotation, abduction, internal rotation
B. External rotation, internal rotation, abduction
C. Internal rotation, abduction, external rotation
D. Abduction, external rotation, internal rotation

Ans. (A) The glenohumeral joint's capsular pattern in a frozen adhesive capsulated shoulder starts with restriction of external rotation, then abduction, followed by internal rotation.

Q 46. The chart review reveals a patient with a condition known as thyrotoxicosis. This condition is due to hyperthyroidism. The disease is characterized by an enlargement of the thyroid gland. What is not another more common name for this disease?

[Medicine Davidson/20th Ed./Pg. 746]

A. Graves' disease
B. Fibrous dysplasia
C. Secondary hyperthyroidism
D. Primary hyperthyroidism

Ans. (B) Fibrous dysplasia is not another name for thyrotoxicosis, as this pertains to an abnormal condition characterized by the fibrous displacement of the osseous tissue within the affected bones. Graves' disease, as well as primary and secondary hyperthyroidism, is also called thyrotoxicosis. The condition of hyperthyroidism is typically caused by secretions of the thyroid gland, which increases the basal metabolism rate, causing an increased demand for food to support metabolic activities.

Q 47. A 21-year-old female sprains her ankle at a basketball game. You are the medical staff member attending the game. You notice that swelling is beginning but she insists on continuing to play. Which of the following modalities would not decrease swelling?

[Electrotherapy/Clayton/AITBS/9th Ed./Pg. 199]

A. Ice massage
B. Cryopressure
C. Ice towel
D. Evaporative coolant

Ans. (D) Evaporative coolants or a spray do not significantly lower tissue temperature below the surface. Evaporative coolants cause a chemical reaction that produces a cool feeling on the outside surface of the skin. Ice massage, cryopressure, and ice towels all decrease swelling by decreasing tissue temperature.

Q 48. A patient with inflammation comes to the clinic with evaluation and treatment orders. Which of the following modalities could be utilized to place chemical substances into the body with direct current to decrease inflammation?

[Electrotherapy/Clayton/9th Ed./Pg. 86]

A. Myoflex with ultrasound
B. Phonophoresis
C. Iontophoresis
D. Ultrasound

Ans. (C) Iontophoresis is a modality in which chemical substances are entered into the body with a direct current to decrease inflammation. Myoflex with ultrasound, phonophoresis, and ultrasound are treatments that may decrease inflammation but are not chemical substances placed into the body with a direct current.

Q 49. You are working with a physical therapist student when performing short-wave diathermy on a 36-year-old female patient. You explain that this treatment is an example of heat

---

Answer   42 D   43 D   44 C   45 A   46 B   47 D   48 C

transferred by energy. Which term listed below correctly identifies this type of heat transfer?

[Electrotherapy Clayton/9th Ed./Pg. 6]

A. Conversion
B. Convection
C. Conduction
D. Radiation

Ans. (B) Convection is the transfer of heat energy by combining mechanisms of fluid and conduction, e.g. diathermy, paraffin. Conversion does not exist. Conduction is heat transferred from one part of the body to another through molecular collision, e.g. hot packs. Radiation is heat transferred in the form of electromagnetic waves without heating the intervening medium, e.g. warming by the sun.

Q 50. You are requested to treat a 56-year-old male in the neurointensive care unit. You find the following results on the patient: no voluntary movement, unresponsive to stimulus, no reflexes, and positive Babinski response. Which most likely describes this patient's condition?

[Neurology Illustrated/Lindsay/3rd Ed./Pg. 82]

A. Cerebrovascular accident
B. Coma
C. Stupor
D. Uncooperative patient

Ans. (B) A patient in a coma would show no voluntary movement, be unresponsive to stimulus, have no reflexes, and exhibit a positive Babinski response. The after-effect of a cerebrovascular accident depends on the location and extent of ischemia. Paralysis, weakness, speech defect, aphasia, and even death may occur. Patients in a stupor would exhibit a state of lethargy and unresponsiveness in which they seem unaware of their surroundings.

Model Question Paper - 15

Q 1. You have a cardiac patient 3 days postoperative referred to cardiac rehab program. The physician refers the patient to physical therapy for you to implement a treatment program. Which of the following treatment programs would be appropriate for this patient?

[Tidy's Physiotherapy/12th Ed./Pg. 245]

A. Ambulating 200 yards in a 5-minute period with no EKG changes or changes in symptoms
B. Lower extremity ergometry x 15 minutes
C. Lower extremity ergometry x 30 minutes
D. Upper extremity ergometry x 15 minutes

Ans. (A) When treating a patient 3 days postoperative, it would be appropriate for the patient to have monitored ambulation with no symptoms. Lower extremity ergometry x 15 or x 30 minutes, and upper extremity ergometry x 15 minutes would be too aggressive to start on a patient 3 days postcardiac surgery.

Q 2. You are performing a treatment program for a neurological patient. You move the patient's extremity through a predetermined range of motion. This motion is shoulder flexion and extension. Then the patient is requested to repeat the movement on her own. Which of the following are you most likely performing on this patient?

[Physical Rehabilitation/Sullivan/5th Ed./Pg. 1343]

A. Kinesthesia
B. Proprioception
C. Graphesthesia
D. Barognosis

Ans. (B) Proprioception tests the patient's ability to determine the direct position sense. Kinesthesia tests the patient's ability to determine movement sensation. Graphesthesia tests the ability of a patient to recognize letters and numbers written on the patient's skin. Barognosis is the ability to determine the weight of an object.

Q 3. A 25-year-old female 6 days post cesarean delivery has been referred to you for training in proper posture and body mechanics. Which of the following would be the proper instructions for body mechanics for a postcesarean patient?

[Tidy's Physiotherapy/12th Ed./Pg. 397]

A. Whenever sitting, the patient should avoid hard chairs because they have poor back support
B. When standing, the patient should relax the abdominal muscles in order not to place any strain upon them
C. When bending over, the patient should keep a flattened lordotic curve in the low back with a wide base of support and legs parallel
D. When getting up from a lying-down position, the patient should roll over to the side, swinging the legs over the edge and getting up slowly

Ans. (D) Proper body mechanics for a post cesarean patient would be to get- up from a lying down position by rolling over to the side, swinging the legs over the edge, and getting up slowly. When sitting, the patient should avoid soft chairs, as they are hard to get-up from and have poor back support. When standing, the patient should keep the chin in and contract the abdominal muscles. When bending over, the patient should keep a curve in the low back with one foot in front of the other.

Q 4. You are in physiology class studying tissue excitation. In regard to the strength/duration curve, which of the following is not a true statement?

[Electrotherapy/Claytons/8th Ed./Pg. 88]

A. It may be considered valuable in testing for nerve degeneration
B. It may be considered valuable in testing for nerve regeneration
C. It shows the relationship of current intensity to the duration of reaching expected threshold
D. It exhibits development and fatigue during a prolonged stimulus

Ans. (D) It is an untrue statement that the strength/duration curve exhibits development and fatigue during a prolonged stimulus. Strength/duration curve is utilized in testing for nerve degeneration and regeneration. It will also show the relationship of the stimulus intensity to duration in reaching an excitation threshold.

Q 5. In a class on physiology of exercise, you are studying the energy needed for muscle contractions. Which of the following statements is false in regard to energy for muscle contractions?

[Human Physiology and Biochemistry/A. K. Jain/2nd Ed./Pg. 448]

A. Energy is produced during aerobic metabolism
B. Energy is produced during anaerobic metabolism
C. Energy may be stored as creatine phosphate
D. Energy is derived from ATP (adenosine triphosphate).

Ans. (C) In regard to energy for muscle contractions, it is false that energy may be stored as creatine phosphate. All other statements are true.

Q 6. You are studying diabetes mellitus and diabetes insipidus in your clinical pathology course. Which of the following statements is not true about diabetes mellitus, but best describes diabetes insipidus?

[Human Physiology and Biochemistry/A. K. Jain/2nd Ed./Pg. 228]

A. It is a disorder of carbohydrate metabolism
B. It results from insulin deficiency

Answer 1 A 2 B 3 D 4 D 5 C

C. It is associated with the pancreas

D. It is associated with the pituitary gland

Ans. (D) The most distinctive feature of diabetes mellitus versus diabetes insipidus is that diabetes insipidus is associated with a pituitary disease, typically a tumor in the pituitary, while diabetes mellitus is associated with the pancreas.

Q 7. Which of the following gestational timeframes is the most susceptible for injury to the fetal cardiovascular system? It is during this time frame that the fetal cardiovascular system produces most congenital defects.

[Tidy's Physiotherapy/12th Ed./Pg. 239]

A. Third Forth

B. Sixth month

C. Between the 21st and 40th days

D. Conception and the 20th day

Ans. (C) The period between the 21st and the 40th day of gestation is the time during prenatal development when the cardiovascular system is beginning its development and is most at risk.

Q 8. You are working with a neurological patient and are concerned about promoting stability. You have to plan a treatment course that includes PNF patterns to increase and promote stability in this patient. What type of PNF pattern listed below would be most appropriate?

[Principal of Exercise Therapy/Dena Gardiner/Pg. 83]

A. Traction   B. Contract-relax

C. Slow reversal   D. Approximation

Ans. (D) Approximation is used to promote stability. Traction is used to promote mobility. Contract-relax is used to increase range of motion. Slow reversal is used to strengthen weakened muscle.

Q 9. You are a physical therapist providing athletic coverage to a high school basketball game. One of the players is injured and begins hemorrhaging. You notice that there is oozing and a gradual seeping of blood from the wounded area. It was easy for you to control the bleeding through elevation of the injured area and applying direct pressure over the wound. Which of the following is the type of hemorrhaging that this patient is most likely experiencing?

[Human Physiology and Biochemistry/A. K. Jain/2nd Ed./Pg. 58]

A. Arterial hemorrhage   B. Venous hemorrhage

C. Capillary hemorrhage   D. Internal hemorrhage

Ans. (C) Capillary hemorrhaging best describes a hemorrhage in which there is oozing and a gradual seeping of blood from the wounded area. This type of hemorrhage can be controlled through elevation of the injured part and direct pressure applied over the wound. Arterial hemorrhage is a condition in which the artery has been damaged or severed. This results in a very rapid flow of bright red blood, which usually escapes in a rhythmical spurting with each heartbeat. Venous hemorrhage is characterized by a rapid state of infusion of dark blood from the wounded area. Internal hemorrhage is unexposed and can only be identified through X-ray or diagnostic techniques.

Q 10. You are a physical therapist practicing in a rural setting with a physical therapist assistant. You receive a phone call late at night and, due to a family emergency, you will be unable to work at the clinic the next day. You have 20 patients scheduled for physical therapy between you and the physical therapist assistant. What would be the most appropriate response to care for these patients?

[5th Ed./Pg. 13,16]

A. Reschedule the patients for your return to work the next day

B. Have the physical therapist assistant treat all the patients, utilizing your progress notes from the prior week

C. Call the physical therapy department some time the next day to inform them of what treatments the patients should receive

D. Provide a thorough summary of each patient and leave it at the department for the physical therapist assistant to begin with the next morning

Ans. (D) Prior to leaving, you should provide a thorough assessment of each patient's condition and the type of treatment to be administered. It would also be appropriate to call in during the day, early if possible, to see if any questions exist.

Q 11. A patient is sent to the physical therapy department with a burn on the right lower extremity from the posterior thigh to below the knee. The patient needs to be positioned to prevent contractures of the knee. Which of the following should be immediately implemented into this patient's treatment program?

[Physical Rehabilitation/Sullivan/5th Ed./Pg. 1106]

A. Exercises to increase the strength of the hamstring muscles

B. Posterior splint with emphasis on extension

C. An anterior splint with emphasis on flexion

D. A whirlpool for wound care

Ans. (B) With a posterior knee burn, a knee flexion contracture would be common. Therefore, a posterior splint with an extension should be the first priority of the therapist to prevent knee flexion contracture.

Q 12. A patient is referred to the physical therapy department status post total hip replacement. The orders read "partial weightbearing utilizing a walker." Which of the following would be the most appropriate pattern given the above information?

[Physical Rehabilitation/Sullivan/5th Ed./Pg. 55]

A. Walker first, then involved lower extremity, then uninvolved extremity is advanced

B. Walker first, then one lower extremity, then the other lower extremity is advanced

C. Walker first, then uninvolved lower extremity, then involved lower extremity is advanced

D. Uninvolved extremity, then the walker, then the involved lower extremity is advanced

Ans. (A) For partial weight bearing, the walker should be advanced first, and then the patient should advance the involved lower extremity, then the uninvolved.

Answer   6 D   7 C   8 D   9 C   10 D   11 B   12 A

Q 13. A patient is referred to physical therapy with a cervical and a vertebral disc disorder. The patient reports no previous history of cervical pain. She had a flare-up approximately 2 weeks ago so she went to see her neurologist. The neurologist has ordered intermittent cervical traction daily along with moist heat, ultrasound, and massage. Note that the patient has no structural abnormalities and slight tenderness to pressure at this time. In implementing this patient's treatment program, which of the following would be the most appropriate set-up of traction?

[Physical Agent is Rehabilitation/Cameroon/Pg. 235]
A. Cervical traction starting at 8 pounds
B. Cervical traction starting at 16 pounds
C. Cervical traction starting at 20 pounds
D. Cervical traction starting at 10 pounds

Ans. (B) Cervical traction should be started with 16 pounds in an attempt to get some separation of the cervical vertebra and the intervertebral disc.

Q 14. You are treating a nursing home patient with a stage-three ulcer on the greater trochanter of the left hip. You are requested to instruct the nursing staff on what would be the most appropriate course of action to avoid future ulcers in other residents. Which of the following would be the most appropriate response?

[Tidy's Physiotherapy/12th Ed./Pg. 283]
A. You are too disgusted to go to the nursing home and they will have to find another therapist
B. You should change the patient's position in bed to relieve weight on bony prominences every 24 hours
C. When lying in bed, the patient should be given a donut cushion to support bony prominences
D. The patient should be checked frequently for red spots and turned in bed at least every 2 hours

Ans. (D) The patient should be checked frequently for red spots or the beginning stages of bedsores. Additionally, he or she should be turned frequently to different positions to prevent further aggravation of a sore. It is commonly recommended that the patient be turned every 2 hours.

Q 15. A patient enters the clinic with acute back pain. Upon testing, you notice that the back pain increases from the low back down the right posterior aspect of the lower extremity. You perform a range of motion assessment, and repeated flexion severely increases this patient's pain. In implementing a treatment program for this patient, which of the following would be the most appropriate exercise initially?
A. Williams' exercises
B. McKenzie exercises
C. Prone lying times 15 minutes
D. Proper posture and body mechanics instruction
[Concise Exercise Therapy/Roshan Lal Meena/1st Ed./Pg. 275]

Ans. (B) The most important treatment technique to start with this patient is McKenzie exercises, since repeated flexion upon range of motion testing increases low back pain. McKenzie exercises emphasize the "extension principle" to reduce back pain. Increased pain upon repeated flexion indicates that the patient should be treated with back extension exercises to reduce symptoms.

Q 16. You implement a gait treatment program for a patient emphasizing the muscle group responsible for deceleration of the limb. You notice through gait evaluation that the patient is having a problem decelerating the unsupported limb. Which of the following muscles would be emphasized in planning this patient's treatment program?

[Joint Structure and Function/Norkin/3rd Ed./Pg. 465]
A. Quadriceps group   B. Hamstring group
C. Gastrocnemius   D. Anterior tibialis

Ans. (B) The hamstring group is responsible for decelerating the unsupported limb and should be emphasized in the treatment of this patient.

Q 17. In determining a target heart rate for a 62-year-old patient, you would use the calculation for maximum heart rate. Which of the following best describes the calculation for maximum heart rate?

[Human Physiology and Biochemistry/A. K. Jain/2nd Ed./Pg. 449]
A. Pulse rate for 60 seconds
B. Count pulse for 15 seconds x 4, plus age
C. (220 plus age)
D. (220 minus age)

Ans. (D) Maximum heart rate is calculated by 220 minus age. This number can be used to help determine target heart rate at which you want the patient to exercise when it is multiplied by 60 to 90%, depending on the level of exercise desired.

Q 18. A patient undergoes open heart surgery at a prestigious heart hospital. The patient is being evaluated 1 day postoperatively for possible placement in the acute inpatient cardiac rehab program. The patient's blood pressure reading indicates hypertension. Which of the following readings would be considered indicative of hypertension?

[Human Physiology and Biochemistry/ A. K. Jain/2nd Ed./Pg. 450]
A. 120/80   B. Above 120/80
C. Above 140/90   D. Under 120/90

Ans. (C) It would be indicative of hypertension if blood pressure readings were above 140/90. Typically, hypertension is indicated when three different readings are all 140/90 or above.

Q 19. A patient comes to you from the hand surgeon with a request to specifically evaluate the anatomical snuffbox. The hand surgeon is concerned that the patient might have suffered an injury to the nerve crossing the anatomical snuffbox. Of the following nerves, which would you need to evaluate?

[Essentials of Orthopaedics and Applied Physiotherapy/Jayant Joshi/1st Ed./Pg. 266]
A. Radial   B. Median
C. Ulnar   D. Musculocutaneous

Ans. (A) The radial nerve, which is the largest branch of the brachial plexus, arising on each side as a continuation of the

---

Answer   13 B   14 D   15 B   16 B   17 D   18 C   19 A posterior cord, is the nerve that passes through the anatomical snuffbox of the wrist. Therefore, if you were evaluating a patient who might have suffered an injury to the nerve crossing the anatomical snuffbox, you would evaluate the radial nerve. The median nerve is one of the terminal branches of the brachial plexus that extends along the radial portions of the forearm and hand and supplies various muscles and the skin of these parts. The ulnar nerve is one of the terminal branches of the brachial plexus that arises on each side from the medial cord of the plexus. The musculocutaneous nerve is one of the terminal branches of the brachial plexus.

Q 20. A patient comes to you status post ankle sprain which is healing well. The patient needs to increase range of motion to resume full activity. Of the following, which movement will take place in the ankle subtalar joint?

[Essentials of Orhtopaedics and Applied/Jayant Joshi/
1st Ed./Pg. 555]

A. Pronation/supination
B. Eversion/inversion
C. Adduction/abduction
D. Dorsiflexion

Ans. (B) At the subtalar joint of the ankle, eversion and inversion movements take place.

Q 21. An 8-year-old male enters the clinic with a diagnosis of fracture of the distal radius. The patient's mother reports that the patient was riding his bicycle down a steep hill when he fell off. The physician sends the patient to you for evaluation because he is concerned about possible nerve damage. A fracture of the distal radius will result in possible nerve damage to which nerve?

[Essentials of Orthopedics and Applied Physiotherapy/
Jayant Joshi/1st Ed./Pg. 266]

A. Musculocutaneous
B. Radial
C. Ulnar
D. Median

Ans. (B) The radial nerve would most likely be injured, as it is in the closest proximity to the distal radius.

Q 22. A patient comes to the clinic with a swollen right thumb. He reports that he was at work operating a press machine when the press closed and caught his thumb. The patient will need joint immobilization to restore range of motion; otherwise he has escaped with minimal injury. The carpometacarpal joint of the thumb is classified as what type of joint?

[Joint Structure and Function/Norkin/3rd Ed./Pg. 277]

A. Uniaxial
B. Biaxial
C. Saddle
D. Hinge

Ans. (C) The carpometacarpal joint in the thumb is unique in that it is classified as a saddle joint. A saddle joint permits no axial rotation but allows flexion, extension, adduction, and abduction. The uniaxial joint is a synovial joint in which movement is only in one axis as with a pivot or hinge joint. A hinge joint is a synovial joint providing a connection in which articular surfaces are closely molded together in a manner that permits extension motion in one place.

Q 23. A muscle is known to have a proximal and distal attachment. It is necessary to know the attachments for

palpation and manual muscle tests. Which of the following is the proximal attachment of a limb muscle?

[Joint Structure and Function/Norkin/3rd Ed./Pg. 96]

A. Tendon
B. Insertion
C. Belly of muscle
D. Origin

Ans. (D) Origin is the proximal attachment of a limb muscle. Tendon, one of many white, glistening fibrous bands of tissue that attach muscle to bone, refers to the tendinous structure. Insertion is the distal attachment of the muscle. The belly is the belly part of the muscle.

Q 24. A patient enters the clinic with what appears to be pinched nerves in the cervical spine area. The patient is reporting radiating symptoms into the left upper extremity that follow no particular dermatome pattern. The patient reports that he is going to have a test in which some type of electrodes are inserted into the muscle to test which nerves are injured. Based on this information, which of the following tests is the patient most likely having?

[Physical Rehabilitation/Sullivan/5th Ed./Pg. 273]

A. Electromyogram
B. Arthroscopy
C. EKG
D. Myelogram

Ans. (A) Electromyogram helps in diagnosing neuromuscular problems by applying surface electrodes or by inserting a needle electrode into the muscle and observing electric activity with an oscilloscope and a loudspeaker. Arthroscopy is the examination of the interior of a joint, performed by inserting a specially designed endoscope through a small incision. An ECG (electrocardiogram. is a graphic record produced by an electrocardiograph. A myelogram is an X-ray film taken after injection of a radiopaque medium into the subarachnoid space to demonstrate any distortions of the spinal cord, spinal nerve roots, and subarachnoid space.

Q 25. Your neuroanatomy professor lectures on the divisions of the brain. The brain is divided into three major divisions. Which of the following is not one of the three major brain regions?

[Tidy's Physiotherapy/12th Ed./Pg. 314]

A. Brainstem
B. Midbrain
C. Cerebellum
D. Cerebrum

Ans. (B) The midbrain, one of the three parts of the brainstem and lying below the cerebrum and just above the pons, is not considered one of the three major brain regions. The three major divisions of the brain region are (1. brainstem, which is the portion of the brain comprising the medulla oblongata, the pons, and the mesencephalon; (2. cerebellum, the part of the brain located in the posterior cranial fossa behind the brainstem; (3. cerebrum, the largest and uppermost section of the brain divided by a central sulcus into the left and right cerebral hemispheres.

Q 26. A pregnant patient is advised to avoid the Valsalva maneuver during her pregnancy. What effect listed below does the Valsalva maneuver have?

[Orthopaedic Physical Assessment/Magee/
5th Ed./Pg. 568]

A. Increase in intrathoracic pressure
B. Decrease in intrathoracic pressure
C. Pressure remains the same, no effect
D. Increase in inspiration needs

Ans. (A) The Valsalva maneuver is a forced expiratory effort against a closed airway, as when an individual holds his or her breath and tightens the muscles in a strenuous effort to move a heavy object or to change position in bed. In pregnancy, the Valsalva maneuver both increases pressure on the pelvic diaphragm and causes fluctuations in venous return to the heart.

Q 27. You are in physiology class studying the difference between erythrocytes and leukocytes in the body. Each one has a primary function to perform so that the body functions normally. Which of the following would be a primary function of erythrocytes in the body?
[Human Physiology and Biochemistry/A. K. Jain/
2nd Ed./Pg. 35]

A. Transport oxygen
B. Carry iron
C. Produce calcium
D. Produce red blood cells

Ans. (A) The main function of erythrocytes, also known as red blood cells, is to transport oxygen in the body, Erythrocytes are biconcave disc that contain hemoglobin confined within a lipid membrane, Erythrocytes originate in the marrow of the long bones.

Q 28. You are continuing your studies in neurology on abnormal reflexes. You are now focusing on the reflex called the flexor withdrawal. The flexor withdrawal integration level is spinal. Where would the stimulus be applied to test the flexor withdrawal?
[Cash's Textbook of Neurology for Physiotherapy/
4th Ed./Pg. 526]

A. Sole of the foot with lower extremity in extension
B. Sole of the foot with lower extremity in flexion
C. Forefoot with the lower extremity in extension
D. Forefoot with the lower extremity in flexion

Ans. (A) The stimulus for testing flexor withdrawal is applied to the sole of the foot with the lower extremity in extended position to start.

Q 29. You are testing the tonic labyrinthine reflex of a patient. You have positioned the patient supine. Which of the following would you consider to be a positive response to this position?
A. Increased extensor tone
B. Increased flexor tone
C. Increased extensor tone in upper extremities and flexor tone
D. Increased flexor tone in upper extremities and extensor tone in lower extremities
[Cash's Textbook of Neurology for Physiotherapy/
Saunder/4th Ed./Pg. 527]

Ans. (A) An increase in extensor tone occurs when the patient's position is supine for the tonic labyrinthine reflex, No specific stimulus is required and the response is dependent upon patient positioning, prone increases flexor tone, side-lying increases extensor tone, and the other sidelying limb increases flexor tone in the nonweight bearing limb.

Q 30. You are testing a patient for the negative support reaction. The integration level for the negative support reaction is the brainstem. You bounce the patient several times on the soles of the feet but you do not allow her to bear weight. Which of the following would you anticipate as the patient's response?
[Cash's Textbook of Neurology Physiotherapy/Saunder/
4th Ed./Pg. 527]

A. Increased extensor tone in lower extremities
B. Increased extensor tone in upper extremities
C. Increased flexor tone in lower extremities
D. Increased extensor tone in upper extremities.

Ans. (C) A positive response to bouncing a patient several times on the soles of the feet but not allowing him or her to bear weight is increased flexor tone in the lower extremities.

Q 31. You have a patient referred to physical therapy with cerebral palsy. Which of the following does not describe what you would typically observe in a cerebral palsy child?
[Cash's Textbook of Neurology for Physiotherapy/Saunders/
4th Ed./Pg. 522]

A. The child may be either passive or stiff
B. The child cannot adjust the body position
C. The child can hold or bring the head into a normal position
D. The child may be classified as either spastic or ataxic

Ans. (C) An incorrect or untrue statement regarding a cerebral palsy child would be that the child can hold or bring the head into a normal position, Typically, a cerebral palsy child cannot hold or bring the head into a normal position, Such children cannot support themselves, Typically, they will demonstrate a scissors gait pattern, They will usually have an exaggerated reflex response, They may be classified as either spastic, ataxic, or athetoid, They may be either passive or stiff and cannot adjust the body position.

Q 32. A physician informs you that he feels that the patient is pretending to be ill to arouse sympathy for his condition. He suspects that the patient is slow to recuperate because he continues to receive benefits from the insurance company during a slow recovery. Which of the following most likely describes this individual?
[Physical Rehabilitation/Sullivan/5th Ed./Pg. 30]

A. Patient is negligent   B. Patient is a hypochondriac
C. Patient is a malingerer   D. Patient is paranoid

Ans. (C) A malingerer is one who pretends to be ill to arouse sympathy or who intentionally slows recuperation from a disorder to continue to receive insurance benefits or other emotional, or social benefits from the disorder If the physical therapist suspects the patient is a malingerer, he or she should discuss the case in a teamwork approach and notify the physician, Negligence is failure to do what another reasonable practitioner would have done under similar circumstances, A hypochondriac is a person with a chronic, abnormal concern about his or her health, A paranoid patient has a mental disorder characterized by an impaired sense of reality and persistent

---

Answer   26 A   27 A   28 A   29 A   30 C   31 C   32 C

delusions,

Q 33. A patient comes to physical therapy for further instructions on crutch ambulation. Upon observation you notice that the patient moves the left crutch first, then the right leg, then the right crutch, then the left leg. Of the following, which type of crutch gait have you most likely observed?

[Physical Rehabilitation/Sullivan/5th Ed./Pg. 549]

A. Three-point gait B. Two-point gait
C. Swing-through D. Four-point gait

Ans. (D) Four-point gait pattern is a slow, stable gait pattern of left crutch, right leg, right crutch, left leg, A three-point gait involves nonweight bearing sequence, The crutch advances first, then the uninvolved leg, then the crutch, A two-point gait requires more balance, The opposite crutch and leg advance simultaneously, A swing-through is used when both lower extremities are involved and a patient swings the crutches, then hops on one leg.

Q 34. A patient is referred to physical therapy several months status post hip burn, The patient reports that he had an allograft over the burn area, Which of the following does this describe?

[Physical Rehabilitation/Sullivan/5th Ed./Pg. 1104]

A. The graft skin is from the same species
B. The graft skin is from the same individual
C. The graft skin is from an animal
D. A surgical incision in the form of the letter Z, the length of the graft

Ans. (A) Allograft is the transfer of skin between the same species, It could involve cadaver skin, An autograft is grafted skin from the same individual A heterograft is a graft from an animal, e.g. a pig, Z-plasty is a surgical revision of a scar or closure of a wound using a Z-shaped incision to reduce contractures of the adjacent skin.

Q 35. You are performing a musculoskeletal examination of a patient's thoracic lumbar spine, Which of the tests listed below would best determine if there is an impingement of the nerve in the thoracic lumbar root level?

*[Orthopedic Physical Assessment Magic/Saunders/
5th Ed./Pg. 561]*

A. Compression test B. Distraction test
C. Ely's test D. Slump test

Ans. (D) Slump test is utilized to determine whether an impingement of the nerve root is sustained in the thoracic lumbar region, Compression test is utilized to test for neurological pathology in the cervical spine at any level distraction test determines the effectiveness of traction, which may be used to alleviate pain, This is a complementary test to the compression test, as it is used to obtain the reverse effect Ely's test checks the L2 to L4 nerve root lever for impingement or for tightness of the rectus femoris.

Q 36. You are performing a neurological evaluation on a patient that has had a vascular injury. The patient has the following impairment: loss of consciousness, coma, no ability to speak, and hemiplegia. Based on this information, in which of the following areas does this vascular involvement occur?

*[Neurology and Neurosurgery Illustrated/Lindsay/
4th Ed./Pg. 244]*

A. Anterior cerebral artery B. Middle cerebral artery
C. Posterior cerebral artery D. Vertebrobasilar artery

Ans. (D) A vertebrobasilar artery involvement will result in loss of consciousness, as well as the patient being comatose or in a vegetative state. The patient will have no ability to speak and may have either hemiplegia or quadriplegia.

Q 37. According to the American Physical Therapy Association Standards of Care, the initial evaluation should include all of the following except?

[Physical Rehabilitation Sullivan/5th Ed./Pg. 4]

A. Diagnosis
B. Social/environment needs
C. Frictional status
D. Medication

Ans. (D) Medication is not required to be listed in an initial evaluation according to the APT a standards of care.

Q 38. A patient is referred to physical therapy with an open wound on the lateral malleolus of the right ankle. He is a spinal cord patient who has developed this wound through improper pressure on the ankle. The physician's order is for a lamp to assist in killing the bacteria in the wound and wound healing. In implementing this patient's treatment program, which of the following lamps would be utilized?

[Electrotherapy/Clayton/8th Ed./Pg. 189]

A. Mercury lamp
B. Pressure mercury vapor lamp
C. Pressure mercury vapor lamp
D. Toilet lamp

Ans. (C) The low-pressure mercury vapor lamp, otherwise known as cold mercury lamp, is utilized in application against the skin to kill bacteria. The hot mercury lamp is a high-pressure mercury vapor lamp used for psoriasis skin conditions. It cannot be placed against the skin. The ultraviolet lamp is used in the control of infectious airborne bacteria and viruses, and in the treatment of psoriasis.

Q 39. Patient is sent to physical therapy with an ulnar nerve injury on the right hand. The patient works at a factory sowing various parts for 8 hours a day. The patient is very motivated with rehabilitation and anxious to be aggressive in physical therapy. Which of the following muscles are you going to emphasize with this patient in physiotherapy?

*[Essentials of Orthopaedic and Applied PT Jayant Joshi/
1st Ed./Pg. 266]*

A. Flexor pollicis longus
B. Flexor carpi ulnaris
C. Flexor digitorum superficialis
D. Flexor carpi radialis

Ans. (B) Flexor carpi ulnaris is innervated by the ulnar nerve. Flexor pollicis longus, flexor digitorum superficialis, and flexor carpi radialis are innervated by the median nerve.

Q 40. A 60-year-old patient has an injury to the brachial plexus as a result of an automobile accident. Muscle testing shows the patient has a fair minus grade of rhomboids, levator scapulae, and serratus anterior. The physician has determined that the patient has injured the dorsal scapular and long thoracic nerves. Which of the following best describes the origin of injury to the brachial plexus?

[Essentials of Orthopaedic and Applied PT Jayant Joshi/ 1st Ed./Pg. 263]

A. From the rami of the plexus
B. From the trunks of the plexus
C. From the lateral cord of the plexus
D. From the medial cord of the plexus

Ans. (A) The dorsal scapular and long thoracic nerves originate from the rami of the plexus. The subclavian nerve originates from the trunk of the plexus. The lateral pectoral and musculocutaneous nerves originate from the lateral cord. The medial pectoral and ulnar nerves originate from the medial cord.

Q 41. A patient is a 22-year-old tennis player with a shoulder injury. You are palpating the external rotators of the shoulder. You are palpating the muscle to determine if tenderness or edema exists. The ideal position for palpation of this muscle as it relates to the joint could best be described by which of the following?

[Orthopaedic Physical/Magee/Sunders/5th Ed./Pg. 330]

A. Loose-packed position   B. Closed-packed position
C. 20° of movement   D. 90° of movement

Ans. (A) The best position for a joint in order to palpate the muscle would be a loose-packed position.

Q 42. You are evaluating a patient status postcerebrovascular injury. Upon evaluation you note that the patient has the following characteristics: paralysis and weakness on the right side, possible motor apraxia, and a decreased discrimination between left and right. These symptoms describe which of the following?

[Neurology and Neurosurgery Illustrated/ Lindsay 4th Ed./Pg. 245]

A. Right hemisphere injury   B. Left hemisphere injury
C. Cerebellar injury   D. Brainstem injury

Ans. (B) A left hemisphere cerebrovascular injury would result in paralysis and weakness on the left side. A cerebellar injury would result in ataxia, dysmetria, asthenia, and tremors. A brainstem injury would result in paralysis bilaterally and loss of consciousness.

Q 43. The physician has ordered electrical stimulation to stimulate a denervated muscle. Which of the following types of electrical current would you most likely select to meet this treatment objective?

[Electrotherapy/Clayton/8th Ed./Pg. 64]

A. Alternating current   B. High-volt current
C. Direct current   D. Interferential stimulation

Ans. (C) Direct current is the only type of current that could be utilized to stimulate a denervated muscle. Direct current is necessary to get a response when stimulating a denervated muscle.

Q 44. You are performing goniometric measurement of the shoulder for external rotation. How should the stationary arm of the goniometer be positioned to appropriately measure this patient?

A. Longitudinally with the shaft of the ulna
B. Longitudinally with the styloid process
C. Parallel or perpendicular to the midline of the floor
D. Longitudinally over the shaft of the humerus

[Physical Rehabilitation/Sullivan/5th Ed./Pg. 171]

Ans. (C) In performing goniometric measurement of the internal or external rotators of the shoulder, the stationary arm should be parallel or perpendicular to the midline of the floor. The moveable arm will then be longitudinally aligned with the shaft of the ulna and the styloid process. The axis for measurement is over the olecranon process.

Q 45. You are assisting in planning the diet of a runner for a prolonged low-intensity running event. You are determining the number of calories required in the conversion process for energy. The number of calories required is different for protein, carbohydrates, and fats. One gram of carbohydrate yields 4 calories. How many grams of fat would yield 9 calories for this runner?

[Human Physiology and Biochemistry for PT and OT A.K. Jain/Arya Publication/2nd Ed./Pg. 479]

A. 1   B. 2.25
C. 3   D. 4

Ans. (A) One gram of fat yields 9 calories. One gram of protein yields 4 calories. One gram of carbohydrate yields 4 calories.

Q 46. You are implementing a treatment program of pelvic traction for a patient with a back disorder. Which of the following percentages would cause distraction of the vertebral bodies with lumbar traction?

[Physical Agents is Rehabilitation/Cameroon/ 2nd Ed/Pg. 236]

A. A 30% of the patient's body weight
B. B. 50% of the patient's body weight
C. C. 25% of the patient's body weight
D. D. 35% of the patient's body weight

Ans. (B) In order for distraction of the bodies to occur under lumbar traction, the therapist must apply traction from 40 to 50% of the body's weight.

Q 47. A physician has prescribed iontophoresis for a patient with acute inflammation. The chemical ion to be utilized in this case by direct current should be negative. Which of the following chemical ions listed below would be appropriate to use for a negative current?

[AITBS/Clayton's/9th Ed./Pg. 86]

A. Hydrocortisone   B. Lidocaine
C. Magnesium   D. Salicylate

Ans. (D) Salicylate is an anti-inflammatory drug that utilizes the negative condition. Hydrocortisone, lidocaine, and magnesium are positive.

Q 48. Which of the following condition may be closely responsible for causing Hallux limitus deformity.

[Thomas C William and Wilkins/1st Ed./Pg. 112]

Answer   40 A   41 A   42 B   43 C   44 C   45 A   46 B   47 D

A. Short 1st metatarsal
B. Elongated 1st metatarsal
C. Hypomobile 1st ray of foot
D. Both B and C

Ans. (D) When 1st metatarsal is elongated during propulsion phase of gait cycle there will be an increase pressure beneath 1st metatarsal head and reacting force with hypomobile 1st ray which will prevent necessary plantar flexion this cause subluxation of MTP joint along with its hallux limitus deformity.

49. Which of the following joint is commonly known as Lisfrancs joint?

[Thomas C William and Wilkins/1st Ed./Pg. 110]

A. 2nd TMT joint of foot
B. Ankel mortise joint
C. Subtalar joint
D. 4th digits DIP joint in foot

Ans. (A) This is fact about the 2nd TMT joint of foot is knowns as Lisfrancs joint.

Q 50. Which of following shoe modification may be helpful to reduce pain and discomfort in patient suffering from stiffness MTP joints and experiencing pan especially during push off phase of gait?

[Thomas C William and Wilkins/
1st Ed./Pg. 224]

A. Thomas bar
B. Addition of rocker bottom
C. Decompression pads
D. None of the above

Ans. (B) Thomas bar is used to support metatarsal neck, decreases pressure beneath metatarsal heads in case of metatarsalgia. Decompression pads are used to distribute pressure away from variety of bony prominences such as bunions/Haglund's deformity. Addition of rocker bottom allows patient to proceed through propulsive period without bending the MTP joints therefore it called be helpful for patient suffering form MTP stiffness or limitations.

Model Question Paper - 16

Q 1. Mechanical advantage (MA) is:
[Textbook of Physiotherapy/Dr BK Nanda's/1st Ed/Pg. 16]
A. The ratio of weight arm (WA) to effort arm (EA)
B. The ratio of input force to out force
C. The ratio of output displacement to input displacement
D. The ratio of effort arm (EA) to weight arm (WA).

Ans. (D) Mechanical advantage (MA) is the ratio of effort arm (EA) to load arm/weight arm (WA)

Q 2. Which of the following is correct regarding to activity limitation?
[Textbook of Physiotherapy/Dr BK Nanda's/1st Ed/Pg. 3]
A. It is due to the impairment.
B. The person who fails to participate in family and community activities/life situations.
C. Individual who fails to perform his normal activities for selfcare and vocation.
D. Both A and C.

Ans. (D) Activity limitation is the stage, where due to the impairment, the individual fails to perform his normal activities for selfcare and vocation.

Q 3. The center of Pressure (COP) is defined as:
[Textbook of Physiotherapy/Dr BK Nanda's/1st Ed/Pg. 5]
A. It is defined as a point that is at the center of the total body pressure.
B. The center of the distribution of the total torque applied to the supporting surface.
C. The center of the distribution of the total force applied to the supporting surface.
D. It is defined as a point that is at the center of the total body mass.

Ans. (C) The center of pressure (COP) is the center of the distribution of the total force applied to the supporting surface. The COP moves continuously around the COM to keep the COM within the support base.

Q 4. Cooling down exercises includes:
[Textbook of Physiotherapy/Dr BK Nanda's/1st Ed/Pg. 4]
A. Performing period of 5–8 minutes.
B. Enhance the recovery with oxidation of metabolic waste of the body.
C. To prevents cardiovascular complications.
D. All of the above.

Ans. (D) Cooling down exercises following vigorous aerobic training, a cool down period of 5–10 minutes is required to enhance the recovery with oxidation of metabolic waste of the body. It prevents cardiovascular complications by promoting gradual return of blood to the heart.

Q 5. Which statements better describes plyometrics exercises:
[Textbook of Physiotherapy/Dr BK Nanda's/1st Ed/Pg. 37]
A. Exercises involving only eccentric contraction of muscles
B. Plyometrics exercises, also known as jump training or plyos
C. Exercises involving eccentric and concentric contraction of muscles
D. Both B and C.

Ans. (D) Plyometric exercises are involving eccentric and concentric contraction of muscles. Plyometrics, also known as jump training or plyos, are exercises in which muscles exert maximum force in short intervals of time.

Q 6. Which of the following is not indications of Frenkel's exercises:
[Textbook of Physiotherapy/Dr BK Nanda's/1st Ed/Pg. 48]
A. Osteoarthritis and lymphedema
B. Parkinson's disease and Wilson's disease
C. Cerebellar ataxia and sensory ataxia
D. Cerebral palsy and multiple sclerosis

Ans. (A) Indications of Frenkel's exercises are cerebellar ataxia, sensory ataxia, stroke cerebral palsy, multiple sclerosis, Wilson's disease, Parkinson's disease and other neurological disorders.

Q 7. Contraindications of suspension therapy is:
[Textbook of Physiotherapy/Dr BK Nanda's/1st Ed/Pg. 52]
A. Acute soft tissue injuries and fractures.
B. Hyper-mobile joints and skin diseases.
C. Open wound and sinuses.
D. All of the above

Ans. (D) Contraindications of suspension Therapy are acute soft tissue injuries and fractures, Hyper-mobile joints, skin diseases, open wound and sinuses.

Q 8. What are the purposes of pulley systems in physiotherapy?
[Textbook of Physiotherapy/Dr BK Nanda's/1st Ed/Pg. 18]
A. For mobilizing joints
B. Lifting body for suspension therapy
C. Both A and B
D. None of the above

Ans. (C) *Use of pulley in physiotherapy:* Pulley systems are used in physiotherapy for mobilizing joints such as shoulder pulley, lifting body for suspension therapy, and for mechanical traction to joints, etc.

Answer   1 D   2 D   3 C   4 D   5 D   6 A   7 D   8 C

Q 9. The term end feels states
[Textbook of Physiotherapy/Dr BK Nanda's/1st Ed/Pg. 33]
A. It is a type of sensation or feeling, which the client/patient experiences, when the joint is at the end of its available active ROM.
B. It is a type of sensation or feeling, which the examiner experiences, when the muscles range is at the end of its available active ROM.
C. It is a type of sensation or feeling, which the examiner experiences, when the joint is at the end of its available passive ROM.
D. All are incorrect

Ans. (C) End feel is a type of sensation or feeling, which the examiner experiences, when the joint is at the end of its available passive range of motion.

Q 10. The buoyancy effect of water in hydrotherapy help in:
[Textbook of Physiotherapy/Dr BK Nanda's/1st Ed/Pg. 56]
A. Minimizes the effects of gravity on weight bearing joints
B. Assists and resists muscles work
C. To reduce edema and stabilizes unstable joints
D. All of the above

Ans. (D) The buoyancy effect of water minimizes the effects of gravity on weight bearing joints, assists and resists muscle work, the hydrostatic pressure exerts a circumferential force that helps to reduce edema and stabilizes unstable joints.

Q 11. Which of the following is not the objective of hydrotherapy:
[Textbook of Physiotherapy/Dr BK Nanda's/1st Ed/Pg. 56]
A. To promote relaxation
B. To reduce muscle girth
C. To strengthen muscles and enhance coordination stability and balance
D. To relieve pain and swelling.

Ans. (B) Objective of hydrotherapy are to relieve pain and swelling, to promote relaxation, to reduce muscle tone (spasticity), to strengthen muscles and enhance coordination stability and balance.

Q 12. Hydromechanics are better defined as:
[Textbook of Physiotherapy/Dr BK Nanda's/1st Ed/Pg. 56]
A. It is the chemical properties and characteristics of the fluid in motion that do not affect movement.
B. It is the chemical properties and characteristics of the fluid in motion that affects movement.
C. It is the physical properties and characteristics of the fluid in motion that do not affect movement.
D. It is the physical properties and characteristics of the fluid in motion that affects movement.

Ans. (D) Hydromechanics are better defined as the physical properties and characteristics of the fluid in motion that affects movement.

Q 13. Which is/are incorrect statement in hydromechanics regarding laminar flow?
[Textbook of Physiotherapy/Dr BK Nanda's/1st Ed/Pg. 56]
A. Laminar flow are the movements where all molecules do not move parallel to each other resulting in typically slow movements.
B. Laminar flow are the movements where all molecules move parallel to each other resulting in typically slow movements.
C. Laminar flow are the movements where all molecules move parallel to each other resulting in typically fast movements.
D. Both A and C

Ans. (D) Laminar flow are the movements where all molecules move parallel to each other resulting in typically slow movements. Laminar flow and turbulent flow are the components of hydromechanics.

Q 14. Choose the correct option for PNF:
[Textbook of Physiotherapy/Dr BK Nanda's/1st Ed/Pg. 59]
A. It stands for proprioceptive neuromuscular facilitation
B. It states that all human beings have potentials that are not fully developed.
C. PNF is a technique that involves stimulation of the proprioceptors for increasing the demand on the neuromuscular mechanism to obtain and facilitate its response for improving function.
D. All are correct

Ans. (D) Proprioceptive neuromuscular facilitation (PNF) is a technique that involves stimulation of the proprioceptors for increasing the demand on the neuromuscular mechanism to obtain and facilitate its response for improving function. It also states that all human beings have potentials that are not fully developed.

Q 15. Which of the following is/are not principles of proprioceptive neuromuscular facilitation?
[Textbook of Physiotherapy/Dr BK Nanda's/1st Ed/Pg. 59]
A. PNF states that normal movement and posture depend on "antagonism" and a balanced interaction of agonists.
B. It states that improvement of the motor ability depends on motor learning.
C. It recognizes that early motor behavior is dominated by the reflex activity.
D. Both A and C

Ans. (A) PNF states that normal movement and posture depend on "synergism" and a balanced interaction of antagonists. It states that improvement of the motor ability depends on motor learning and recognizes that early motor behavior is dominated by the reflex activity.

Q 16. Assertion: PNF is based on the principles of motor learning and motor control.
[Textbook of Physiotherapy/Dr BK Nanda's/1st Ed/Pg. 56]

Reason: PNF uses specific patterns of movement and sensory input to facilitate the neuromuscular system, which can improve motor learning and motor control.
A. Both the assertion and reason are true, and the reason provides a valid explanation for the assertion.
B. Both the assertion and reason are true, and but reason is not valid explanation for the assertion.
C. Assertion is true but reason is false
D. Both assertion and reason are false

Ans. (A) Follow the *Textbook of Physiotherapy/Dr BK Nanda's/1st Ed/Pg. 56.*

Answer 9 C   10 D   11 B   12 D   13 D   14 D   15 A   16 A

Q 17. What are the goals of dynamic reversal/slow reversal?
[Textbook of Physiotherapy/Dr BK Nanda's/1st Ed/Pg. 65]
A. To decrease muscle tone.
B. To increase strength and endurance.
C. To increase active range of motion.
D. All are correct

Ans. (D) The goals of dynamic reversal/slow reversal to increase active range of motion, to increase strength and endurance, to decrease muscle tone.

Q 18. Correct statements about direct treatment:
[Textbook of Physiotherapy/Dr BK Nanda's/1st Ed/Pg. 67]
A. Also known as contract-relax/Hold-relax
B. It is resisted isotonic/isometric contraction of the restricting muscles followed by relaxation and movement into the increased range.
C. Both A and B
D. All are incorrect

Ans. (C) Contract-relax/Hold-relax (direct treatment): Resisted isotonic/isometric contraction of the restricting muscles (antagonists) followed by relaxation and movement into the increased range.

Q 19. What is the chopping pattern?
[Textbook of Physiotherapy/Dr BK Nanda's/1st Ed/Pg. 69]
A. It is two-dimensional movements referred to as spiral and diagonal patterns are used to improve activities like running, throwing, changing directions.
B. It is three-dimensional movements referred to as spiral and diagonal patterns are used to improve activities like running, throwing, changing directions.
C. It is traditional PNF pattern involving cross over stepping of the lower extremities is used in functional training for the lower extremity.
D. Both B and C

Ans. (B) Chopping pattern is three-dimensional movements referred to as spiral and diagonal patterns are used to improve activities like running, throwing, changing directions, etc.

Q 20. Braiding pattern is:
[Textbook of Physiotherapy/Dr BK Nanda's/1st Ed/Pg. 69]
A. Two-dimensional movements referred to as spiral and diagonal patterns are used to improve activities like running, throwing, changing directions.
B. Three-dimensional movements referred to as spiral and diagonal patterns are used to improve activities like running, throwing, changing directions.
C. Traditional PNF pattern involving cross over stepping of the lower extremities is used in functional training for the lower extremity.
D. Both B and C

Ans. (C) Braiding pattern/technique: This traditional PNF pattern involving cross over stepping of the lower extremities is used in functional training for the lower extremity. This movement requires both D1 and D2 patterning from each hip when performing multiple steps.

Q 21. The relative contribution of different phases in the gait cycle is:
[Textbook of Physiotherapy/Dr BK Nanda's/1st Ed/Pg. 70]
A. Stance phase: 60% of the gait cycle.
B. Swing phase: 40% of the gait cycle.
C. Double support: 20% of the gait cycle.
D. All are correct

Ans. (D) The relative contribution of different phases in the gait cycle are: Stance phase: 60% of the gait cycle, swing phase: 40% of the gait cycle, double support: 20% of the gait cycle.

Q 22. The swing phase consists:
[Textbook of Physiotherapy/Dr BK Nanda's/1st Ed/Pg. 70]
A. Early swing
B. Mid-swing
C. Late swing
D. All

Ans. (D) Swing phase: 40% of the gait cycle it consists early swing, mid-swing and late swing.

Q 23. Which is wrong about stance phase?
[Textbook of Physiotherapy/Dr BK Nanda's/1st Ed/Pg. 70]
A. It is 40% of the gait cycle
B. It consists heel strike
C. It consists of 50% of the gait cycle
D. All of the above

Ans. (C) Stance phase: 60% of the gait cycle it consists respectively heel strike, foot flat, mid-stance and foot off.

Q 24. Assertion: The use of walking aids can improve the gait pattern of individuals with impaired mobility.
[Textbook of Physiotherapy/Dr BK Nanda's/1st Ed/Pg. 77]
Reason: Walking aids provide stability and support, reducing the risk of falls and improving overall confidence during walking.
A. Both the assertion and reason are true, and the reason provides a valid explanation for the assertion.
B. Both the assertion and reason are true, and but reason is not valid explanation for the assertion.
C. Assertion is true but reason is false
D. Both assertion and reason are false

Ans. (A) The assertion and reason are both correct. Walking aids are commonly used to assist individuals with impaired mobility in maintaining their balance, stability and improving their gait pattern. The reason given for the assertion is also accurate, as walking aids provide support and reduce the risk of falls, thus increasing confidence during walking.

Q 25. Which of the following is NOT a type of pathological gait?
[Textbook of Physiotherapy/Dr BK Nanda's/1st Ed/Pg. 78]
A. Crouch gait
B. Rhythmic gait
C. Trendelenburg gait
D. Scissors gait

Ans. (B) Rhythmic gait, on the other hand, is not a recognized type of pathological gait. However, it is possible for an individual with a pathological gait to have a rhythmic pattern to their walking due to compensatory movements or muscle imbalances.

Answer 17 D 18 C 19 B 20 C 21 D 22 D 23 C 24 A 25 B

Q 26. Which of the following is a characteristic of Trendelenburg gait?
[Textbook of Physiotherapy/Dr BK Nanda's/1st Ed/Pg. 78]
A. Stiff-legged gait with foot drop
B. Circumduction of the affected limb
C. Excessive knee flexion during the swing phase
D. Lateral trunk lean towards the affected side during the stance phase of gait

Ans. (D) Trendelenburg gait is a pathological gait that is characterized by a lateral trunk lean towards the affected side during the stance phase of gait. This is due to weakness of the hip abductor muscles on the contralateral side, which normally stabilize the pelvis during single-leg stance.

Q 27. In which condition 2-point gait is applied?
[Textbook of Physiotherapy/Dr BK Nanda's/1st Ed/Pg. 75]
A. Mild arthritis of the unilateral knee joint
B. Weakness of one leg
C. Unilateral lower limb amputation
D. Bilateral lower limb weakness

Ans. (D) 2-point crutch gait: This gait pattern is similar to the four point gait. However, it is less stable as only two points of floor contact are maintained and the use of such gait requires better balance. This pattern more closely simulates normal gait, i.e., lower extremity along with opposite upper extremity move together along with the crutch.

Q 28. Which of the following statement correct about 4-point crutch gait?
[Textbook of Physiotherapy/Dr BK Nanda's/1st Ed/Pg. 75]
A. This gait pattern is used when there is a lack of coordination, poor balance, and muscle weakness in both lower extremities.
B. In this gait pattern, one crutch is advanced and then the opposite leg is advanced.
C. Both A and B
D. It is used in unilateral lower limb amputation

Ans. (C) 4-point crutch gait: This gait pattern is used when there is a lack of coordination, poor balance, and muscle weakness in both lower extremities. In this gait pattern, one crutch is advanced and then the opposite leg is advanced.

Q 29. Determinants of gait is?
[Textbook of Physiotherapy/Dr BK Nanda's/1st Ed/Pg. 72]
A. Walking width
B. Lateral pelvic tilt
C. Rotation of pelvis in transverse plane
D. All of the above

Ans. (D) Determinants of gait are knee ankle and foot interactions, Lateral pelvic tilt rotation of pelvis in transverse plane, knee flexion during stance phase, physiological valgus of knee and lateral displacement of the pelvis.

Q 30. General contraindications of massage is:
[Textbook of Physiotherapy/Dr BK Nanda's/1st Ed/Pg. 72]
A. Varicose veins
B. After long walk
C. Respiratory problems
D. After the sports activity

Ans. (A) Varicose veins and atherosclerosis are local contraindications of massage. General contraindications of massage are severe spasticity, high fever, renal diseases, cardiac diseases, deep X-ray therapy/radiotherapy, generalized osteoporosis.

Q 31. Assertion: Massage can be an effective treatment for reducing pain and improving function in individuals with musculoskeletal injuries.
[Textbook of Physiotherapy/Dr BK Nanda's/1st Ed/Pg. 83]
Reason: Massage helps to increase blood flow and promote relaxation, which can reduce pain and improve range of motion in affected areas.
A. Both the assertion and reason are true, and the reason provides a valid explanation for the assertion.
B. Both the assertion and reason are true, and but reason is not valid explanation for the assertion.
C. Assertion is true but reason is false
D. Both assertion and reason are false

Ans. (A) Massage is a commonly used for the treatment of musculoskeletal injuries. The assertion that it can be effective for reducing pain and improving function is supported by research studies. Massage can help to increase blood flow to affected areas, which can reduce pain and promote healing.

Q 32. Which of the following massage techniques involves using rapid tapping or chopping movements with the hands?
[Textbook of Physiotherapy/Dr BK Nanda's/1st Ed/Pg. 81]
A. Effleurage
B. Tapotement
C. Petrissage
D. Wringing

Ans. (B) Tapotement/percussion is a massage technique that involves using rapid tapping or chopping movements with the hands. It is often used to stimulate the muscles and increase circulation. Wringing, on the other hand, involves using squeezed, twisted, and then released, using both the hands.

Q 33. Which of the following is not a classification of massage:
[Textbook of Physiotherapy/Dr BK Nanda's/1st Ed/Pg. 80]
A. Effleurage
B. Petrissage
C. Taping
D. None of the above

Ans. (C) Taping is a technique used in physiotherapy, but it is not a classification of massage. The classifications of massage commonly include effleurage, petrissage, friction, tapotement, and vibration.

Q 34. Which of the following massage techniques involves using back-and-forth movements over the skin without applying pressure?
[Textbook of Physiotherapy/Dr BK Nanda's/1st Ed/Pg. 82]
A. Friction
B. Petrissage
C. Both A and B
D. Effleurage

Ans. (D) Effleurage is a massage technique that involves using back-and-forth movements over the skin without applying pressure. It is often used as a warm-up or cool-down technique and is effective in promoting relaxation and increasing blood flow to the muscles. Petrissage involves kneading or squeezing the muscles, friction involves using deep circular movements to release adhesions.

Answer   26 D   27 D   28 C   29 D   30 A   31 A   32 B   33 C   34 D

Q 35. Which type of massage is commonly used in sports medicine to prevent and treat injuries?
[Textbook of Physiotherapy/Dr BK Nanda's/1st Ed/Pg. 81]
A. Trigger point therapy
B. Swedish massage
C. Myofascial release
D. Deep tissue massage

Ans. (C) Myofascial release technique is indicated to lengthen muscle and fascia, increase mobility between fascia layers, and break adhesions. It also decreases pain and increases flexibility (ROM).

Q 36. Which of the following pair is incorrectly match to normal ranges of motion of thoracolumbar spine. Movement range of motion (in degrees)?
[Textbook of Physiotherapy/Dr BK Nanda's/1st Ed/Pg. 87]
A. Flexion—80
B. Extension—20–30
C. Lateral flexion (right)—35
D. Rotation (left)—80–90

Ans. (D) Ranges of motion of thoracolumbar spine are flexion—80, extension—20–30, lateral flexion (right)—35, rotation (left)—45.

Q 37. The stability of the lumbar spine is not maintained by the:
[Textbook of Physiotherapy/Dr BK Nanda's/1st Ed/Pg. 87]
A. Iliolumbar ligament
B. Posterior longitudinal ligaments (PLL)
C. Inter transverse ligament
D. Quadratus lumborum

Ans. (D) The stability of the lumbar spine is maintained by the strong ligaments like **iliolumbar ligament** that stabilizes the lumbosacral joints, the **inter-transverse ligament**, that helps to limit lateral flexion, the anterior and **posterior longitudinal ligament.**

Q 38. Choose correct option about the zygapophyseal joints.
[Textbook of Physiotherapy/Dr BK Nanda's/1st Ed/Pg. 87]
A. It is the joint of L1 to L4
B. It favors flexion and extension and limits lateral flexion and rotation.
C. Both A and B
D. The lowest amount of flexion takes place at this joint.

Ans. (C) The greatest amount of flexion takes place at the lumbosacral joints, The zygapophyseal joints of L1 to L4 lie primarily in the sagittal plane, which prefer flexion and extension and limits lateral flexion and rotation.

Q 39. What is the normal range for the lumbosacral angle in adults?
[Textbook of Physiotherapy/Dr BK Nanda's/1st Ed/Pg. 87]
A. 10–20   B. 30–40
C. 60–70   D. 90

Ans. (B) The 1st sacral segment, which is inclined slightly anteriorly and inferiorly, forms an angle with the horizontal, called the lumbosacral angle. The normal range for this angle in adults is 30–40 degrees.

Q 40. Which of the following movements is most limited in the thoracic spine?
[Textbook of Physiotherapy/Dr BK Nanda's/1st Ed/Pg. 88]
A. Flexion   B. Extension
C. Lateral rotation   D. Rotation

Ans. (C) Lateral flexion. The thoracic spine is most limited in lateral flexion, or side bending, due to the presence of the ribs.

Q 41. Which of the following exercises is most appropriate for a patient with cervical spondylosis who experiences neck pain during forward bending?
[Textbook of Physiotherapy/Dr BK Nanda's/1st Ed/Pg. 99]
A. Biceps curls   B. Cervical manipulation
C. Shoulder blade squeezes   D. Neck retraction exercise

Ans. (D) Chin tucks. Chin tucks/neck retraction exercise can help to correct forward head posture and reduce strain on the neck muscles during forward bending, which can alleviate neck pain in patients with cervical spondylosis.

Q 42. Choose the incorrect statement regarding cervical nerves and cervical vertebrae:
[Textbook of Physiotherapy/Dr BK Nanda's/1st Ed/Pg. 89]
A. The spinal nerves emerges between C7 vertebrae and T1 vertebrae are not cervical nerve
B. There are eight cervical nerves C1–C8.
C. There are only seven cervical vertebrae (C1–C7)
D. All cervical nerves except C8 emerge above their corresponding vertebrae, while the C8 nerve emerges below the C7 vertebra

Ans. (A) The **cervical nerves** are the **spinal nerves** from the **cervical vertebrae** in the cervical segment of the **spinal cord.** Although there are seven cervical vertebrae (C1–C7), there are eight cervical nerves C1–C8. All cervical nerves except C8 emerge above their corresponding vertebrae, while the C8 nerve emerges below the C7 vertebra.

Q 43. Which of the following is categories of cervical spondylotic myelopathies?
[Textbook of Physiotherapy/Dr BK Nanda's/1st Ed/Pg. 90]
A. Brown-Sequard syndrome and transverse lesion syndrome
B. Brachialgia and cord syndrome
C. Motor syndrome and central cord syndrome
D. All of the above

Ans. (D) Categories of cervical spondylotic myelopathies exist such as Brown-Sequard syndrome and transverse lesion syndrome, brachialgia and cord syndrome, motor syndrome and central cord syndrome, transverse lesion syndrome.

Q 44. In case of vertebral artery involvement patient may complain of:
[Textbook of Physiotherapy/Dr BK Nanda's/1st Ed/Pg. 90]
A. Dizziness   B. Retro-ocular pain
C. Sleep disorder   D. Both A and B

Ans. (D) In case of vertebral artery involvement patient may complain of **dizziness, tinnitus, blurring of vision** and **retro-ocular pain.**

Answer   35 C   36 D   37 D   38 C   39 B   40 C   41 D   42 A   43 D   44 D

Q 45. Which of the following is correctly match:
[Textbook of Physiotherapy/Dr BK Nanda's/1st Ed/Pg. 99]
A. Tight erector spinae—the lower crossed syndrome
B. Deep neck flexors—the upper cross syndrome
C. Weak serratus anterior—the lower crossed syndrome
D. Tight iliopsoas—the upper cross syndrome

Ans. (A) The upper cross syndromes are Weak deep neck flexors, tight pectorals, tight upper trapezius and levator scapulae and weak lower trapezius.

Q 46. Mechanical back pain include:
[Textbook of Physiotherapy/Dr BK Nanda's/1st Ed/Pg. 106]
A. Lumber nerve compression
B. Degenerated disc/vertebrae (spondylosis)
C. Traumatic injury
D. All of the above

Ans. (B) Musculoskeletal/mechanical back pain: It include muscle strain, muscle spasm, degenerated disc/vertebrae (spondylosis), spondylitis, herniated disc (PIVD), spinal canal stenosis, spondylolysis, spondylolisthesis, compression fracture, etc.

Q 47. Wrong statements regarding straight leg raise test:
[Textbook of Physiotherapy/Dr BK Nanda's/1st Ed/Pg. 110]
A. Also known as sciatic nerve tension tests
B. Also known as Lasegue test/Fajersztajn test
C. Normal value of SLR is 80–90°
D. Both A and B

Ans. (B) Straight leg raise test (sciatic nerve tension tests): The normal value of SLR is 80–90°. Lasegue test/Fajersztajn test, it is the pain coming from stretch of hamstrings muscles.

Q 48. What is the primary goal of Williams flexion exercises?
[Textbook of Physiotherapy/Dr BK Nanda's/1st Ed/Pg. 126]
A. To increase mobility of the lumbar spine
B. To increase flexibility of the hip extensors
C. SLR training
D. Both A and B

Ans. (A) The primary goal of Williams flexion exercises to increase the mobility of the lumbar spine.

Q 49. Which of the following is NOT a variation of the Williams flexion exercise?
[Textbook of Physiotherapy/Dr BK Nanda's/1st Ed/Pg. 127]
A. Knee-to-chest stretch
B. Pelvic tilt
C. Single knee-to-chest stretch
D. Cobra pose

Ans. (D) Knee-to-chest stretch, pelvic tilt, single knee-to-chest stretch are the variations of the William flexion exercises.

Q 50. Assertion: Lumbar canal stenosis is a condition that can result in compression of the nerve roots in the lower back, leading to pain, numbness, and weakness in the legs.
[Textbook of Physiotherapy/Dr BK Nanda's/1st Ed/Pg. 128]

Reason: Lumbar canal stenosis is often caused by degenerative changes in the spine, such as arthritis, which can lead to the narrowing of the spinal canal.
A. Both the assertion and reason are true, and the reason provides a valid explanation for the assertion.
B. Both the assertion and reason are true, and but reason is not valid explanation for the assertion.
C. Assertion is true but reason is false
D. Both assertion and reason are false

Ans. (A) The assertion and reason are both true and are related, as the narrowing of the spinal canal is what leads to the compression of the nerve roots in the lower back. Lumbar canal stenosis is a condition that can result in compression of the nerve roots in the lower back, leading to symptoms such as pain, numbness, and weakness in the legs. The condition is often caused by degenerative changes in the spine, such as arthritis, which can lead to the narrowing of the spinal canal.

Answer   45 A   46 B   47 B   48 A   49 D   50 A

Model Question Paper - 17

Q 1. Which of the following is incorrect regarding the telescopic sign?

[Textbook of Physiotherapy/Dr BK Nanda's/1st Ed/Pg. 137]

A. Telescopic sign is found to be present in dislocated hip.
B. The tested side hip and knee are bent at 90°
C. This sign found to be present in dislocated shoulder.
D. During test patient complains of increased pain.

Ans. (C) Telescopic sign is found to be present in dislocated hip. The patient is made to lie supine or flat on their back on an examination table. The tested side hip and knee are bent at 90°. During test patient complains of increased pain.

Q 2. Ortolani test used to diagnose?

[Textbook of Physiotherapy/Dr BK Nanda's/1st Ed/Pg. 138]

A. Patellar dislocation
B. Osgood-Schlatter disease
C. Meniscal tear
D. Congenital hip joint dysplasia

Ans. (D) The confirms Ortolani test to diagnose of congenital hip joint dysplasia.

Q 3. Which of the following conditions may associated with a positive Ober's test?

[Textbook of Physiotherapy/Dr BK Nanda's/1st Ed/Pg. 138]

A. Patellar tendinitis
B. IT band syndrome
C. Plantar fasciitis
D. Hip joint dysplasia

Ans. (B) Iliotibial (IT) band tightness indicates positive Ober's test

Q 4. What is the purpose of the Thomas test?

[Textbook of Physiotherapy/Dr BK Nanda's/1st Ed/Pg. 138]

A. To evaluate the flexibility of the hip flexors
B. To determine the presence of tightness in the hamstring muscles
C. To assess the strength of the quadriceps muscle
D. To evaluate the range of motion in the ankle joint

Ans. (A) To evaluate the flexibility of the hip flexors This test helps to diagnose hip flexor tightness/contracture. The patient is asked to lie supine on examination bed with both legs hanging over the side of the examination bed.

Q 5. How is Patrick's test performed?

[Textbook of Physiotherapy/Dr BK Nanda's/1st Ed/Pg. 139]

A. By having the patient actively move their hip joint through a range of motion
B. By applying downward pressure on the hip joint while the patient is lying down
C. By palpating the hip joint for signs of tenderness or inflammation
D. By passively moving the patient's knee through a range of motion and assessing for pain or clicking at the hip joint

Ans. (D) Patrick's test performed by passively moving the patient's leg through a range of motion and assessing for pain or clicking in the hip joint. The test is performed to evaluate hip and sacroiliac joint diseases. The patient is made to lie supine on examination bed. Both the legs are tested alternately.

Q 6. Assertion: Piriformis syndrome is a common cause of sciatica.

[Textbook of Physiotherapy/Dr BK Nanda's/1st Ed/Pg. 139]

Reason: Only due to the piriformis muscle compress the sciatic nerve and causing pain of sciatica.

A. Both the assertion and reason are true, and the reason provides a valid explanation for the assertion.
B. Both the assertion and reason are true, and but reason is not valid explanation for the assertion.
C. Assertion is true but reason is false
D. Both assertion and reason are false

Ans. (C) The assertion is true, but the reason is false. Piriformis syndrome is indeed a common cause of sciatica, but the reason given is not entirely accurate. While it is true that the piriformis muscle can compress the sciatic nerve and cause symptoms, this is not the only possible mechanism of injury.

Q 7. Medical management used in piriformis syndrome:

[Textbook of Physiotherapy/Dr BK Nanda's/1st Ed/Pg. 140]

A. NSAIDs
B. Steroids
C. Antidepressants
D. Pilocarpine

Ans. (A) Medical management for piriformis syndrome are NSAIDs, muscle relaxants.

Q 8. Which of the following is incorrect about snapping hip syndrome?

[Textbook of Physiotherapy/Dr BK Nanda's/1st Ed/Pg. 144]

A. Also known as dancer's hip
B. It is characterized by snapping/popping sensation felt when the hip is flexed and extended
C. It is accompanied by pain in the hip, which decreases with rest.
D. It causes due to extreme thickening of the iliofemoral ligament of hip joint

Ans. (D) Snapping hip syndrome, called as dancer's hip, is a medical condition characterized by snapping/popping sensation felt when the hip is flexed and extended, accompanied by pain in the hip, which decreases with rest. The cause is usually attributed to extreme thickening of the tendons in the hip region.

Answer   1 C   2 D   3 B   4 A   5 D   6 C   7 A   8 D

Q 9. Which of the following exercises is recommended for patients with Ischial bursitis?
[Textbook of Physiotherapy/Dr BK Nanda's/1st Ed/Pg. 147]
A. Hip flexor stretches
B. Running
C. Sit-ups
D. Jumping jacks
Ans. (A) Static stretching of hamstrings, gluteus maximus may be performed several times a day to improve flexibility of hamstring/gluteus maximus muscle and to reduce pressure on the bursa.

Q 10. Osteonecrosis is known as:
[Textbook of Physiotherapy/Dr BK Nanda's/1st Ed/Pg. 147]
A. Vascular necrosis
B. Avascular necrosis
C. Natural death of bone
D. Septic necrosis
Ans. (B) Avascular necrosis (AVN), also known as osteonecrosis, is characterized by variable areas of dead trabecular bone and bone marrow, extending to and including the subchondral plate in the head of the femur. It also known as aseptic necrosis.

Q 11. Which of the following is the most common type of dislocation in hip?
[Textbook of Physiotherapy/Dr BK Nanda's/1st Ed/Pg. 148]
A. Posterior dislocation in hip
B. Anterior dislocation in hip
C. Central fracture dislocation in hip
D. All of the above
Ans. (A) Posterior dislocation of hip is the most common dislocation in hip. The affected lower limb, remains in a position of flexion, adduction, and medial rotation. Sciatic nerve palsy may be present in such dislocations.

Q 12. Which of the following test is not used to diagnosed the congenital dislocation of hip (CDH)?
[Textbook of Physiotherapy/Dr BK Nanda's/1st Ed/Pg. 152]
A. Barlow test
B. Ortolani's test
C. Galeazzi test
D. Patrick's test
Ans. (D) Patrick's test is performed to evaluate hip and sacroiliac joint diseases but Barlow test Ortolani's test and Galeazzi test may use used to diagnosed the congenital dislocation of hip (CDH)/developmental dysplasia of hip.

Q 13. What is the hip arthroplasty?
[Textbook of Physiotherapy/Dr BK Nanda's/1st Ed/Pg. 148]
A. It is the posterior dislocation of hip joint
B. It is the anterior dislocation of the hip joint
C. It is the surgical reconstruction of the hip joint
D. It is the plastic surgery of hip joint
Ans. (C) Hip arthroplasty is the surgical reconstruction of the hip joint, which has lost its mobility and function due either to pathologies involving the hip such as fusion (as occurs in ankylosing spondylitis), AVN, unbearable pain.

Q 14. How to test for patellar instability?
[Textbook of Physiotherapy/Dr BK Nanda's/1st Ed/Pg. 162]
A. To measuring the Q-angle
B. To applying the Thomas test
C. To applying the Osgood-Schlatter test
D. To performing the Plica test
Ans. (A) Measurement of Q-angle, apprehension test for patella are the test of patellar instability.

Q 15. McMurray test is for the:
[Textbook of Physiotherapy/Dr BK Nanda's/1st Ed/Pg. 163]
A. Patellar instability
B. Meniscus injury
C. Hip dislocation
D. Posterior cruciate ligament injury
Ans. (B) McMurray test is for the meniscus injury.

Q 16. Which of the following test can not performed for the anterior cruciate ligament (ACL) injury?
[Textbook of Physiotherapy/Dr BK Nanda's/1st Ed/Pg. 163]
A. Lachman test
B. Pivot shift test
C. Sag sign/Godfrey test
D. Apprehension test
Ans. (C) Sag sign/Godfrey test is for posterior cruciate ligament injury in which patient supine, knee flexed to 90, heel supported by the examiner.

Q 17. Which of the following is correctly match:
[Textbook of Physiotherapy/Dr BK Nanda's/1st Ed/Pg. 166]
A. Test for posterolateral knee instability—Dial test
B. Tests for Plica syndrome—Swain test
C. Test for anterior rotator instability of knee—Varus stress test
D. Tests for anterior cruciate ligament (ACL) injury—Slocum's test
Ans. (A) Tests for Plica syndrome are Hughston's Plica test, Plica Stutter test. Test for anterior rotator instability of knee is Slocum's test: The Slocum's test, which is a modification of anterior drawer test. Tests for anterior cruciate ligament (ACL) injury are anterior drawer test, Lachman test and Pivot shift test. These tests with positive is an indication of tear of ACL.

Q 18. Osgood Schlatter disease is a traction apophysitis at the level of the tibial tuberosity due to:
[Textbook of Physiotherapy/Dr BK Nanda's/1st Ed/Pg. 173]
A. Repetitive strain on the secondary ossification lateral of the tibial tuberosity
B. Repetitive strain on the primary ossification medially of the tibial tuberosity
C. Repetitive stress on the secondary ossification center of the tibial tuberosity
D. Repetitive strain on the secondary ossification center of the tibial tuberosity
Ans. (D) Osgood Schlatter disease is a traction apophysitis at the level of the tibial tuberosity due to repetitive strain on the secondary ossification center of the tibial tuberosity.

Answer   9 A   10 B   11 A   12 D   13 C   14 A   15 B   16 C   17 A   18 D

Q 19. What is Osgood Schlatter disease?
[Textbook of Physiotherapy/Dr BK Nanda's/1st Ed/Pg. 174]
A. It is a greater tuberosity of humerus fracture
B. It is the inflammation of ACL
C. It is the apophysitis of tibial tuberosity
D. It is the apophysitis of greater trochanter of hip

Ans. (C) Osgood Schlatter disease is a traction apophysitis at the level of the tibial tuberosity due to repetitive strain on the secondary ossification center of the tibial tuberosity.

Q 20. Risk factors for ACL injuries is not include:
[Textbook of Physiotherapy/Dr BK Nanda's/1st Ed/Pg. 175]
A. Poor fitness.
B. Using poorly maintained sports equipment
C. Improper foot wear
D. Male are more prone than females

Ans. (D) Risk factors for ACL injuries are poor fitness, using poorly maintained sports equipment, playing on artificial turf surfaces, improper foot wear and females are three times more prone to sustain an injury than males.

Q 21. Females are three times more prone to sustain an ACL injury than males due to:
[Textbook of Physiotherapy/Dr BK Nanda's/1st Ed/Pg. 175]
A. Anatomical configuration
B. Muscle strength and hormonal influences
C. Only A
D. Both A and B

Ans. (D) Females are three times more prone to sustain an injury than males due to anatomical configuration, muscle strength and hormonal influences, resulting in ligament laxity.

Q 22. Which of the following is NOT the types of meniscal tears?
[Textbook of Physiotherapy/Dr BK Nanda's/1st Ed/Pg. 183]
A. Radial and oblique tear
B. Straight and multidirectional tear
C. Horizontal and bucket handle tear
D. Bucket handle tear

Ans. (B) Types of meniscal tears: (A) Radial tear, (B) Oblique tear, (C) Longitudinal tear, (D) Complex degenerative tear, (E) Horizontal tear, (F) Bucket handle tear.

Q 23. Which of the following is NOT the aim of physiotherapy in meniscus injury?
[Textbook of Physiotherapy/Dr BK Nanda's/1st Ed/Pg. 183]
A. Hot pack is applied within the first 10 minutes
B. Cryotherapy is applied for 20 minutes at every 2 hourly intervals
C. To improve knee function and to reduce pain.
D. Both B and C

Ans. (A) Cryotherapy is applied for 20 minutes at every 2 hourly intervals within the first 48–72 hours not the hot packs. After acute pain subsided, knee rehabilitation is started.

Q 24. The main goal of physiotherapy in plica syndrome is:
[Textbook of Physiotherapy/Dr BK Nanda's/1st Ed/Pg. 187]
A. To minimize the ROM and increase the strength of the muscles.

B. Stretching of hamstrings and strengthening of quadriceps isometrically
C. Stretching of rhomboid minor muscles
D. Strengthening of biceps isometrically

Ans. (B) The main goal of physiotherapy in plica syndrome is to reduce pain, maximize the ROM and increase the strength of the muscles and gentile stretching of hamstrings and strengthening of quadriceps isometrically.

Q 25. Which of the following is not the contraindications for total knee replacement:
[Textbook of Physiotherapy/Dr BK Nanda's/1st Ed/Pg. 187]
A. Painful solid knee fusion   B. Neuropathic joints
C. Severe osteoporosis   D. Rheumatoid arthritis

Ans. (D) Contraindications for total knee replacement are neuropathic joints (Charcot's joint). Joint infection, painful solid knee fusion (as a complication of reflex sympathetic dystrophy). Systemic infection and severe osteoporosis, etc.

Q 26. Ankle joint is also called:
[Textbook of Physiotherapy/Dr BK Nanda's/1st Ed/Pg. 192]
A. Talocrural joint
B. Talofibular joint
C. Calcaneofibular joint
D. Talocalcaneal joint

Ans. (A) Ankle joint also called talocrural joint is the articulation between the talus and distal tibia and fibula. The proximal joint surface is composed of the concave surfaces of distal tibia and fibular malleoli.

Q 27. Which phenomena will happen when the ankle joint are dorsiflexed?
[Textbook of Physiotherapy/Dr BK Nanda's/1st Ed/Pg. 192]
A. The talus glides anteriorly, and the fibula moves proximally and laterally away from the tibia.
B. The talus glides posteriorly, and the fibula moves laterally and proximally away from the tibia.
C. The talus glides posteriorly, and the fibula moves distally and laterally away from the tibia.
D. The talus glides posteriorly, and the fibula moves proximally and laterally away from the tibia.

Ans. (D) During dorsiflexion of ankle, the talus glides posteriorly, and the fibula moves proximally and laterally away from the tibia.

Q 28. What will happen during plantar flexion of the ankle joint?
[Textbook of Physiotherapy/Dr BK Nanda's/1st Ed/Pg. 192]
A. The talus glides anteriorly, and the fibula moves proximally and laterally towards to the tibia.
B. The talus glides anteriorly, and the fibula moves distally, slightly anteriorly and toward to the tibia.
C. The talus glides posteriorly, and the fibula moves distally and laterally away from the tibia.
D. The talus glides posteriorly, and the fibula moves proximally and laterally away from the tibia.

Ans. (B) During plantar flexion the talus glides anteriorly, and the fibula moves distally, slightly anteriorly and toward the tibia.

Answer   19 C   20 D   21 D   22 B   23 A   24 B   25 D   26 A   27 D   28 B

Q 29. Talocalcaneal joint, is composed of:
[Textbook of Physiotherapy/Dr BK Nanda's/1st Ed/Pg. 192]
A. Posterior, middle, and anterior articulations between the talus and calcaneus.
B. Anterior, middle, and posterior articulations between the talus and calcaneus.
C. Posterior, lateral, and anterior articulations between the talus and calcaneus.
D. Anterior, lateral and anteroposterior articulations between the talus and calcaneus.

Ans. (A) Talocalcaneal joint, is composed of posterior, middle, and anterior articulations between the talus and calcaneus also called subtalar joint.

Q 30. Incorrect statement regarding Thompson's test for ankle joint:
[Textbook of Physiotherapy/Dr BK Nanda's/1st Ed/Pg. 193]
A. This test examines the integrity of the tendo-Achilles.
B. It is used to identify rupture of tendo-Achilles.
C. The test is positive, when there is no plantar flexion of the ankle.
D. This test is also known as the external rotation test.

Ans. (D) The external rotation test is known as Kleiger's test. Thompson's test/Simmond's test: This test examines the integrity of the Achilles tendon. It is used to identify rupture of tendo-Achilles. This test is positive, when there is no plantar flexion of the ankle, when the calf muscles are squeezed.

Q 31. In sprain of ankle ligaments physiotherapy management PRICE stands for:
[Textbook of Physiotherapy/Dr BK Nanda's/1st Ed/Pg. 197]
A. P-Protections, R-Rest, I-Ice, C-Compression, E-Elevation
B. P-Protections, R-Rest, I-Ice, C-Compression, E-Elongation
C. P-Precautions, R-Rest, I-Ice, C-Compression, E-Elevation
D. P-Protections, R-Rest, I-Ice, C-Conservation, E-Elevation

Ans. (A) In physiotherapy management PRICE is P-Protections, R-Rest, I-Ice, C-Compression, E-Elevation.

Q 32. Which of the following statements about flat foot deformity is TRUE?
[Textbook of Physiotherapy/Dr BK Nanda's/1st Ed/Pg. 201]
A. Flat foot deformity is a condition where the medial longitudinal arch of the foot is abnormally high
B. Flat foot deformity can be caused by a variety of factors including genetics, injury, and neuromuscular conditions
C. Flat foot deformity is only seen in adults and cannot be diagnosed in children
D. Flat foot deformity is a common condition that does not require any intervention

Ans. (B) Flat foot deformity, also known as pes planus, is a condition where the arch of the foot is abnormally low or absent. This can be caused by a variety of factors including genetics, injury, and neuromuscular conditions such as cerebral palsy or muscular dystrophy.

Q 33. Which of the following statements about pes cavus deformity is FALSE?
[Textbook of Physiotherapy/Dr BK Nanda's/1st Ed/Pg. 204]
A. Pes cavus deformity is a condition where the medial longitudinal arch of the foot is abnormally high
B. Pes cavus deformity can be caused by nerve damage or muscle weakness
C. Pes cavus deformity is always accompanied by pain in the foot and ankle
D. Pes cavus deformity can cause difficulty with balance and walking

Ans. (C) Pes cavus deformity, also known as high arches, is a condition where the arch of the foot is abnormally high. This can be caused by a variety of factors, including nerve damage or muscle weakness. Pes cavus deformity can cause difficulty with balance and walking, as well as an increased risk of foot and ankle injuries. While pain can be a symptom of pes cavus deformity, it is not always present.

Q 34. Assertion: Morton's disease is caused by compression or irritation of the interdigital nerves in the ball of the foot.
[Textbook of Physiotherapy/Dr BK Nanda's/1st Ed/Pg. 205]
Reason: The most common location for Morton's disease is between the 3rd and 4th metatarsal bones.
A. Both the assertion and reason are true, and the reason provides a valid explanation for the assertion.
B. Both the assertion and reason are true, and but reason is not valid explanation for the assertion.
C. Assertion is true but reason is false
D. Both assertion and reason are false

Ans. (A) The assertion is correct in stating that Morton's disease is caused by compression or irritation of the interdigital nerves in the ball of the foot. This compression or irritation can be caused by a variety of factors, including wearing tight or narrow shoes, high heels, or participating in activities that put pressure on the ball of the foot. The reason is also correct in stating that the most common location for Morton's disease is between the 3rd and 4th metatarsal bones. This is because the interdigital nerves that are affected by Morton's disease run between these two bones.

Q 35. Which of the following conditions can not affect scapulohumeral rhythm?
[Textbook of Physiotherapy/Dr BK Nanda's/1st Ed/Pg. 209]
A. Frozen shoulder
B. Rotator cuff tear
C. Biceps tendonitis
D. Fracture of clavicle

Ans. (D) Various conditions can affect scapulohumeral rhythm, including frozen shoulder, rotator cuff tear, and biceps tendonitis, etc.

Answer   29 A   30 D   31 A   32 B   33 C   34 A   35 D

Q 36. Choose the correct statement regarding the sulcus test:
[Textbook of Physiotherapy/Dr BK Nanda's/1st Ed/Pg. 215]
A. The presence of sulcus/indentation inferior to acromion is the positive test.
B. In this test the examiner resists patient's forward shoulder flexion, with the patient's forearm in supination.
C. It is due to laxity of the inferior glenohumeral ligament and coracohumeral ligament.
D. It is used to assess the glenohumeral joint for superior instability.

Ans. (A) The presence of sulcus/indentation inferior to acromion is the positive test. The sulcus test is used to assess the glenohumeral joint for inferior instability, due to laxity of the superior glenohumeral ligament and coracohumeral ligament.

Q 37. The presentations of rotator cuff injury may NOT include:
[Textbook of Physiotherapy/Dr BK Nanda's/1st Ed/Pg. 216]
A. Weakness of the involved muscle.
B. Severe pain at the time of injury.
C. Stiffness
D. It painless during the time of injury

Ans. (D) The site of injury has an important influence on possible dysfunctions. The presentations of this disorder include: Severe pain at the time of injury. Pain at night. Limitation of movement (pain with overhead activities). Positive painful arc sign. Weakness of the involved muscle. Stiffness (frozen shoulder).

Q 38. Which of the following is NOT the goal of physiotherapy in rotator cuff tear?
[Textbook of Physiotherapy/Dr BK Nanda's/1st Ed/Pg. 216]
A. Regaining proprioception and movement automatism through neuromotor rehabilitation.
B. Reduction of pain and muscle spasm around shoulder and neck.
C. Strengthening the muscles that stabilize the shoulder.
D. Reduce scapulohumeral mobility.

Ans. (D) The goals of physiotherapy in rotator cuff tear/injury are: Reduction of pain and muscle spasm around shoulder and neck. Improvement of scapulohumeral mobility. Strengthening the muscles that stabilize the shoulder. Regaining proprioception and movement automatism through neuromotor rehabilitation. Improvement of function.

Q 39. What is the most common type of shoulder dislocation?
[Textbook of Physiotherapy/Dr BK Nanda's/1st Ed/Pg. 219]
A. Anterior
B. Posterior
C. Superior
D. Inferior

Ans. (A) Anterior shoulder dislocation is the most common type of shoulder dislocation, accounting for approximately 95% of all dislocations. It occurs when the head of the humerus bone pops out of the glenoid fossa of the scapula bone and moves forward.

Q 40. Assertion: Strengthening exercises should be avoided in the initial phase of rehabilitation after shoulder dislocation.
[Textbook of Physiotherapy/Dr BK Nanda's/1st Ed/Pg. 223]
Reason: They can lead to recurrent dislocation.
A. Both assertion and reason are true, but the reason is not the correct explanation for the assertion.
B. Both assertion and reason are true, and the reason is the correct explanation for the assertion.
C. Assertion is true but reason is false
D. Both assertion and reason are false

Ans. (B) While strengthening exercises may increase the risk of recurrent dislocation if performed improperly, they are an important part of the rehabilitation process. However, they should be introduced gradually and under the supervision of a qualified healthcare professional to ensure proper form and progression.

Q 41. Assertion: In the management of frozen shoulder, pain relief is the primary goal of physiotherapy.
[Textbook of Physiotherapy/Dr BK Nanda's/1st Ed/Pg. 228]
Reason: Once pain is relieved, range of motion can be easily restored through stretching exercises.
A. Both assertion and reason are true, but the reason is not the correct explanation for the assertion.
B. Both assertion and reason are true, and the reason is the correct explanation for the assertion.
C. Assertion is true but reason is false
D. Both assertion and reason are false

Ans. (A) Pain relief is an important goal of physiotherapy in the management of frozen shoulder, but it is not the primary goal. The primary goal is to restore range of motion in the affected shoulder, as this is the main limitation experienced by patients with frozen shoulder. Stretching exercises are a key component for frozen shoulder, but they may need to be supplemented with other modalities such as mobilization under anesthesia or corticosteroid injections, depending on the severity of the condition.

Q 42. Elbow joint is also known as:
[Textbook of Physiotherapy/Dr BK Nanda's/1st Ed/Pg. 231]
A. Humeroulnar joint
B. Trochlea ginglymoid joint
C. Humeroradial joint
D. Glenohumeral joint

Ans. (B) The elbow joint is a hinged compound synovial joint that consists of the humeroulnar and the humeroradial joints. It is also known as trochlea ginglymoid joint, as it can flex and extend like a hinge (ginglymoid).

Q 43. Which of the following is correct option regarding the tennis elbow?
[Textbook of Physiotherapy/Dr BK Nanda's/1st Ed/Pg. 233]
A. It is a tendinopathy involving the extensor muscles of the forearm
B. It is a tendinopathy involving the flexor muscles of the forearm
C. It is painful condition not associated with elbow
D. It is known as medial epicondylitis

Ans. (A) Tennis elbow called lateral epicondylitis is the most common overuse syndrome/cumulative trauma disorder of the upper limb. It is a tendinopathy involving the extensor muscles of the forearm, at their origin on the lateral epicondyle of the humerus.

Answer   36 A   37 D   38 D   39 A   40 B   41 A   42 B   43 A

Q 44. Epicondylitis NOT diagnosed by:
[Textbook of Physiotherapy/Dr BK Nanda's/1st Ed/Pg. 234]
A. By physical examination
B. By imaging studies such X-ray MRI, ultrasound
C. By assessing the patient's medical history and symptoms
D. By Slocum's test

Ans. (D) Epicondylitis is diagnosed by a combination of physical examination, imaging studies such as X-ray, MRI, or ultrasound, and by assessing the patient's medical history and symptoms. Slocum's test is used to diagnosed for the ACL injury.

Q 45. What is the purpose of the grip strength test in the diagnosis of epicondylitis?
[Textbook of Physiotherapy/Dr BK Nanda's/1st Ed/Pg. 234]
A. To assess the patient's pain level during gripping
B. To assess the patient's range of motion in the affected elbow joint
C. To assess the patient's grip strength specifically in relation to the affected elbow joint
D. To assess the patient's overall hand strength

Ans. (C) The grip strength test is used to assess the patient's grip strength specifically in relation to the affected elbow joint. This can help in diagnosing epicondylitis and monitoring progress during treatment.

Q 46. Which of the following tests is commonly used to diagnose medial epicondylitis of elbow joint?
[Textbook of Physiotherapy/Dr BK Nanda's/1st Ed/Pg. 239]
A. Maudsley's test
B. Cozen's test
C. Mill's test
D. Golfer's elbow test

Ans. (D) Golfer's elbow test is commonly used to diagnose medial epicondylitis, also known as Golfer's elbow. It involves resisted wrist flexion while the elbow is in a slightly flexed position.

Q 47. What is the recommended duration of rest for patients with lateral epicondylitis of elbow joint?
[Textbook of Physiotherapy/Dr BK Nanda's/1st Ed/Pg. 235]
A. 1–2 weeks
B. 3–4 months
C. 1–2 years
D. 1–2 days

Ans. (D) 1–2 weeks of rest is recommended for patients with lateral epicondylitis, followed by a gradual return to activity. Prolonged rest and immobilization can actually worsen symptoms and delay recovery.

Q 48. The objectives of physiotherapy in the chronic stage lateral epicondylitis of elbow joint:
[Textbook of Physiotherapy/Dr BK Nanda's/1st Ed/Pg. 235]
A. To induce inflammation and pain
B. To stretch the scar over the common extensor origin
C. Modalities like high-intensity laser therapy are used
D. To strengthen the common Flexors.

Ans. (A) The objectives of physiotherapy in the chronic stage lateral epicondylitis of elbow joint are to reduce inflammation and pain. To stretch the scar over the common extensor origin. To strengthen the common extensors. To improve function. To educate the patient on activity modification and pain control. To promote activity/sports specific training.

Q 49. Medial epicondylitis (Golfer's elbow) develops due to:
[Textbook of Physiotherapy/Dr BK Nanda's/1st Ed/Pg. 235]
A. Overload stress on the extensor muscles of hand and the medial collateral ligament of the elbow
B. Overload stress on the flexor muscles of hand and the lateral collateral ligament of the elbow.
C. Overload stress on the only extensor muscles of hand.
D. Overload stress on the elbow joint

Ans. (B) Golfer's elbow, known as medial epicondylitis or pitcher's elbow causes pain, inflammation, and tenderness over the medial aspect of elbow and forearm. It develops due to stress overload on the flexor muscles of hand and the medial collateral ligament of the elbow.

Q 50. Assertion: Range of motion exercises should be avoided in the early stages of postoperative management of medial epicondylitis.
[Textbook of Physiotherapy/Dr BK Nanda's/1st Ed/Pg. 241]

Reason: Range of motion exercises can exacerbate pain and inflammation in the early stages of postoperative management of medial epicondylitis.
A. Both assertion and reason are true, but the reason is not the correct explanation for the assertion.
B. Both assertion and reason are true, and the reason is the correct explanation for the assertion.
C. Assertion is false but reason is true
D. Both assertion and reason are false

Ans. (C) The assertion is false, but the reason is true. Range of motion exercises are actually important in the early stages of postoperative management of medial epicondylitis to prevent joint stiffness and promote healing.

Model Question Paper - 18

Q 1. Degree of freedom possible in the wrist joint?
[Textbook of Physiotherapy/Dr BK Nanda's/1st Ed/Pg. 242]
A. Three
B. Two
C. One
D. Four

Ans. (B) The wrist joint is a condyloid type of synovial joint having two degrees of freedom, i.e., flexion/extension in the sagittal plane and radial deviation/ulnar deviation in the frontal plane.

Q 2. Clinical tests for wrist joint not include:
[Textbook of Physiotherapy/Dr BK Nanda's/1st Ed/Pg. 246]
A. Carpal compression test
B. Square sign test
C. Phalen's test
D. Mill's test

Ans. (D) Clinical tests for wrist joint are carpal compression test, square sign test, Phalen's test, reverse Phalen's test, Hoffmann–Tinel sign. Mill's test used to diagnose medial epicondylitis of elbow joint?

Q 3. Which type splint is preferred in carpel tunnel syndrome?
[Textbook of Physiotherapy/Dr BK Nanda's/1st Ed/Pg. 246]
A. A thumb spica splint
B. Outrigger splint
C. Sugar-tong splint
D. Dorsal splints

Ans. (D) Customized volar or dorsal splints are provided with neutral position of wrist joint. Dorsal based splint is preferred, as there is no contact pressure on the CT, as occurs in volar splints.

Q 4. Which of the following tendons are most commonly affected in De Quervain's disease?
[Textbook of Physiotherapy/Dr BK Nanda's/1st Ed/Pg. 247]
A. Adductor tendons
B. Abductor tendons
C. Flexor tendons
D. All of the above

Ans. (B) The abductor tendons are most commonly affected in De Quervain's disease. These tendons are located on the side of the wrist and thumb and are responsible for moving the thumb away from the hand.

Q 5. What is the primary cause of Dupuytren's contracture?
[Textbook of Physiotherapy/Dr BK Nanda's/1st Ed/Pg. 250]
A. Infection
B. Genetics
C. Repetitive hand movements
D. Trauma to the hand

Ans. (B) Genetics is the primary cause of Dupuytren's contracture. It is an inherited condition found in the hand due to thickening of the palmar fascia (palmar aponeurosis), leading to flexion contracture of fingers. The condition was originally described by Clive in 1808.

Q 6. Which of the following incorrect option regarding scoliosis?
[Textbook of Physiotherapy/Dr BK Nanda's/1st Ed/Pg. 256]
A. It is a deformity of spine
B. In this deformity where spine is bent anteriorly
C. Its causing significant cosmetic issues and functional problems.
D. In this deformity where spine is bent laterally

Ans. (B) Scoliosis is a deformity of spine, where the spine is bent laterally. This is the most common deformity of spine, causing significant cosmetic issues and functional problems.

Q 7. Clinical features of an individual with scoliosis may presents:
[Textbook of Physiotherapy/Dr BK Nanda's/1st Ed/Pg. 256]
A. Muscular problem in trunk and upper limbs that affect the spinal cord.
B. Body bent to one side with uneven shoulders and pelvis.
C. An individual bent with tilted forearm and hip
D. Presence of cyst that affect the spinal cord

Ans. (D) The individual with scoliosis presents with some mention features like body bent to one side with uneven shoulders and pelvis, presence of rib humps on the convex side of the curve, back pain and neuromuscular problem in trunk and lower limbs in progressive conditions that affect the spinal cord.

Q 8. Recommending exercise to correct scoliosis in physiotherapy?
[Textbook of Physiotherapy/Dr BK Nanda's/1st Ed/Pg. 260]
A. Chest PT
B. Core muscle strengthening exercise
C. Swimming and walking
D. Practicing deep breathing exercise

Ans. (B) Spinal extension exercise in prone lying and quadruped posture pelvic bridging exercise, core muscle strengthening exercises and pilates exercise should teach the client.

Q 9. Which of the following tests is commonly used to assess scoliosis?
[Textbook of Physiotherapy/Dr BK Nanda's/1st Ed/Pg. 256]
A. Adam's forward bend test
B. Straight leg raise
C. Tinel's sign
D. Spurling's test

Ans. (A) Adam's forward bend test. This test is performed in sitting or standing to establish, whether the scoliosis is structural/functional (flexible).

Answer   1 B   2 D   3 D   4 B   5 B   6 B   7 D   8 B   9 A

Q 10. Which type of orthosis is use for scoliosis affecting the whole spine?
[Textbook of Physiotherapy/Dr BK Nanda's/1st Ed/Pg. 256]
A. CPM (continuous passive motion)
B. CTLSO (Milwaukee brace)
C. HKAFO (hip-knee-ankle-foot orthosis)
D. AFO (ankle foot orthosis)

Ans. (B) Orthosis for scoliosis: The orthoses selected for patients with scoliosis depends on the parts of spine affected. For scoliosis affecting the whole spine, CTLSO (Milwaukee brace) is considered.

Q 11. What is amputation?
[Textbook of Physiotherapy/Dr BK Nanda's/1st Ed/Pg. 264]
A. It is the intentional surgical removal of a limb or part of limb of body.
B. It is the surgical removal of any body part
C. It is the surgical removal of visceral organs
D. Both B and C

Ans. (A) Amputation is the intentional surgical removal of a limb or part of a limb / part of body. For limb, it is done through the bone(s) or through a joint.

Q 12. Which of the following pair is correctly match?
[Textbook of Physiotherapy/Dr BK Nanda's/1st Ed/Pg. 265]
A. Duputryen's amputation—it is amputation of the foot
B. Gritti-Stoke's amputation—amputation of the leg through the knee.
C. Hey's amputation—amputation of the arm at the shoulder joint.
D. Syme's amputation—amputation at 1.3 cm proximal to the ankle joint line.

Ans. (B) Gritti-Stoke's amputation: Amputation of the leg through the knee, using an oval anterior flap. **Duputryen's amputation:** Amputation of the arm at the shoulder joint. **Hey's amputation:** Amputation of the foot between the tarsus and metatarsus. **Syme's amputation:** Disarticulation of the foot with removal of both malleoli, 0.6 cm proximal to the ankle joint line.

Q 13. Which of the following pair is incorrectly match?
[Textbook of Physiotherapy/Dr BK Nanda's/1st Ed/Pg. 265]
A. Above knee stump length is—23–27 cm from greater trochanter of femur.
B. Below knee stump length is—12–17 cm from the knee.
C. Above elbow stump length is—30–35 cm from the elbow.
D. Below elbow stump length is—16–18 cm from the olecranon process of ulna.

Ans. (C) Above knee stump length: 23–27 cm from greater trochanter of femur, below knee stump length is: 12–17 cm from the knee, above elbow stump length 20 cm from the shoulder, below elbow stump length 18 cm from the olecranon process of ulna.

Q 14. Pre-prosthetic rehabilitation focuses on?
[Textbook of Physiotherapy/Dr BK Nanda's/1st Ed/Pg. 266]
A. Ambulation with temporary prosthesis
B. Ambulation with permanent prosthesis and positioning of the stump

C. It focuses on wound healing and pain control
D. Both B and C

Ans. (A) Pre-prosthetic rehabilitation focuses on: Ambulation with temporary prosthesis and using a pair of axillary crutches, positioning of the stump.

Q 15. Boyd's amputation well referred as:
[Textbook of Physiotherapy/Dr BK Nanda's/1st Ed/Pg. 266]
A. It is amputation of the arm at the shoulder joint
B. It is amputation at the level of the ankle
C. It is amputation of the leg through the knee
D. Amputation of toe is known as Boyd's amputation

Ans. (B) Boyd's amputation refers to amputation at the level of the ankle, with preservation of the calcaneus and heel pad and consequent fixation of the calcaneus to tibia.

Q 16. What is best treatment procedure of arthritis as per the international classification of function (ICF) model?
[Textbook of Physiotherapy/Dr BK Nanda's/1st Ed/Pg. 271]
A. Activity limitation → Impairment → Participation limitation
B. Impairment → Activity limitation → Participation limitation
C. Impairment → Participation limitation → Activity limitation
D. Participation limitation → Activity limitation → Impairment

Ans. (B) The stages of international classification of function (ICF) model are impairment → Activity limitation → Participation limitation. So that the patient lives a painless life with maintenance and restoration of function and overall improved quality of life.

Q 17. Which vitamin deficiency may cause ataxia?
[Textbook of Physiotherapy/Dr BK Nanda's/1st Ed/Pg. 471]
A. Vitamin A   B. Vitamin D
C. Vitamin K   D. Vitamin E

Ans. (D) Ataxia is the term for a group of neurological diseases (diseases related to the nervous system) that affect movement and coordination. Vitamin deficiencies such as, Vitamin E deficiency which may cause ataxia and dysarthria.

Q 18. Which of the following is NOT a typical symptom of coccydynia?
A. Pain in the lower back
B. Pain during bowel movements
C. Numbness or tingling in the legs
D. Piercing pain in the tail bone
[Textbook of Physiotherapy/Dr BK Nanda's/1st Ed/Pg. 481]

Ans. (C) Coccydynia is the inflammation of the coccyx or tailbone. It results from a change of posture during late stages of pregnancy. Numbness or tingling in the legs are not the symptoms of coccydynia.

Q 19. Which of following is not common causes for osteoarthritis (OA) of knee:
[Textbook of Physiotherapy/Dr BK Nanda's/1st Ed/Pg. 272]
A. Heredity   B. Gender
C. Hypertension   D. Repetitive stress and injuries

Ans. (C) Common causes for osteoarthritis (OA) of knee heredity, gender, age, women aged 55 years and older are more likely than men to develop OA of the knee, repetitive stress injuries, etc.

Answer   10 B   11 A   12 B   13 C   14 A   15 B   16 B   17 D   18 C   19 C

Q 20. Segmental breathing involves:
[Textbook of Physiotherapy/Dr BK Nanda's/1st Ed/Pg. 511]
A. Focusing on specific areas of the chest or abdomen during inhalation and exhalation
B. Rapidly alternating between deep inhalations and forceful exhalations
C. Holding the breath for as long as possible and then exhaling slowly
D. Contracting the abdominal muscles during inhalation and relaxing them during exhalation

Ans. (A) Segmental breathing is performed on a segment of a lung, or a section of the chest wall that needs increased ventilation or movement.

Q 21. Which one of the following most common deformity due to involvement of medial compartment of knee?
[Textbook of Physiotherapy/Dr BK Nanda's/1st Ed/Pg. 273]
A. Pes varum   B. Genu valgum
C. Genu varum   D. Pes valgus

Ans. (C) Deformity in the form of genu varum (most common deformity due to involvement of medial compartment of knee).

Q 22. Symptoms of joint locking and buckling occur due to:
[Textbook of Physiotherapy/Dr BK Nanda's/1st Ed/Pg. 273]
A. Damage to stabilizing menisci and ligaments.
B. Over movement of patella bone
C. Tightness of posterior capsule
D. Both A and C

Ans. (A) Symptoms of joint locking and buckling may also occur due to damage of stabilizing menisci and ligaments.

Q 23. Pursed lip breathing is a technique that involves:
A. Taking slow, deep breaths through the nose
B. Taking short, shallow breaths through the mouth
C. Inhaling through the nose and exhaling through pursed lips as if blowing out a candle
D. Exhaling forcefully through the mouth
[Textbook of Physiotherapy/Dr BK Nanda's/1st Ed/Pg. 514]

Ans. (C) To breathe slowly and deeply through the nose, and then breathe out gently through lightly pursed lips this breathing technique is known as pursed lip breathing technique.

Q 24. Can traction apply on a patient who is suffering from OA?
[Textbook of Physiotherapy/Dr BK Nanda's/1st Ed/Pg. 273]
A. Yes sure
B. Never
C. It may cause more severity
D. It is not the part of physiotherapy management.

Ans. (A) Traction to the knee either manually or by using weight and pulley system is found to be helpful, in the chronic stage, particularly in stage-3 and stage-4, where significant joint space reduction and deformity like varus/valgus is present.

Q 25. Abnormal limb synergies are:
[Textbook of Physiotherapy/Dr BK Nanda's/1st Ed/Pg. 362]
A. It is the patterns of movement which develop from poor diet
B. It is the patterns of movement that develop after a stroke
C. It is the patterns of movement that are commonly seen in athletes
D. It is the patterns of movement that develop as a result of poor posture

Ans. (B) Abnormal limb synergies are patterns of movement that develop after a stroke or other neurological injury. These abnormal synergies patterns could be either flexor or extensor types, which make the movements purposeless in such patients. Spastic patterns seen in the patients have components from the abnormal flexor and extensor synergies.

Q 26. The symmetric tonic neck reflex is commonly seen in patients with hemiplegia involves?
[Textbook of Physiotherapy/Dr BK Nanda's/1st Ed/Pg. 363]
A. Flexion of the arm and leg on the same side as the head in response to turning the head to one side
B. Extension of the neck results in flexion of the arms and flexion of the legs
C. Flexion of the neck results in flexion of the arms and extension of the legs
D. Flexion of the arm and leg on the opposite side of the head in response to turning the head to one side

Ans. (C) Symmetric tonic neck reflex (STNR): Flexion of the neck results in flexion of the arms and extension of the legs extension of the neck results in extension of the arms and flexion of the legs.

Q 27. What is the purpose of a median sternotomy?
[Textbook of Physiotherapy/Dr BK Nanda's/1st Ed/Pg. 542]
A. To access the heart and surrounding blood vessels
B. To remove a portion of the sternum for bone grafting
C. To repair a herniated disc in the cervical spine
D. To access the lungs for bronchoscopy procedures

Ans. (A) Median sternotomy is a surgical procedure used to access the heart and surrounding structures for various cardiac procedures, such as coronary artery bypass grafting, valve replacement, and repair of congenital heart defects.

Q 28. Psoriatic arthritis is a type of:
[Textbook of Physiotherapy/Dr BK Nanda's/1st Ed/Pg. 280]
A. Osteoarthritis
B. Rheumatoid arthritis
C. Inflammatory arthritis
D. Infectious arthritis

Ans. (C) Psoriatic arthritis (PsA) (also called as arthritis psoriatica, arthropathic psoriasis, or psoriatic arthropathy) is a type of inflammatory arthritis that develops in between 6 and 42% of people who have the chronic skin condition psoriasis.

Q 29. Which of the following laboratory tests is most specific for the diagnosis of psoriatic arthritis?
[Textbook of Physiotherapy/Dr BK Nanda's/1st Ed/Pg. 281]
A. Rheumatoid factor (RF)
B. Anti-cyclic citrullinated peptide (anti-CCP) antibodies
C. HLA-B27 gene test
D. No definitive test to diagnose psoriatic arthritis

Ans. (D) There is no definitive test to diagnose psoriatic arthritis. Physical examinations, health history, blood tests, and X-rays (pencil in cup deformity) help to diagnose psoriatic arthritis, differentiating it from other similar conditions like RA.

Answer   20 A   21 C   22 A   23 C   24 A   25 B   26 C   27 A   28 C   29 D

Q 30. Syphilitic arthritis is caused by infection with the bacterium:
[Textbook of Physiotherapy/Dr BK Nanda's/1st Ed/Pg. 281]
A. *Treponema pallidum*
B. *Borrelia burgdorferi*
C. *Mycobacterium tuberculosis*
D. *Staphylococcus aureus*

Ans. (A) Syphilitic arthritis is a sexually transmitted infection caused by the bacterium *Treponema pallidum*.

Q 31. Which of the strategy of physiotherapy may not use in chronic arthritis?
[Textbook of Physiotherapy/Dr BK Nanda's/1st Ed/Pg. 279]
A. Pulsed ultrasound/IFT/TENS
B. Galvanic stimulation to inhibited muscles.
C. Hydrotherapy.
D. Isometric exercise to postural muscles, like glutei, quadriceps, etc.

Ans. (B) Faradic stimulation instead of galvanic stimulation use to inhibited muscles in chronic arthritis.

Q 32. Incorrect statement regarding ankylosing spondylitis (AS)?
[Textbook of Physiotherapy/Dr BK Nanda's/1st Ed/Pg. 283]
A. It is a type of autoimmune disease
B. It is mostly affect spine and sacroiliac joints
C. It also associated with pathology of gastrointestinal (GI) tract
D. It is seropositive chronic inflammatory autoimmune disease

Ans. (D) Ankylosing spondylitis (AS) is a seronegative chronic inflammatory autoimmune disease of the spine and sacroiliac joints. It may be associated with pathology involving a number of extra-articular structures, such as the eye, gastrointestinal (GI) tract, skin, lungs, kidneys, and heart.

Q 33. What is avulsion fracture?
[Textbook of Physiotherapy/Dr BK Nanda's/1st Ed/Pg. 288]
A. The bone breaks into several pieces.
B. Fracture without breaking of skin.
C. Bone fragment is separated from the main mass of bone.
D. It also known as fissured fracture

Ans. (C) Avulsion fracture: In this fracture a bone fragment is separated from the main mass of bone.

Q 34. Hangman fracture also known as:
[Textbook of Physiotherapy/Dr BK Nanda's/1st Ed/Pg. 289]
A. Traumatic spondylolisthesis of the axis
B. Traumatic ankylosing spondylitis
C. Fissured fracture
D. Transverse fracture

Ans. (A) Hangman fracture, also known as traumatic spondylolisthesis of the axis, is a fracture which involves the pars interarticularis of C2 on both sides, and is a result of hyperextension and distraction.

Q 35. What is Whiplash?
[Textbook of Physiotherapy/Dr BK Nanda's/1st Ed/Pg. 289]
A. An ankle injury
B. A spine injury
C. A neck injury
D. A meniscal tear injury

Ans. (C) Whiplash is a neck injury due to forceful, rapid back-and forth movement of the neck, like the cracking of a whip. Whiplash injury is commonly caused by rear-end car accidents.

Q 36. Smith's fracture is better defined as:
[Textbook of Physiotherapy/Dr BK Nanda's/1st Ed/Pg. 296]
A. It is an extra-articular fracture of the distal radius featuring a volar displacement of the distal fragment.
B. It is an intra-articular fracture involving the lower end of radius with dislocation of radiocarpal joints.
C. A fracture which involves an incomplete longitudinal break
D. It is a fracture which involves fracture to one or both malleoli of ankle joint

Ans. (A) Smith's fracture: It is an extra-articular fracture of the distal radius featuring a volar displacement or angulation of the distal fragment.

Q 37. Which of the following is NOT a symptom of a lower brachial plexus injury?
[Textbook of Physiotherapy/Dr BK Nanda's/1st Ed/Pg. 443]
A. Weakness or paralysis of the hand
B. Radioulnar synostosis.
C. Horner's syndrome
D. Loss of sensation in the hand

Ans. (B) A lower brachial plexus injury can cause weakness or paralysis of the hand, loss of sensation in the hand, and Horner's syndrome (drooping eyelid, small pupil, and lack of sweating on the affected side of the face).

Q 38. Which of the following correct option regarding Dupuytren's fracture?
[Textbook of Physiotherapy/Dr BK Nanda's/1st Ed/Pg. 308]
A. It also known as Smith's fracture
B. It is the fractures around the foot or ankle
C. It is an intra-articular fracture involving the lower end of radius with dislocation of radiocarpal joints
D. It is a fracture which involves an incomplete longitudinal break

Ans. (B) A Pott's fracture also called as Dupuytren's fracture. It is the fractures around the foot or ankle which involves fracture to one or both malleoli (lateral and medial).

Q 39. Which nerve roots are typically affected in Klumpke's palsy?
[Textbook of Physiotherapy/Dr BK Nanda's/1st Ed/Pg. 450]
A. C5-C6
B. C7-T1
C. C8-T1
D. C6-C7

Ans. (D) Klumpke's palsy is one obstetric brachial plexus injury, which is named after Augusta Dejerine-Klumpke usually the 8th cervical (C8) and 1st thoracic (T1) roots are injured.

Q 40. Which of the following is NOT a factor used to determine the severity of burn injury?
[Textbook of Physiotherapy/Dr BK Nanda's/1st Ed/Pg. 311]
A. Depth of burn
B. Location of burn
C. Age of the patients
D. Percentage of burn

Ans. (B) While the location of the burn can affect the functional outcomes and cosmetic appearance of the patient, it is not used to determine the severity of the burn injury. The factors used are the depth and percentage of burn, as well as the age of the patient.

Answer   30 A   31 B   32 D   33 C   34 A   35 C   36 A   37 B   38 B   39 D

Q 41. What is partial thickness burn?
[Textbook of Physiotherapy/Dr BK Nanda's/1st Ed/Pg. 311]
A. The burn which involves damage the capillaries and free nerve endings in the dermis.
B. The burn which involve only the epidermal layer of the skin.
C. The burn which involve all layer of the skin
D. The burn which involve only portions of dermis

Ans. (A) Partial thickness burn: This is the burn involving the epidermis and portions of dermis. It involves damage to capillaries and free nerve endings in the dermis.

Q 42. Which of the following body regions represents 1% of the total body surface area in the "rule of nines"?
[Textbook of Physiotherapy/Dr BK Nanda's/1st Ed/Pg. 313]
A. Genitalia
B. Foot
C. Face
D. Hand

Ans. (A) According to rule of nine the genitalia represents 1% of the total body surface area.

Q 43. Which of the following is not the aims of physiotherapy in late stage of burn?
[Textbook of Physiotherapy/Dr BK Nanda's/1st Ed/Pg. 315]
A. To prevent from the development of strong keloids
B. To improve muscle strength, endurance, balance, coordination.
C. Muscle strengthening exercises using Therabands or dumbbell.
D. PNF techniques.

Ans. (A) Prevention of development of strong scar/keloids and, tightness/contracture/deformity is the aims of physiotherapy in early stage of burn.

Q 44. Which type of exercises are typically prescribed in the early stage of burn recovery?
[Textbook of Physiotherapy/Dr BK Nanda's/1st Ed/Pg. 315]
A. Isometrics exercises
B. Isotonic exercises
C. Passive range motion exercises
D. Active range of motion exercises

Ans. (C) In the early stage of burn recovery, passive range of motion exercises are typically prescribed to maintain joint mobility without putting stress on the healing tissue.

Q 45. Cerebral palsy (CP) is the most chronic childhood disease also known as:
[Textbook of Physiotherapy/Dr BK Nanda's/1st Ed/Pg. 315]
A. Little baby disease
B. Little's disease
C. Little's child disease
D. None of the above

Ans. (B) Cerebral palsy (CP) is the most chronic childhood disease today. The condition was first described by an English physician Sir Francis William Little in 1861, and is known as Little's disease.

Q 46. Which level of the GMFCS classification system is characterized by the ability to walk with hand-held mobility devices?
[Textbook of Physiotherapy/Dr BK Nanda's/1st Ed/Pg. 322]
A. GMFSC Level I
B. GMFSC Level II
C. GMFSC Level III
D. GMFSC Level IV

Ans. (C) Level III of the GMFCS classification system is characterized by the ability to walk with hand-held mobility devices, but the inability to walk independently. Children at this level may also use a wheelchair for longer distances.

Q 47. Which type of gait is commonly observed in individuals with dyskinetic cerebral palsy?
[Textbook of Physiotherapy/Dr BK Nanda's/1st Ed/Pg. 322]
A. Scissoring gait
B. Athetoid dance gait
C. Crouch gait
D. Jump knee gait

Ans. (B) Athetoid gait is commonly observed in individuals with dyskinetic cerebral palsy. This gait is characterized by involuntary movements and a lack of coordination, resulting in an unsteady and irregular gait pattern.

Q 48. At what age can cerebral palsy be diagnosed?
[Textbook of Physiotherapy/Dr BK Nanda's/1st Ed/Pg. 339]
A. At birth
B. Between 6 months and 2 years
C. Between 2 and 5 years
D. At any age

Ans. (B) Cerebral palsy can be diagnosed between 6 months and 2 years of age. This is because this is when motor milestones are typically achieved, and delays or abnormalities can be identified.

Q 49. What is the primary goal of orthotic management for individuals with cerebral palsy?
[Textbook of Physiotherapy/Dr BK Nanda's/1st Ed/Pg. 351]
A. To correct gait patterns
B. To prevent muscles atrophy
C. To improve strength and flexibility
D. To improve sensory disability

Ans. (A) The primary goal of orthotic management for individuals with cerebral palsy is to improve overall function and independence. This can include improving gait patterns, providing support for weak or unstable joints, and reducing pain and discomfort.

50. Commonly not used positions during 2nd stage of labor.
[Physiotherapy in Obstetrics and Gynaecology/1990/Margaret Polden/Jaypee]
A. Lithotomy
B. Dorsal (recumbent)
C. Long sitting
D. Lateral and semi-recumbent

Ans. (C) Because in second stage of labor certain upright positions such as squatting position and sitting position, may correlate with perineal trauma and greater blood loss.

Answer   40 B   41 A   42 B   43 A   44 C   45 B   46 C   47 B   48 B   49 A   50 C

Model Question Paper - 19

Q 1. When can postoperative physiotherapy after SEMLS begin?
[Textbook of Physiotherapy/Dr BK Nanda's/1st Ed/Pg. 354]
A. Immediately after surgery B. 1 week after surgery
C. 2 week after surgery   D. 4 week after surgery

Ans. (A) Postoperative physiotherapy after SEMLS can begin immediately after surgery, with a focus on pain management, early mobilization, and preventing complications.

Q 2. Choose the incorrect statement regarding to stroke:
[Textbook of Physiotherapy/Dr BK Nanda's/1st Ed/Pg. 358]
A. It is an acute onset of neurological dysfunction due to abnormality in cerebral circulation
B. Also known as cerebral vascular accident
C. Another name of stroke is apoplexy
D. Patient complain insomnia

Ans. (D) According to WHO, stroke is defined as "acute onset of neurological dysfunction due to abnormality in cerebral circulation". Stroke is also known as "cerebral vascular accident (CVA)", "brain attack", or "apoplexy."

Q 3. Which type of stroke occurs when a blood vessel in the brain ruptures?
[Textbook of Physiotherapy/Dr BK Nanda's/1st Ed/Pg. 359]
A. Cryptogenic strokes
B. Transient ischemic attack (TIA)
C. Hemorrhagic strokes
D. Ischemic strokes

Ans. (C) In hemorrhagic strokes a blood vessel ruptures in the brain.

Q 4. Which of the following is NOT one of the vascular territories affected by stroke?
[Textbook of Physiotherapy/Dr BK Nanda's/1st Ed/Pg. 359]
A. Anterior cerebral artery
B. The brachial artery
C. Middle cerebral artery
D. Posterior cerebral artery

Ans. (B) The brachial artery is not one of the vascular territories affected by stroke.

Q 5. What is the most common cause of stroke affecting the anterior cerebral artery?
[Textbook of Physiotherapy/Dr BK Nanda's/1st Ed/Pg. 359]
A. Atherosclerosis
B. Embolism
C. Hypertension
D. Arteriovenous malformation (AVM)

Ans. (B) Embolism is the most common cause of stroke affecting the anterior cerebral artery (ACA).

Q 6. Which cranial nerve is commonly affected in Weber syndrome?
[Textbook of Physiotherapy/Dr BK Nanda's/1st Ed/Pg. 360]
A. Cranial nerve II
B. Cranial nerve III
C. Cranial nerve IV
D. Cranial nerve V

Ans. (B) Weber syndrome is characterized by a lesion in the midbrain which affects the oculomotor nerve (cranial nerve III). This results in weakness or paralysis of the muscles that control eye movement, leading to symptoms such as drooping eyelids and difficulty moving the eyes.

Q 7. Abnormal limb synergies can result in which of the following impairments?
[Textbook of Physiotherapy/Dr BK Nanda's/1st Ed/Pg. 360]
A. Decreased muscle tone
B. Increased range of motion
C. Increased control of movement
D. Decreased ability to perform functional activities

Ans. (D) Abnormal limb synergies can result in decreased ability to perform functional activities.

Q 8. Perceptual dysfunction can result in which of the following impairments?
[Textbook of Physiotherapy/Dr BK Nanda's/1st Ed/Pg. 364]
A. Apraxia
B. Loss of sensation
C. Decreased muscles strength
D. Increased joint mobility

Ans. (A) Difficulty with motor planning (apraxia), the left (dominant hemisphere) has a primary role in sequencing of movement. The individuals with left CVA (i.e., right hemiplegia) with frontal and posterior parietal lesions may present with deficits in motor planning (apraxia).

Q 9. Which of the following is NOT one of Brunnstrom's stages of recovery?
[Textbook of Physiotherapy/Dr BK Nanda's/1st Ed/Pg. 367]
A. Stage 1: Flaccidity
B. Stage 2: Rigidity
C. Stage 3: Synergies
D. Stage 4: Coordination

Ans. (B) Stage 2: Spasticity is one of Brunnstrom's stages of recovery. However, spasticity is a common feature that can occur during some of the stages.

Answer   1 A   2 D   3 C   4 B   5 B   6 B   7 D   8 A   9 B

Q 10. Which of the following is a contraindication for conventional exercises in the acute stage of neurological conditions?

[Textbook of Physiotherapy/Dr BK Nanda's/1st Ed/Pg. 372]

A. Mild muscles weakness
B. Mild muscles spasticity
C. Confusion or disorientation
D. Hemiplegia

Ans. (C) Confusion or disorientation is a contraindication for conventional exercises in the acute stage of neurological conditions. The patient should be able to follow commands and cooperate with the exercises.

Q 11. What is the role of the physiotherapist in neurodevelopmental therapy (NDT)?

[Textbook of Physiotherapy/Dr BK Nanda's/1st Ed/Pg. 381]

A. To provide hands-on facilitation to help the patient learn new movement patterns
B. To design exercise programs that target specific muscle groups
C. To prescribe medication to manage pain
D. To monitor the patient's vital signs during therapy sessions

Ans. (A) The role of the physiotherapist in NDT is to provide hands-on facilitation to help the patient learn new movement patterns and promote motor learning.

Q 12. Which of the following classification systems assesses both sensory and motor function in spinal cord injury patients?

[Textbook of Physiotherapy/Dr BK Nanda's/1st Ed/Pg. 389]

A. ASIA impairment scale
B. Frankel classification
C. ISNCSCI
D. Modified Ashworth scale

Ans. (C) The ISNCSCI is a comprehensive assessment of both motor and sensory function in SCI patients. It evaluates the patient's ability to move and feel below the level of injury, and it is the most widely used classification system for SCI. It is also sometimes referred to as the International Standards for Neurological Classification of Spinal Cord Injury.

Q 13. Brown-Sequard syndrome is a type of spinal cord injury that results in:

[Textbook of Physiotherapy/Dr BK Nanda's/1st Ed/Pg. 390]

A. Loss of sensory function on one side and loss of motor function on the opposite side below the level of injury.
B. Loss of motor function on one side and loss of sensory function on the opposite side below the level of injury.
C. Complete loss of motor function below the level of injury.
D. Complete loss of sensory function below the level of injury.

Ans. (B) Brown-Sequard syndrome is a type of spinal cord injury that affects only one side of the spinal cord. It results in loss of motor function on one side and loss of sensory function on the opposite side below the level of injury. This occurs because the pathways for motor and sensory function crossover at different levels of the spinal cord.

Q 14. What is Rood's approach in stroke?

[Textbook of Physiotherapy/Dr BK Nanda's/1st Ed/Pg. 384]

A. A manual therapy technique
B. A therapeutic exercise approach
C. A cognitive behavioral therapy approach
D. A surgical approach

Ans. (B) Rood's approach is a therapeutic exercise approach that was developed by Margaret Rood, a pioneer in the field of physiotherapy. It involves the use of sensory stimulation and motor patterns to improve muscle function and movement in patients with neurological conditions such as stroke.

Q 15. Which of the following tools may use to assess the severity of spinal cord injury?

[Textbook of Physiotherapy/Dr BK Nanda's/1st Ed/Pg. 395]

A. ASIA Impairment Scale
B. Functional independence measure
C. Berg balance scale
D. Goniometer

Ans. (A) The ASIA Impairment Scale is a tool used to assess the severity of spinal cord injury based on motor and sensory function. It classifies spinal cord injury into five categories: (A) complete injury, (B) incomplete injury, (C) incomplete injury with motor function preserved, (D) incomplete injury with sensory function preserved, and (E) normal.

Q 16. Which of the following is a commonly used crutch gait for patients with spinal cord injury who have weaker upper extremity strength?

[Textbook of Physiotherapy/Dr BK Nanda's/1st Ed/Pg. 408]

A. Two-point gait
B. Swing-to gait
C. Four-point gait
D. None of the above

Ans. (C) The four-point gait involves advancing one crutch followed by the opposite lower extremity, then advancing the other crutch followed by the opposite lower extremity. This gait is often used for patients with spinal cord injury who have weaker upper extremity strength or less stable balance.

Q 17. Parkinson's disease is characterized by the degeneration of which type of neurons in the brain?

[Textbook of Physiotherapy/Dr BK Nanda's/1st Ed/Pg. 412]

A. Dopaminergic neuron
B. Serotonergic neurons
C. Cholinergic neurons
D. GABAergic neurons

Ans. (A) Parkinson's disease is a neurodegenerative disorder that is characterized by the progressive loss of dopaminergic neurons in the substantia nigra, a region of the brain involved in motor control.

Q 18. What is pallidotomy?

[Textbook of Physiotherapy/Dr BK Nanda's/1st Ed/Pg. 419]

A. This is a surgical procedure used to treat tremor.
B. A neurosurgical procedure used to destroy a small area of braincells.
C. It is surgical procedure to remove uterine contents
D. Both A and B

Ans. (B) Pallidotomy: A neurosurgical procedure, where a tiny electrical probe is placed in the globus pallidus (one of the basal nuclei of the brain), which is then heated to 80°C for 60 seconds, to destroy a small area of braincells.

Answer   10 C   11 A   12 C   13 B   14 B   15 A   16 C   17 A   18 B

Q 19. What is cauda equina syndrome?
[Textbook of Physiotherapy/Dr BK Nanda's/1st Ed/Pg. 391]
A. A musculoskeletal condition that affects the lower back
B. A cardiovascular condition that affects the heart
C. A respiratory condition that affects the lungs
D. A neurological condition that affects the spinal cord

Ans. (D) Cauda equina syndrome is a rare but serious neurological condition that affects the nerve roots of the spinal cord. It is caused by compression of the cauda equina, a bundle of nerves located at the base of the spinal cord.

Q 20. What happens during the primary phase of traumatic brain injury?
[Textbook of Physiotherapy/Dr BK Nanda's/1st Ed/Pg. 420]
A. The brain undergoes a series of chemical changes that can cause further damage
B. The brain experiences direct damage from the initial impact
C. The brain swells as a result of the injury
D. The patient experiences a loss of consciousness

Ans. (B) The primary phase of TBI occurs immediately following the initial impact and involves direct damage to the brain tissue as a result of the mechanical forces involved in the injury.

Q 21. What is a concussion?
[Textbook of Physiotherapy/Dr BK Nanda's/1st Ed/Pg. 420]
A. A type of brain injury caused by a lack of oxygen to the brain
B. A type of brain injury caused by a viral or bacterial infection
C. A type of brain injury caused by a sudden blow to the head or body
D. A type of brain injury caused by bleeding in the brain

Ans. (C) Concussions are a common type of mild traumatic brain injury and can occur as a result of a sports injury, motor vehicle accident, fall, or other types of trauma.

Q 22. Incorrect statement regarding multiple sclerosis:
[Textbook of Physiotherapy/Dr BK Nanda's/1st Ed/Pg. 427]
A. It is a chronic complex neurodegenerative disease of the CNS.
B. It is autoimmune in nature.
C. It is affecting function of multiple systems of the body
D. It is a chronic gastrointestinal disease of the digestive system of the body

Ans. (D) Multiple sclerosis is a chronic complex neurodegenerative disease of the central nervous system (CNS), widely believed to be autoimmune in nature, characterized by chronic inflammation, demyelination, gliosis and neuronal loss in brain, spinal cord, and optic nerves, affecting function of multiple systems of the body.

Q 23. What are the common age groups affected with multiple sclerosis?
[Textbook of Physiotherapy/Dr BK Nanda's/1st Ed/Pg. 427]
A. Infants
B. 1–10 years
C. 20–40 years
D. After the 60 years

Ans. (C) In India, no largescale studies are available regarding the incidence and prevalence of multiple sclerosis. The common age groups affected are individuals between the ages of 20 and 40 years and the disease rarely affect children and adults over the age of 50 years.

Q 24. What is decorticate posture?
[Textbook of Physiotherapy/Dr BK Nanda's/1st Ed/Pg. 422]
A. A type of postural deviation caused by a spinal cord injury
B. A type of postural deviation caused by a musculoskeletal disorder
C. A type of postural deviation caused by a respiratory condition
D. A type of postural deviation caused by a brain injury

Ans. (D) Decorticate posture is a type of abnormal postural deviation that can occur after a brain injury. It is characterized by pathology is in the cortex, the neck and legs remain in extension, hips medially rotated and feet plantar flexed with upper limbs in flexor pattern.

Q 25. Which is best physiotherapy technique may use to improve pelvic floor muscle function in patients with PID?
[Textbook of Physiotherapy/Dr BK Nanda's/1st Ed/Pg. 496]
A. Spinal manipulation
B. Myofascial release therapy
C. TENS
D. Kegel exercises

Ans. (D) Kegel exercises are a type of pelvic floor muscle exercise that can be used to improve pelvic floor muscle function in patients with PID. These exercises involve contracting and relaxing the muscles that support the pelvic organs.

Q 26. What is the characteristic sign of pseudo-hypertrophic muscular dystrophy?
[Textbook of Physiotherapy/Dr BK Nanda's/1st Ed/Pg. 428]
A. Muscles wasting
B. Muscles hypertrophy
C. Joint and pain stiffness
D. Vision problems

Ans. (B) Pseudo-hypertrophic muscular dystrophy, also known as Duchenne muscular dystrophy, is characterized by muscle hypertrophy or enlargement, especially in the calves. This is due to the accumulation of fatty tissue within the muscle fibers, which makes them appear larger than normal.

Q 27. Which of the following is a potential complication of PID?
[Textbook of Physiotherapy/Dr BK Nanda's/1st Ed/Pg. 496]
A. Decreased risk of infertility
B. Increased risk of uterine cancer
C. Ectopic pregnancy
D. Reduced risk of ovarian cysts

Ans. (C) Ectopic pregnancy is a potential complication of PID. PID can cause scarring of the fallopian tubes, which can lead to a fertilized egg implanting outside of the uterus. This can be a life-threatening condition that requires immediate medical attention.

Answer 19 D 20 B 21 C 22 D 23 C 24 D 25 D 26 B 27 C

Q 28. Which one of is the incorrect option regarding Landouzy-Dejerine disease?

[Textbook of Physiotherapy/Dr BK Nanda's/1st Ed/Pg. 434]

A. It is also known as facioscapulohumeral muscular dystrophy (FSHD).

B. It is an is an inherited and progressive muscle disorder

C. It is a congenital muscular dystrophy

D. Both A and B

Ans. (C) Facioscapulohumeral muscular dystrophy (FSHD) is an inherited and progressive muscle disorder. Initially, it affects the muscles of the face, shoulders, and upper arms with progressive weakness affecting the leg and trunk muscles.

Q 29. Physiotherapy management in myotonic dystrophy consists of:

[Textbook of Physiotherapy/Dr BK Nanda's/1st Ed/Pg. 435]

A. Gait training with/or without orthosis and walking aids.

B. Low intensity strength and endurance training

C. Breathing exercises

D. All of the above

Ans. (D) Relaxed passive exercises, breathing exercises, low intensity strength and endurance training, balancing exercises, gait training with/or without orthosis and walking aids, functional training.

Q 30. Which type of motor neuron disease affects the muscles involved in speech and swallowing?

[Textbook of Physiotherapy/Dr BK Nanda's/1st Ed/Pg. 439]

A. Amyotrophic lateral sclerosis

B. Progressive bulbar palsy

C. Primary lateral sclerosis

D. Spinal muscular atrophy

Ans. (B) Progressive bulbar palsy (PBP). It affects brainstem. The condition causes frequent choking spells, difficulty in swallowing, speaking, eating, etc. It may be associated with ALS also. The survival time from start of symptoms is 6 months to 3 years.

Q 31. Which of the following best imaging tests used to diagnose spinal muscular atrophy?

[Textbook of Physiotherapy/Dr BK Nanda's/1st Ed/Pg. 440]

A. Ultrasound

B. X-ray

C. Computed tomography (CT) scan

D. Magnetic resonance imaging

Ans. (D) MRI can be used to evaluate the structure and function of the muscles and nerves in patients with SMA. It can help to identify muscle atrophy, spinal cord abnormalities, and other signs of the condition.

Q 32. Assertion: Grade 1 nerve injuries according to Sunderland's classification involve damage to the myelin sheath of the nerve fiber.

[Textbook of Physiotherapy/Dr BK Nanda's/1st Ed/Pg. 440]

Reason: Grade 1 nerve injuries are the mildest form of nerve injury and usually involve a complete recovery

A. Both the assertion and reason are true, and but reason is not valid explanation for the assertion.

B. Both the assertion and reason are true, and reason provides valid explanation for the assertion.

C. Assertion is true but reason is false

D. Both assertion and reason are false

Ans. (C) Assertion is true but reason is false grade I temporary paralysis of a nerve caused by lack of blood flow or compression/stretching of the affected nerve with no loss of structural continuity. There is disruption of myelin. Complete recovery is possible, but not guaranteed.

Q 33. Which of the following pair is incorrectly match?

[Textbook of Physiotherapy/Dr BK Nanda's/1st Ed/Pg. 445]

A. C5 nerve root is responsible for—innervation of the wrist extensors.

B. C6 nerve root is responsible for—affected area of thumb and index finger.

C. C7 nerve root is responsible for—innervation of the triceps muscle.

D. C8 nerve root is responsible for—affected area of ulnar two fingers

Ans. (A) C5 nerve root is responsible for the innervation of the skin over the upper arm (deltoid region) not the wrist extensors.

Q 34. Assertion: Bell's palsy is a condition that causes sudden weakness or paralysis of the facial muscles.

[Textbook of Physiotherapy/Dr BK Nanda's/1st Ed/Pg. 440]

Reason: Bell's palsy is usually caused by a viral infection that affects the facial nerve.

A. Both the assertion and reason are true, and but reason is not valid explanation for the assertion.

B. Both the assertion and reason are true, and reason provides valid explanation for the assertion.

C. Assertion is true but reason is false

D. Both assertion and reason are false

Ans. (B) Both assertion and reason are true and reason is the correct explanation of the assertion. Bell's palsy occurs when the seventh cranial nerve becomes swollen or compressed, resulting in facial weakness or paralysis. The viruses/bacteria that have been linked to the development of Bell's palsy include herpes simplex, which causes cold sores and genital herpes.

Q 35. Which of the following is NOT a common sign or symptom of Erb's palsy?

[Textbook of Physiotherapy/Dr BK Nanda's/1st Ed/Pg. 439]

A. Weakness or paralysis in the affected arm

B. Lack of movement in the shoulder or elbow

C. Numbness or tingling in the hand or fingers

D. Abnormal curvature of the spine

Ans. (D) Abnormal curvature of the spine. Erb's palsy typically affects the upper limb, causing weakness or paralysis in the affected arm, as well as reduced movement in the shoulder and elbow joints. Sensory symptoms such as numbness or tingling may also be present.

Answer 28 C 29 D 30 B 31 D 32 C 33 A 34 B 35 D

Q 36. How is Guillain-Barré syndrome typically diagnosed?
[Textbook of Physiotherapy/Dr BK Nanda's/1st Ed/Pg. 468]
A. Through imaging tests such as X-rays and MRIs
B. Through a physical examination and medical history
C. Through nerve conduction studies and electromyography
D. Through blood tests for specific antibodies

Ans. (C) Through nerve conduction studies and electromyography. Nerve conduction studies and electromyography can help identify nerve damage and determine the severity of Guillain-Barré syndrome.

Q 37. What is the underlying cause of Friedreich's ataxia?
[Textbook of Physiotherapy/Dr BK Nanda's/1st Ed/Pg. 468]
A. Inflammation of the spinal cord
B. Genetic mutations affecting frataxin production
C. Traumatic brain injury
D. Autoimmune diseases

Ans. (B) Genetic mutations affecting frataxin production. Friedreich's ataxia is caused by genetic mutations affecting the production of frataxin, a protein involved in the function of mitochondria in cells.

Q 38. What is diastasis recti?
[Textbook of Physiotherapy/Dr BK Nanda's/1st Ed/Pg. 488]
A. A type of musculoskeletal pain common during pregnancy and childbirth
B. A form of postpartum depression that can be treated with physical therapy and exercise
C. A separation of the abdominal muscles which can lead to a bulging or "doming" appearance of the belly
D. A condition in which the pelvic floor muscles weaken, leading to incontinence and other symptoms

Ans. (C) A separation of the abdominal muscles, which can lead to a bulging or "doming" appearance of the belly. Physiotherapy during the postnatal period can help manage diastasis recti through exercises aimed at strengthening the abdominal muscles and improving overall core stability.

Q 39. Which of the following is a common complication after radical mastectomy?
[Textbook of Physiotherapy/Dr BK Nanda's/1st Ed/Pg. 493]
A. Stiffness of shoulder
B. Carpal tunnel syndrome
C. Plantar fasciitis
D. Achilles tendonitis

Ans. (A) Shoulder stiffness is a common complication after radical mastectomy, as the surgery can disrupt the muscles and ligaments that support the shoulder joint. Physiotherapy interventions such as range of motion exercises, manual therapy can help prevent and treat shoulder stiffness.

Q 40. Which of the following is the primary focus of exercise training in pulmonary rehabilitation?
[Textbook of Physiotherapy/Dr BK Nanda's/1st Ed/Pg. 525]
A. Increasing muscle strength
B. Improving cardiovascular fitness
C. Increasing lung infection
D. Increasing the pO_2 in blood

Ans. (B) The primary focus of exercise training in pulmonary rehabilitation is to improve cardiovascular fitness. This is achieved through aerobic exercise, which increases heart and lung function and improves oxygen delivery to the body.

Q 41. Which of the following is an absolute contraindication to resistance training during cardiac rehabilitation?
[Textbook of Physiotherapy/Dr BK Nanda's/1st Ed/Pg. 533]
A. Severe pulmonary hypertension
B. Uncontrolled hypertension
C. Controlled atrial fibrillation
D. Recent heart surgery

Ans. (B) Resistance training, which involves the use of weights or other resistance devices, can place a significant strain on the cardiovascular system. Patients who have recently undergone heart surgery may not be able to tolerate this level of stress and are therefore considered an absolute contraindication to resistance training during cardiac rehabilitation.

Q 42. Which of the following is a potential side effect of physiotherapy intervention in abdominal surgeries?
[Textbook of Physiotherapy/Dr BK Nanda's/1st Ed/Pg. 540]
A. Increased pain and discomfort
B. Reduced mobility
C. Increased risk of postoperative complications
D. Decreased pain and discomfort

Ans. (D) Physiotherapy intervention in abdominal surgeries is typically well-tolerated and does not typically result in increased pain or discomfort, reduced mobility, or increased risk of postoperative complications.

Q 43. Which of the following is a physiotherapy technique that can help improve mobility after abdominal or thoracic surgery?
[Textbook of Physiotherapy/Dr BK Nanda's/1st Ed/Pg. 545]
A. Isometric muscle contractions
B. Passive range of motion exercises
C. Deep breathing exercises
D. Static stretching exercises

Ans. (B) After abdominal or thoracic surgery, patients may experience limited mobility due to pain and discomfort, as well as the effects of anesthesia. Passive range of motion exercises involve gently moving a patient's limbs and joints to improve mobility without causing discomfort or further injury.

Q 44. What is the role of professional organizations in promoting professional ethics in physiotherapy?
[Textbook of Physiotherapy/Dr BK Nanda's/1st Ed/Pg. 554]
A. To provide continuing education and training to healthcare providers
B. To develop and enforce ethical standards for the profession
C. To advocate for policies that promote patient welfare
D. All of the above

Ans. (D) Professional organizations such as the World Confederation for Physical Therapy and national physiotherapy associations play a critical role in promoting ethical practices among healthcare providers.

Answer 36 C 37 B 38 C 39 A 40 B 41 B 42 D 43 B 44 D

Q 45. What is the importance of data management and analysis in managing a physiotherapy department?
[Textbook of Physiotherapy/Dr BK Nanda's/1st Ed/Pg. 560]
A. To identify areas for improvement in patient care and department operations
B. To maintain compliance with regulatory requirements
C. To manage department budgets and finances
D. All of the above

Ans. (A) The importance of data management and analysis in managing a physiotherapy department is to identify areas for improvement in patient care and department operations.

Q 46. According to motor program theory, what is a motor program?
[Textbook of Physiotherapy/Dr BK Nanda's/1st Ed/Pg. 568]
A. A set of instructions for emotional response
B. A set of instructions for movement
C. A set of instructions for sensory feedback
D. A set of instructions for cognitive processing

Ans. (B) Motor program theory suggests that movements are planned in advance and stored in the central nervous system as a motor program. This program contains a set of instructions for movement, such as the sequence and timing of muscle contractions needed to perform a specific task.

Q 47. What is the goal of neurodevelopmental treatment (NDT) examination in physiotherapy?
[Textbook of Physiotherapy/Dr BK Nanda's/1st Ed/Pg. 586]
A. To identify the specific diagnosis of the patient
B. To prescribe exercises for the patient
C. To identify the underlying impairments that contribute to functional limitations
D. To measure the patient's pain level

Ans. (B) The goal of NDT examination in physiotherapy is to identify the underlying impairments that contribute to functional limitations, and to develop a treatment plan to address those impairments.

Q 48. Which of the following is NOT a common characteristic of Dr Vojta's trigger points?
[Textbook of Physiotherapy/Dr BK Nanda's/1st Ed/Pg. 594]
A. Referral pain to a specific area
B. Palpable knot or band in the muscle

C. Local twitch response when stimulated
D. Reduced range of motion in the affected joint

Ans. (D) Dr Vojta has described 18 trigger points 9 points on left half of the body and 9 points on right half of the body. While trigger points may cause pain and other symptoms in the affected area, they are not typically associated with reduced range of motion in the joint.

Q 49. Which of the following pair is incorrectly match regarding to grades of Maitland mobilization techniques?
[Textbook of Physiotherapy/Dr BK Nanda's/1st Ed/Pg. 600]
A. **Grade I:** High velocity thrusts to anatomical limit.
B. **Grade II:** Large amplitude movement within the available ROM.
C. **Grade III:** Large amplitude movement that moves into stiffness
D. **Grade IV:** Small amplitude movement stretching into stiffness

Ans. (A) Grade I: Maitland mobilization techniques is small amplitude movement at the beginning of the available range of movement (small amplitude out of resistance) not the high velocity thrusts to anatomical limit.

Q 50. Which of the following is incorrect statement regarding to transverse friction massage (TFM)?
[Textbook of Physiotherapy/Dr BK Nanda's/1st Ed/Pg. 603]
A. It is a technique devised by Cyriax
B. This type of massage is indicated in acute ligament, tendon, or muscle injuries.
C. It is contraindicated in bacterial and rheumatoid type tendinitis
D. It is the type Swedish massage

Ans. (D) Transverse friction massage (TFM) is a technique devised by Cyriax, whereby repeated cross-grain massage is applied to muscle, tendon, or ligament to increase the mobility and extensibility of individual musculoskeletal tissues and to help prevent and treat inflammatory scar tissue. it is contraindicated in bacterial and rheumatoid type tendinitis, tenosynovitis, tenovaginitis, skin ulcers/blisters/psorias, bursitis and hematoma (large).

Model Question Paper - 20

Q 1. A collegiate basketball physical training specialist would like to know which of his players has the most muscular power. Which of the following is the most valid test for monitoring a basketball player's muscular power?

[Essentials of Exercise Physiology/William D. McArdle and Katch/2nd Ed/Pg. 182]

A. Vertical jump test
B. 1 RM bench press
C. 100 m sprint
D. 15 RM squat

Ans. (A) Vertical jump is very specific to basketball, which involves vertical jumping during play, and it is the best test to stimulate the physical movements and energy demands of a real game.

Q 2. According to the body mass index (BMI), which of the following athletes are considered obese?

[Essentials of Exercise Physiology/William D. McArdle and Katch/2nd Ed/Pg. 162]

A. Body builder with BMI of 32.9
B. Shot–putter with BMI of 28.0
C. Basketball player with BMI of 25.0
D. Power lifter with BMI of 29.4

Ans. (A) BMI is calculated as weight in kilograms divided by height squared in meters. Up to the BMI value of 29.9, the athlete is put under the classification 'Overweight'. If the BMI is between 30–34.9, it is classified as Class I obesity.

Q 3. A 16-year-old high school track participant returns to physical therapy after a physician's appointment. The patient indicates that MRI revealed a tear in medical meniscus of left knee. As you look back on the initial examination, which of the following special tests would you expect to have been positive?

[Therapeutic Exercise/Kisner/7th Ed/Pg. 824]

A. Lachman
B. Pivot shift
C. McMurray
D. Apprehension

Ans. (C) McMurray test is used to confirm the meniscal lesion in which the patient is in supine position with the knee completely flexed, the examiner then laterally rotates the tibia and extends the knee to the full range of motion to test the medial meniscus. If there is a loose fragment of the medial meniscus, this action causes a snap or click that is often accompanied by pain.

Q 4. A physical therapist examines a patient diagnosed with an acute posterior cruciate sprain. The mechanism of injury for the posterior cruciate ligament is:

[Essential Orthopaedics/Maheshwari/6th Ed/Pg. 149]

A. A forceful landing on the anterior tibia with the knee hyperflexed.
B. An anteriorly directed force applied to the tibia when the foot is fixed
C. A valgus force applied to the knee when the foot is fixed
D. Hyperextension, medial rotation of leg with lateral rotation of body

Ans. (A) A forceful landing on the tibial tubercle while the knee is at 90 degrees may drive the tibia backwards on the femur rupturing the posterior cruciate ligament.

Q 5. Which of the following muscle fiber types would be more beneficial for a power lifter?

[Therapeutic Exercise/Kisner/7th Ed/Pg. 171]

A. Type I
B. Type II a
C. Type II b
D. Type III

Ans. (C) Power lifting is the activity requiring near maximal performance, in which most of the motor units are called to play with fast twitch units especially type II b fibers making more significant contribution to the efforts.

Q 6. Maximum oxygen consumption (VO_{2max}) is expressed in terms of the following:

[Essentials of Exercise Physiology/William D. McArdle and Katch/2nd Ed/Pg. 196]

A. mL/kg per minute
B. L/g per minute
C. mL/g per minute
D. mL/kg per hour

Ans. (A) Maximum oxygen consumption is usually expressed relative to body weight, as milliliters of oxygen per kilogram of body weight per minute (mL/kg per minute).

Q 7. The term 'over training' is otherwise called as:

[Therapeutic Exercise/Kisner/7th Ed/Pg. 204]

A. Burnout
B. Over fatigue
C. Staleness
D. All of the above

Ans. (D) Over training syndrome is the condition resulting from over training. Many alternative terms have been suggested for over training including staleness, burnout, chronic over work, physical overstrain and over fatigue.

Q 8. Dynamic stretching is most similar to which of the following?

[Essentials of Exercise Physiology/William D. McArdle and Katch/2nd Ed/Pg. 491]

A. Specific warm up
B. General warm up
C. Easy stretch
D. Static stretch

Ans. (A) Dynamic stretching is similar to specific warm-up and movements used help to prepare the athlete for competition by allowing him or her to increase sport specific flexibility.

Answer   1 A   2 A   3 C   4 A   5 C   6 A   7 D   8 A

Q 9. Following the hold-relax with agonist contraction PNF stretch for the hamstring, increased flexibility is due to which of the following?
I. Autogenic inhibition
II. Reciprocal inhibition
III. Crossed-extension inhibition
IV. Stretch inhibition

[Therapeutic Exercise/Kisner/7th Ed/Pg. 103]
A. I and III only
B. I and II only
C. I, II and III only
D. II and IV only

Ans. (B) The hold-relax with agonist contraction is the most effective PNF stretching technique due to facilitation via both reciprocal (activation of hip flexors) and antagonist inhibition (activation of hamstrings).

Q 10. The key elements of endurance training program is characterized by:
[Essentials of Exercise Physiology/William D. McArdle and Katch/2nd Ed/Pg. 346]
A. Low intensity, high repetitions and a prolonged time period
B. High intensity, low repetitions and a prolonged time period
C. Low intensity, low repetitions and a prolonged time period
D. Low intensity, high repetitions and a shorter time period

Ans. (A) Endurance training is characterized by having a muscle contract and lift or lower a light load for many repetitions or sustain a muscle contraction for an extended period of time.

Q 11. The level of strength can be determined by using the following devices except:
[Essentials of Exercise Physiology/William D. McArdle and Katch/2nd Ed/Pg. 392]
A. Cable tensiometer
B. Dynamometer
C. Nautilus apparatus
D. Cyber isokinetic dynamometer

Ans. (C) Nautilus apparatus is used for providing resistance training to strengthen the muscles

Q 12. Following statements are true regarding eccentric isokinetic exercise, *except*:
[Essentials of Exercise Physiology/William D. McArdle and Katch/2nd Ed/Pg. 406]
A. Implemented only after functional ROM has been restored
B. Performed at slower velocities up to 180° per second for athletes
C. Introduced only after maximal effort concentric isokinetic exercise can be performed
D. Appropriate to use in the early phase of rehabilitation program

Ans. (D) Eccentric isokinetic exercise is only appropriate in the final phase of rehabilitation program to continue to challenge individual muscle groups when isolated deficits in strength and power persist.

Q 13. Following are the examples of plyometric warm-up drills, *except*:
[Therapeutic Exercise/Kisner/7th Ed/Pg. 921]
A. Lunging
B. Zigzag hop
C. Skipping
D. Marching

Ans. (B) Zigzag hop is a type of lower body plyometric drill, which involves multiple hops and jumps, repeated movements and may be viewed as a combination of jumps in place and standing jumps.

Q 14. An isotonic resistance training consists of three sets of 10 repetitions, which are performed at 100%, 75% and 50% of the ten-repetition maximum is known as:
[Therapeutic Exercise/Kisner/7th Ed/Pg. 226]
A. Oxford technique
B. Delorme technique
C. DAPRE technique
D. All of the above

Ans. (A) Oxford technique is just opposite to Delorme technique in which the weight is taken off rather than added on. This method is probably less effective and is seldom used in sports medicine.

Q 15. Following statements are true about plyometric training except:
[Essentials of Exercise Physiology/William D McArdle and Katch/2nd Ed/Pg. 407]
A. Plyometric volume is expressed as the number of repetitions and sets performed during a given training session
B. Plyometric follows the principles of progressive overload
C. Mini-trampolines are commonly used for beginning plyometrics
D. The critical weight for an athlete to avoid high-volume high intensity plyometric exercise is 80 kg so as to overcome the risk of injury

Ans. (D) Athletes who weigh more than 220 lb (100 kg) may be at the increased risk for injury when performing plyometric exercises. Greater weight increases compressive force on joints, thereby predisposing these joints to injury.

Q 16. Rehabilitation programs are influenced by the following factors, *except*:
[Therapeutic Exercise/Kisner/7th Ed/Pg. 224]
A. The severity of injury
B. The stage of tissue healing
C. Strength of injured muscle of the limb
D. Joint swelling

Ans. (C) Rehabilitation should not be focused on strength of injured muscle group, instead all muscles of the limb need to be exercised concentrating on those that are weaker. However, the limitations imposed by the injury or surgery should be observed.

Answer   9 B   10 A   11 C   12 D   13 B   14 A   15 D   16 C

Q 17. Which is the weakest part of growth plate in which separation usually occurs in the event of an injury?
[Therapeutic Exercise/Kisner/7th Ed/Pg. 177]
A. Resting layer
B. Zone of proliferating cells
C. Zone of hypertrophied cells
D. Zone of provisional calcification

Ans. (C) Zone of hypertrophied cells are the weakest part of the growth plate and are the area through which separation usually occurs in the event of an injury.

Q 18. Which somatotypes of an athlete is suitable for marathon running?
[Essentials of Exercise Physiology/William D. McArdle and Katch/2nd Ed/Pg. 174]
A. Endomorphs
B. Viscerotonic
C. Mesomorphs
D. Ectomorphs

Ans. (D) The ectomorphs has a high proportion of skin and nerves on a small skeletal frame, with very little subcutaneous fat and tend to make good marathon runners.

Q 19. Which of the following exercises are to be prescribed towards the final stage of injury rehabilitation when the athlete demonstrates pain free range of motion and has 90% of power strength and endurance of opposite leg and feels stable both clinically and subjectively?
[Therapeutic Exercise/Kisner/7th Ed/Pg. 247]
A. Circuit training program
B. Sport specific skills
C. DAPRE techniques
D. Extrinsic exercises

Ans. (B) Sport specific skills with progressively complex drills are incorporated during the final stage of rehabilitation. The exercises are designed to improve proprioception and co-ordination and it should be adapted to the specific needs of the athlete's particular position in a sport.

Q 20. An athlete's current condition or level of preparedness to begin a new or revised program is known as:
[Essentials of Exercise Physiology/William D. McArdle and Katch/2nd Ed/Pg. 188]
A. Training status
B. Training background
C. Exercise history
D. Exercise technique experience

Ans. (A) Training status is an important consideration when designing training program, which includes an evaluation of any current or previous injuries that may affect training.

Q 21. Which group of athletes is more prone for sternoclavicular joint sprain?
[Therapeutic Exercise/Kisner/7th Ed/Pg. 558]
A. Cricketers
B. Wrestlers
C. Tennis players
D. Swimmers

Ans. (B) The most common injury to the sternoclavicular joint is sprain, which occurs particularly in such activities as football and wrestling.

Q 22. What defect is known as bankart lesion in shoulder joint?
[Essential Orthopaedics/Maheshwari/6th Ed/Pg. 90]
A. Defect of posterolateral glenoid labrum
B. Defect of anterior glenohumeral ligaments and glenoid labrum
C. Defect of inferior glenoid labrum
D. Defect of posteroinferior glenoid labrum

Ans. (B) Bankart's lesion is an injury involving the anterior glenohumeral ligaments and glenoid labrum, which become separated from the articular surface of the anterior glenoid neck during a traumatic anterior dislocation.

Q 23. Homan's sign indicates:
[Essential Orthopaedics/Maheshwari/6th Ed/Pg. 44]
A. Thrombophlebitis of posterior tibial vein
B. Tarsal tunnel compression syndrome
C. Achilles tendon ruptures
D. 1st ray mobility

Ans. (A) Homan's sign: Patient sits with legs off the edge of the table and both feet in a slight plantarflexed position. Examiner compresses or squeezes calf muscle and the patient complain of pain in case of thrombophlebitis.

Q 24. Which nerve will get injured during the late cocking phase of the throwing motion?
[Therapeutic Exercise/Kisner/7th Ed/Pg. 569]
A. Spinal accessory
B. Long thoracic nerve
C. Suprascapular nerve
D. Axillary nerve

Ans. (C) The mechanism of injury is due to the traction produced on the nerve during the late cocking phase of the throwing motion. This motion causes nerve entrapment at the spinoglenoid notch that result in isolated infraspinatus palsy.

Q 25. In posterior tennis elbow which muscle gets affected?
[Essential Orthopaedics/Maheshwari/6th Ed/Pg. 302]
A. Flexor carpi radialis origin
B. Pronator teres origin
C. Triceps insertion
D. Anconeus insertion

Ans. (C) Medial tennis elbow typically presents with pain over the flexor pronator mass and posterior tennis elbow with pain over the triceps insertion.

Q 26. Why throwing athletes develop medial epicondylitis?
[Therapeutic Exercise/Kisner/7th Ed/Pg. 642]
A. Distraction
B. Compression
C. Varus stress
D. Valgus stress

Ans. (D) Throwing athletes tend to develop medial tendinosis (epicondylitis) because of the valgus stress experienced.

Q 27. Which type of athletes is more prone for ulnar nerve injury?
[Therapeutic Exercise/Kisner/7th Ed/Pg. 386]
A. Throwing athletes
B. Football players
C. Cross-country skiing
D. Badminton players

Ans. (A) Athletic injuries to the ulnar nerve are most common in the throwing athletes.

Answer   17 C   18 D   19 B   20 A   21 B   22 B   23 A   24 C   25 C   26 D   27 A

Q 28. Which one among these is a pure motor neuropathy?
[Essentials of Exercise Physiology/William D. McArdle and Katch/2nd Ed/Pg. 305]
A. Anterior interosseus syndrome
B. Pronator syndrome
C. Both A and B
D. Radial tunnel syndrome

Ans. (A) Anterior interosseous syndrome is a pure motor neuropathy of the muscles supplied by the anterior interosseous nerve.

Q 29. Intersection syndrome is related to excessive friction between which contacting soft tissues?
[Therapeutic Exercise/Kisner/7th Ed/Pg. 661]
A. Abductor pollicis longus, extensor pollicis brevis and extensor carpi radialis longus, extensor carpi radialis brevis
B. Extensor pollicis longus, extensor pollicis brevis and extensor carpi radialis longus, extensor carpi radialis brevis
C. Extensor pollicis longus, abductor pollicis longus and extensor carpi radialis longus extensor carpi radialis brevis
D. Extensor pollicis brevis, adductor pollicis and extensor carpi radialis longus, extensor carpi radialis brevis

Ans. (A) The abductor pollicis longus and extensor pollicis brevis muscles cross the extensor carpi radialis longus and extensor carpi radialis brevis tendons several centimeters proximal to extensor retinaculum. Excessive friction between contacting soft tissues is described in weightlifters, skiers and racquetball players.

Q 30. Improperly treated proximal interphalangeal joint injuries to fingers can lead to:
[Therapeutic Exercise/Kisner/7th Ed/Pg. 663]
A. Coach's finger
B. Trainer's finger
C. Athlete's finger
D. Player's finger

Ans. (A) The proximal interphalangeal joint is especially vulnerable to injury in athletic competition. They are treated on the side line by the coach, trainer or the player himself. They return to competition with unprotected use of finger, long before healing takes place. The result is, in 2–3 weeks time, a painful, stiff and deformed finger develops termed as coacher's finger.

Q 31. Avulsion fracture of pisiform bone results from rupture of which structure?
[Therapeutic Exercise/Kisner/7th Ed/Pg. 658]
A. Flexor carpi ulnaris
B. Pisohamate ligament
C. Pisotriquetral ligament
D. All of the above

Ans. (D) All these structures are attached to the pisiform bone and are responsible for its avulsion fracture when stretched.

Q 32. The term "Catch-up Clunk" is referred to which pathological condition?
[Therapeutic Exercise/Kisner/7th Ed/Pg. 386]
A. Lunotriquetral ligament injuries
B. Ulnar midcarpal instability
C. Torn triangular fibrocartilage complex
D. Scapholunate injuries

Ans. (B) In ulnar midcarpal instability, patient complains of ulnar sided pain and a clunk that occurs with ulnar deviation and pronation. This term represents abnormally flexed proximal carpal row "catching-up" as it reduces into the extended position late in ulnar deviation.

Q 33. To improve strength and speed after a pelvis, hip or thigh injury which of the following rehabilitation techniques would likely be used?
[Therapeutic Exercise/Kisner/7th Ed/Pg. 215]
A. Proprioceptive neuromuscular facilitation
B. Kinesthetics
C. Plyometrics
D. Functional exercises

Ans. (C) Plyometric exercises are those that allow a muscle to obtain its maximum strength or produce a maximum amount of force as rapidly as possible.

Q 34. Which of the following studies is the most sensitive and specific for diagnosis of a femoral neck stress fracture?
[Essential Orthopaedics/Maheshwari/6th Ed/Pg. 302]
A. Bone scan
B. MRI
C. Radiography
D. Arthrography

Ans. (B) Femoral neck stress fracture is classified into compression-side, tension-side and displaced types and usually results from overstraining and can occur in almost any sport. MRI is most sensitive and specific for diagnosis than a bone scan.

Q 35. Nontraumatic trochanteric bursitis is commonly seen in which sports activity?
[Therapeutic Exercise/Kisner/7th Ed/Pg. 748]
A. Running
B. Volley ball
C. Basket ball
D. Tennis

Ans. (A) Repetitive snapping of the tensor fascia over the prominent greater trochanter with the trochanteric bursa wedged between these two structures can lead to inflammation of the bursa.

Q 36. Exercises that are often used to determine if an athlete is ready to return to a higher level of activity or sports competition are called as:
[Therapeutic Exercise/Kisner/7th Ed/Pg. 169]
A. Functional exercises
B. Cardiovascular exercises
C. Kinesthetic exercises
D. Plyometric exercises

Ans. (A) Functional activities include everything from walking to sport-specific drills. These are often timed and are only limited by the imagination.

Answer   28 A   29 A   30 A   31 D   32 B   33 C   34 B   35 A   36 A

Q 37. Benchwarmers bursitis is referred to as:
[Therapeutic Exercise/Kisner/7th Ed/Pg. 748]
A. Trochanteric bursitis
B. Iliopectineal bursitis
C. Iliac bursitis
D. Ischial bursitis

Ans. (D) Benchwarmers bursitis occurs due to sitting for a prolonged period of time, especially with the leg crossed or on a hard surface leading to tenderness over the ischial bursa.

Q 38. Off balance position from a long jump or from a basket ball rebound leads to the injury of:
[Therapeutic Exercise/Kisner/7th Ed/Pg. 773]
A. Quadriceps/patellar tendon
B. Hamstrings
C. Gastrosoleus
D. Tendo-Achilles

Ans. (A) Complete rupture of the quadriceps or patellar tendon is a major injury which occurs when the athlete lands in an off balance position from a long jump or from a basketball rebound.

Q 39. Why stress fracture is common in female athletes?
[Essential Orthopaedics/Maheshwari/6th Ed/Pg. 156]
A. Narrow tibial width
B. Osteoporosis
C. Cavus foot
D. Planus foot

Ans. (A) Tibial stress fracture are most frequently encountered in the posteromedial cortex or compression side.

Q 40. The mechanism of adductor strain is:
[Therapeutic Exercise/Kisner/7th Ed/Pg. 748]
A. Eccentric adductor muscle contraction with concurrent hip internal rotation and adduction
B. Eccentric adductor muscle contraction with concurrent hip internal rotation and abduction
C. Eccentric adductor muscle contraction with concurrent hip external rotation and abduction
D. Concentric adductor muscle contraction with concurrent hip external rotation and abduction

Ans. (D) Adductor strains are more common strain injuries in hockey, with a reported injury rate as high as 0.43/1000 hours.

Q 41. Jumper's knee refers to tendonitis involving:
[Therapeutic Exercise/Kisner/7th Ed/Pg. 793]
A. Patellar tendon
B. Quadriceps tendon
C. Both A and B
D. Quadriceps strain

Ans. (C) Jumper's knee refers to tendinitis involving either the patellar tendon, the quadriceps tendon or both.

Q 42. Which nerve is compressed in Ski-boot syndrome?
[Therapeutic Exercise/Kisner/7th Ed/Pg. 772]
A. Medial plantar nerve
B. Superficial peroneal nerve
C. Lateral plantar nerve
D. Deep peroneal nerve

Ans. (D) Compression of the deep peroneal nerve occurs at the inferior edge of the extensor retinaculum, is commonly seen in football and basketball players, runners and athletes who wear tight fitting shoes or boots.

Q 43. Normal calcaneal inclination angle is:
[Joint Structure and Function/Cynthia C. Norkin/6th Ed/Pg. 415]
A. 5°
B. 10°
C. 15°
D. 20°

Ans. (C) Calcaneal inclination angle is formed by plane of support and the calcaneal inclination axis and helps to evaluate whether pronation or supination of foot is excess.

Q 44. Which structure plays an important role in stabilizing the thoracic spine during loading and resist anterior shear loads?
[Therapeutic Exercise/Kisner/7th Ed/Pg. 449]
A. Costovertebral joints
B. Ligamentum flavum
C. Facet joints
D. Supraspinous and interspinous ligament

Ans. (C) Facet joints are direct source of pain and are important stabilizing structures and resist anterior shear loads while the disc carries the remaining and contributes to the overall stability of the spine.

Q 45. According to "Laws of Freyette" in atlantoaxial joint:
[Therapeutic Exercise/Kisner/7th Ed/Pg. 419]
A. Rotation and side bending occurs together
B. Rotation and side bending does not occur together
C. Only side bending takes place
D. Only rotation takes place

Ans. (B) Rotation and side bending occur to opposite sides at the occipito-atlanto-articulation; the only segment in the spine where rotation and side bending do not occur together is the atlantoaxial articulation because the ring-like structure of atlas allows only rotation to occur.

Q 46. Cervical cord neuropraxia results from:
[Essential Orthopaedics/Maheshwari/6th Ed/Pg. 63]
A. Spinal stenosis
B. Congenital fusion of vertebra
C. Cervical instability
D. All of the above

Ans. (D) Undergoing cause associated with these conditions decreases the anteroposterior diameter of the spinal canal and cause neuropraxia to the nerves that exists from the foramen.

Q 47. Biomechanical function of rib cage related to thoracic spine is to:
[Joint Structure and Function/Cynthia C. Norkin/6th Ed/Pg. 163]
A. Increase the mobility of the spine
B. Protect the spine
C. Allow displacement during trauma
D. Decrease the transverse diameter of the thoracic spine

Ans. (B) Rib cage protects the spine, stiffens and strengthens the spine, increases resistance to displacement, increases thoracic spine transverse dimension and adds to the spines strength and energy absorbing capacity during trauma.

Answer 37 D   38 A   39 A   40 D   41 C   42 D   43 C   44 C   45 B   46 D   47 B

Q 48. Swayback increases the risk of which condition in lumbar spine?
[Joint Structure and Function/Cynthia C. Norkin/6th Ed/Pg. 462]
A. Spondylosis
B. Disc herniation
C. Spondylolysis
D. All of the above

Ans. (D) Swayback, i.e., hyperlordotic posturing of the low back may be flexible or fixed which increases the shear load in the facet joints and disc leading to the related pathologies.

Q 49. The type of anxiety experienced by the athlete would proportionately reduce his performance requiring high amount of information processing is known as?
[Therapeutic Exercise/Kisner/7th Ed/Pg. 31]
A. Somatic anxiety
B. Cognitive anxiety
C. Trait anxiety
D. Psychic arousal

Ans. (B) Cognitive anxiety is a psychological state-involving task-irrelevant mental processes that are negative in nature, flood attention and can deter performance proportionately, especially activities requiring high amounts of information processing.

Q 50. A somatopsychic technique by which psychological and physical arousal are self-regulated through the control of skeletal muscle tension is knows as?
[Therapeutic Exercise/Kisner/7th Ed/Pg. 110]
A. Autogenic training
B. Counter conditioning
C. Systematic desensitization
D. Progressive muscular relaxation

Ans. (D) Progressive muscular relaxation technique is employed by the athletes to achieve an appropriate level of psychic vigor and physiological arousal before performance. In this technique, by going through a series of alternate muscular tension and relaxing phases, the athlete learns to become aware of somatic tension and thereby to control it. Theoretically, the technique exerts its effect by means of a process termed reciprocal inhibition, stating that a relaxed body will promote a relaxed mind.

EU GSPR Authorised Reprsentative
Logos Europe, 9 rue Nicolas Poussin
1700, La Rochelle, France
Phone: +33 (0) 6 67 93 73 78
E-mail: contact@logoseurope.eu

www.ingramcontent.com/pod-product-compliance
Ingram Content Group UK Ltd.
Pitfield, Milton Keynes, MK11 3LW, UK
UKHW051942150726
7214IPUK00020B/384